OCCUPATIONAL THERAPY IN
Community-Based Practice Settings

OCCUPATIONAL THERAPY IN
Community-Based
Practice Settings

MARJORIE E. SCAFFA, PhD, OTR, FAOTA

Department of Occupational Therapy
University of South Alabama
Mobile, Alabama

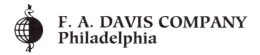

F. A. DAVIS COMPANY
Philadelphia

F. A. Davis Company
1915 Arch Street
Philadelphia, PA 19103

Printed in the United States of America

Last digit indicates print number: 10 9 8 7 6

Publisher: Margaret Biblis
Senior Editor: Lynn Borders Caldwell
Developmental Editors: Sharon Lee & Christa Fratantoro
Cover Designer: Louis Forgione

As new scientific information becomes available through basic and clinical research, recommended treatments and drug therapies undergo changes. The author and publisher have done everything possible to make this book accurate, up to date, and in accord with accepted standards at the time of publication. The author, editors, and publisher are not responsible for errors or omissions or for consequences from application of the book, and make no warranty, expressed or implied, in regard to the contents of the book. Any practice described in this book should be applied by the reader in accordance with professional standards of care used in regard to the unique circumstances that may apply in each situation. The reader is advised always to check product information (package inserts) for changes and new information regarding dose and contraindications before administering any drug. Caution is especially urged when using new or infrequently ordered drugs.

Library of Congress Cataloging-in-Publication Data

Scaffa, Marjorie E.
  Occupational therapy in community-based practice settings / Marjorie E. Scaffa.
    p.   cm.
  Includes bibliographical references and index.
  ISBN 10:0-8036-0559-5 (pbk.)   ISBN 13:978-0-8036-0559-6
  1. Occupational therapy.   2. Community health services.   I. Title.
RM735 .S27 2001
615.8'515—dc21

00-065594

*To all those special people
who see what others ignore,
embrace what others fear,
and create new paths that others can follow.*

Foreword

Twenty-five years ago I collaborated on my first publication with one of my mentors, Florence Cromwell. The paper described preparation of occupational therapy students to work in community settings (Cromwell and Kielhofner, 1976). I had the good fortune of working with a mentor who appreciated that much of the future of occupational therapy would be in community practice. A quarter century ago, this was still a new idea.

In the intervening period a number of changes in health care, health demographics, and funding of health services have made community-based practice not only common, but the most promising direction for the future of practice in occupational therapy.

It gives me great satisfaction to see that one of my former students has gone on to edit the first comprehensive volume in community practice. It is even more gratifying to note the scope and quality of chapters that make up this ambitious volume. Community practice means much more than physical placement in a community setting. Importantly, it represents (as Scaffa notes in Chapter 2) a different paradigm of care than that seen in traditional hospital and rehabilitation settings. The therapist working in the community most likely works in an organization whose philosophy, reimbursement, and expectations for practice are much different from traditional medically defined settings. Moreover, the voices and viewpoints of those served will often carry much more weight than in a traditional setting. Therapists who wish to be effective in community practice must be prepared to take on new roles, to take unusual risks, and to envision service in creative ways. Thus, although community practice is not as anomalous as it was 25 years ago, it still represents new territory for most of occupational therapy.

Marjorie Scaffa and her colleagues have assembled a remarkable set of resources for the occupational therapist in community practice. The scope and depth of the chapters make this at once an authoritative work on community practice and an invaluable collection of resources.

Gary Kielhofner, DrPH, OTR

Cromwell, F.S., and Kielhofner, G. (1976). An educational strategy for occupational therapy community service. *American Journal of Occupational Therapy, 30,* 629–633.

Preface

This book is the culmination of one aspect of my professional journey that started when I was an undergraduate major in psychology with a minor in health and continued on in an entry-level master's program to become an occupational therapist. During my years as an occupational therapy student at Virginia Commonwealth University, I was introduced to the Model of Human Occupation and became increasingly excited about the potential for practice in nonmedical settings. When given the opportunity to choose a topic for a paper, I wrote about occupational therapy's role in community health, and the seeds of what would later become this book were sown.

As a practicing occupational therapist, I gained experience in a variety of settings but was most energized and excited by home health practice. Providing services in the home enabled me to become part of the person's daily life context in which he or she participated in self-care, work, and leisure. I was impressed by how much more meaningful occupations were to individuals and their families in real-life environments.

It occurred to me that if occupation could restore function and enhance the quality of life for individuals with disabilities and their families, then maybe it could also be used to prevent disability and promote health. Thus began my quest for a doctorate in health education with a focus on family and community health. I quickly realized that much of what I had learned in occupational therapy would be useful in prevention and health promotion but that I needed to become acculturated to the mind-set and conceptual framework of a health educator, which was quite different from that of an occupational therapy practitioner. I was exposed to planning, implementing, and evaluating preventive interventions directed at groups and populations rather than rehabilitative interventions directed at individuals.

At this point in my professional journey, I began to feel frustrated, confused, and in some ways disenfranchised. I was a misfit in occupational therapy and in health education because I belonged totally to neither—I was a hybrid without a home. After several years of soul-searching, I began to assimilate both of my professional identities, which enabled me to envision, edit, and write this book. It is clearly and straightforwardly an occupational therapy text with an appreciation of the importance of community as the context for health.

Some readers may praise this book as groundbreaking in the discipline; however, it is more accurately a return to occupational therapy as practiced at Hull House in the early 1900s. Some readers may criticize this book as being superficial, reflecting fairly traditional community-based settings for occupational therapy practice and ignoring some very promising emerging roles for practitioners. It is true that this text was constrained by the literature and supporting documentation currently available. However, efforts were made throughout the text to speculate about the direction of future practice and to encourage clinically based occupational therapy practitioners to join their colleagues in community-based practice settings.

This book is, hopefully, a useful discussion of the issues related to present day community practice in occupational therapy and a description of a variety of settings in which this practice occurs. It is designed as a textbook for entry-level students but will also prove useful to practitioners wishing to facilitate a transition from medical model practice to community-based practice. I am grateful for this opportunity to participate in and contribute to the profession's expanding role in prevention, health promotion, and community health.

Marjorie E. Scaffa

Acknowledgments

This book would not have been possible if not for the time and talent provided by my colleagues/contributors, who shared my vision, commitment, and excitement of community-based practice, and by my administrative assistant, Cherie McGee, who kept me organized and who protected my writing time from interruptions. I am also indebted to the fine staff at F. A. Davis, including Lynn Borders Caldwell, Sharon Lee, Christa Fratantoro, and Margaret Biblis, and to freelancer Maryann Foley for their exceptional guidance and assistance with this project.

To paraphrase the noted physicist, Werner Heisenberg, *the most innovative developments in human thinking often occur when two divergent ideas collide.* This is most assuredly true of this book which represents, in part, an attempt to integrate my two professional selves. I am especially grateful to my mentors, Dr. Gary Kielhofner in occupational therapy, Dr. Robert Gold and Dr. Glen Gilbert in health education, and Dr. Pat C. Covey, Vice President for Academic Affairs at the University of South Alabama, for helping me find my professional path, a path with a heart.

And last, but certainly not least, to my family, particularly my mother, Doris R. Scaffa, for teaching me at a very young age the joy and value of an education, and for inspiring in me a love of reading and learning. And to my husband, S. Blaise Chromiak, MD, who believed in me and this book, even when I doubted myself, for the countless hours he spent reviewing drafts and discussing with me the ideas contained in this book. He has traveled with me on this journey and sometimes carried me along the way. His love continues to inspire me to reach for the stars and beyond, and I am grateful with all my heart.

Contributors

Felecia Moore Banks, MEd, OTR
Department of Occupational Therapy
Howard University
Washington, DC

Robin E. Bowen, EdD, OTR, FAOTA
Occupational Therapy Education Program
Rockhurst College
Kansas City, Missouri

Brent H. Braveman, MEd, OTR
Director of Clinical Services
University of Illinois at Chicago
Chicago, Illinois

Carol A. Brownson, MSPH
Division of Health Behavior Research
Washington University in St. Louis
School of Medicine
St. Louis, Missouri

S. Blaise Chromiak, MD
Family Physician
Mobile, Alabama

Sharon Desmond, PhD
Department of Health Education
University of Maryland
College Park, Maryland

Linda Gray, OTR
Department of Occupational Therapy
University of South Alabama
Mobile, Alabama

Gary Kielhofner, DrPH, OTR, FAOTA
Department of Occupational Therapy
University of Illinois at Chicago
Chicago, Illinois

Kathy G. Lemcool, MA, OTR
Department of Occupational Therapy
University of South Alabama
Mobile, Alabama

Penelope A. Moyers, EdD, OTR, FAOTA
School of Occupational Therapy
University of Indianapolis
Indianapolis, Indiana

Michael Pizzi, MS, OTR, CHES, FAOTA
President
Wellness Lifestyles, Inc.
Bronxville, New York

S. Maggie Reitz, PhD, OTR, FAOTA
Department of Occupational Therapy
Towson University
Towson, Maryland

Vanessa Russell, OTR
Department of Occupational Therapy
University of South Alabama
Mobile, Alabama

Marjorie E. Scaffa, PhD, OTR, FAOTA
Department of Occupational Therapy
University of South Alabama
Mobile, Alabama

Marian Scheinholtz, MS, OT/L
Mental Health Program Manager
American Occupational Therapy Association
Bethesda, Maryland

Supriya Sen, MS, OTR
Department of Occupational Therapy
University of Illinois at Chicago
Chicago, Illinois

Anne Shordike, MOT, OTR
Department of Occupational Therapy
Eastern Kentucky University
Richmond, Kentucky

Virginia C. Stoffel, MS, OTR, FAOTA
Department of Occupational Therapy
University of Wisconsin–Milwaukee
Milwaukee, Wisconsin

Nancy Van Slyke, EdD, OTR
Department of Occupational Therapy
University of South Alabama
Mobile, Alabama

Donna A. Wooster, MS, OTR, BCP
Department of Occupational Therapy
University of South Alabama
Mobile, Alabama

Photographs supplied by:
Jeanenne Dallas, MA, OTR/L
Instructor, Program in Occupational
  Therapy
Washington University in St. Louis School
  of Medicine

Reviewers

S. Kay Ashworth, MAT, OTR/L
Program Director and Professor
Department of Occupational Therapy
    Assistant
Sinclair Community College
Dayton, Ohio

Rebecca R. Bahnke, OTR/L
Program Director
Occupational Therapy Assistant Program
Parkland College
Champaign, Illinois

Carol A. Brownson, MSPH
Division of Health Behavior Research
Washington University School of Medicine
Saint Louis, Missouri

Julie Carson, MA, OTR
Program Director
Department of Occupational Therapy
St. Mary of the Woods College
St. Mary of the Woods, Indiana

E. Nelson Clark, MS, OTR/L
Lt. Com. MSC, USN Retired
Currently Part-Time Drug and Alcohol
    Counselor
Hollidaysburg, Pennsylvania

Jeanenne Dallas, MA, OTR/L
Instructor and Community Practice
    Therapist
Program in Occupational Therapy
Washington University School of Medicine
Saint Louis, Missouri

Stephen L. Heater, OTR, EdD, FAOTA
Dean, Waldron College of Health
    and Human Services
Radford University
Radford, Virginia

Gary Kielhofner, DrPH, OTR, FAOTA
Professor and Head, Department
    of Occupational Therapy
Professor, School of Public Health
University of Illinois at Chicago
Chicago, Illinois

Heather J. Moulton, MS, MPH, OTR/L
Faculty
Graduate Program in Occupational
    Therapy
Department of Occupational Therapy
Mercy College
Dobbs Ferry, New York

**Karin J. Opacich, PhD (cand.), OTR/L,
    FAOTA**
Occupational Therapy Program
    Developer/Director
North Park University
Chicago, Illinois

S. Maggie Reitz, PhD, OTR, FAOTA
Associate Professor and Chairperson
Department of Occupational Therapy
Towson University
Towson, Maryland

**Sharan L. Schwartzberg, EdD, OTR,
    FAOTA**
Professor and Chair
Tufts University
Boston School of Occupational Therapy
Medford, Massachusetts

Ruth Zemke, PhD, OTR, FAOTA
Professor and Graduate Program
    Coordinator
Department of Occupational Science
    and Occupational Therapy
University of Southern California
Los Angeles, California

Contents

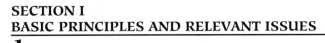

4 THEORETICAL FRAMEWORKS FOR COMMUNITY-BASED PRACTICE   51

S. Maggie Reitz, PhD, OTR, FAOTA,
and Marjorie E. Scaffa, PhD, OTR, FAOTA

5 LEGISLATION AND POLICY ISSUES   85

Nancy Van Slyke, EdD, OTR

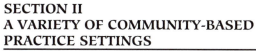

**SECTION II
A VARIETY OF COMMUNITY-BASED
PRACTICE SETTINGS**

*Brent H. Braveman, MEd, OTR; Supriya Sen, MS, OTR;
and Gary Kielhofner, DrPH, OTR, FAOTA*

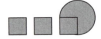

SECTION III
LOOKING AHEAD

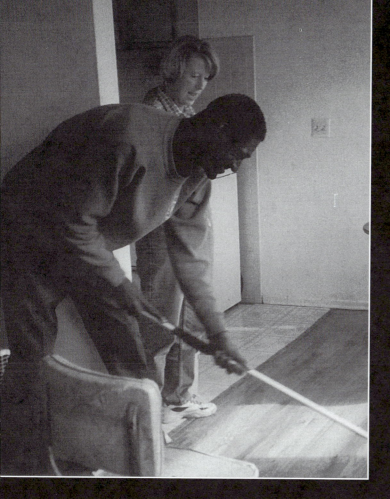

Basic Principles and
Relevant Issues

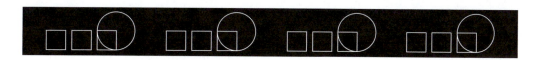

1 CHAPTER

Community-Based Practice: Occupation in Context

Marjorie E. Scaffa, PhD, OTR, FAOTA

■ OUTLINE

INTRODUCTION
THE NATURE OF DISABILITY
TRANSITIONS IN HEALTH CARE
COMMUNITY-BASED PRACTICE
    Definitions of Terms
    Historical Perspectives
    Trends in Practice Settings
    Roles in Community-Based Practice

OCCUPATIONAL THERAPY ROLES
    Role Descriptions
    Characteristics of Effective Community-
        Based Occupational Therapy
        Practitioners

Case manager   Disability
Community   Entrepreneur
Community-based practice   Health
Community-based rehabilitation   Health agent
Community-based service   Occupational performance
Community health promotion   Paradigm shift
Community model   Systems perspective
Consultant

LEARNING OBJECTIVES

This chapter is designed to enable the reader to:
- Define the term "disability," discussing the impact on the profession of broadening the concept to include populations not typically served by occupational therapy.
- Describe the trends in practice settings for occupational therapy practitioners over the past 25 years.
- Identify key characteristics of the community model of service.
- Describe the history of community-based practice in occupational therapy.
- Describe the variety of roles for occupational therapy practitioners in community-based practice.
- Describe the characteristics of effective community-based practitioners.
- Define the term "community," identifying the types of health services that can be provided in community settings.
- Identify the key issues related to the "deinstitutionalization" of the occupational therapist.

We know what we are, but we know not what we may be.

Shakespeare

 ## *INTRODUCTION*

In 1961, Mary Reilly presented the Eleanor Clarke Slagle Lecture titled "Occupational Therapy Can Be One of the Great Ideas of 20th Century Medicine" (Reilly, 1962). As we enter the 21st century, this pronouncement is truer today than ever, requiring only a slight modification in time frame. Reilly (1962) asked the question "Is occupational therapy a sufficiently vital and unique service for medicine to support and society to reward?" In today's health-care marketplace, occupational therapy must look beyond the support of the medical community and redefine its mission and role with a much broader scope.

More than 30 years later, in the foreword of Christianson and Baum's text *Occupational Therapy: Enabling Function and Well-Being,* Gail Fidler (1997) reaffirmed this notion by stating that occupational therapy should be reconceptualized as a health science rather than a medical science. The pressing problems in today's society will not be solved by medicine alone, but rather by systems of intervention, including health care, social services, community coalitions, and public policy. The philosophy and scope of expertise of occupational therapy offer unique solutions to societal problems. As a profession, occupational therapy can be true to its philosophical roots while still expanding its perspective, roles, and services to meet the health needs of individuals, families, communities, and society. The "essential worth" of occupational therapy will be demonstrated in how the profession meets these challenges and provides leadership in solving the many social problems that impact health.

Paula Steib, in an *OT Week* article (February 13, 1997), described 10 trends in health care that have emerged during the past decade. These trends included:

1. The proliferation of managed care
2. The passing of the Americans with Disabilities Act in 1990
3. The rise in computer use and access to the Internet
4. The increased competition in the health-care marketplace and greater consumer empowerment in health care
5. A focus on outcomes research
6. An increase in community-based services
7. An increase in school services due to the Individuals with Disabilities Education Act
8. A greater emphasis on case management
9. Expanded acceptance of alternative medicine
10. A dramatic increase in the numbers of new occupational therapy personnel

Many of these trends are interrelated and affect occupational therapy practice in significant ways. The rise of managed care and its increased emphasis on cost containment have promoted the shift to community-based services as a way to lower health-care costs. The impact of legislation, such as the Americans with Disabilities Act (ADA) of 1990 with its mandates for accommodations and the Individuals with Disabilities Education Act (IDEA) with its emphasis on early intervention, provides new roles for occupational therapy practitioners in health care as advocates, case managers, and community organizers.

The use of computers and related Internet resources in occupational therapy practice, administration, and research has made the profession more mobile, with diminished attachment to specific service delivery sites. More informed and empowered consumers have the ability to choose and demand occupational therapy services for health promotion and disability prevention, as well as for treatment. Occupational therapists may no longer need to rely on referrals strictly from the medical community. Outcomes research, which is currently being conducted in institutional settings, also needs to be conducted in community-based settings to ensure that services in the community are both effective and efficient. At the same time, occupational therapy services in the community quite possibly are more efficacious and more cost effective than services provided in hospital settings.

The increased acceptance of alternative medicine by the general public and the traditional medical community, the establishment of a center for the study of alternative and complementary medicine at the National Institutes of Health, and an enhanced emphasis on health promotion and disease prevention are all compatible with occupational therapy philosophy and practice. Occupational therapy professionals can create new realms of practice that incorporate health promotion and disability prevention strategies. The expanding workforce of practitioners provides the personnel needed to develop new niches for occupational therapy and infuse services into these newly emerging community-based settings.

At the 1997 American Occupational Therapy Annual Conference in Orlando, Florida, three past Slagle lecturers, Gail Fidler, Carolyn Baum, and Susan Fine, updated their original presentations and added a present-day message. Their messages were compelling and had an almost urgent tone. Fidler, after 50 years as an occupational therapist, urged practitioners to expand beyond traditional rehabilitation and form new alliances with professionals in social work, education, and psychology. Baum applauded the profession for being in the forefront of the movement toward more client-centered care. She advocated that occupational therapy practitioners expand their services and include welfare recipients and the homeless as part of their clientele. Fine urged practitioners to go out and create new career opportunities. She stated that the profession needed to form a new paradigm that responded to the new realities in health care.

This chapter provides an overview of community-based practice for occupational therapy. It broadens the scope of the term "disability," presenting transitions in health care as a basis for a paradigm shift. The chapter reviews the historical perspectives of community-based practice, highlighting the dramatic shift in practice settings currently employing occupational therapy practitioners and identifying the various roles associated with community-based practice. The chapter also describes occupational therapy roles and characteristics necessary for effective community-based occupational therapy practice.

 ## THE NATURE OF DISABILITY

Occupational therapy has long focused its services on individuals with disabilities. However, the definition of disability has been very narrowly defined, thus limiting the populations served. A broader view of the term **disability** to include other populations typically ignored by occupational therapy practitioners is needed. The *American Heritage College Dictionary* (1997, p. 394) defines disability as:

1. the condition of being disabled; incapacity;
2. a disadvantage or deficiency, esp. a physical or mental impairment that impedes normal achievement;
3. something that hinders or incapacitates.

Any individual, family, group, organization, or community that demonstrates a limitation that prevents or hinders the ability to maximize its potential is then a candidate for occupational therapy services. Consider using the notation "dis-ability" to denote this broader definition. Homeless shelters, abused and battered spouses and children, violent gangs, and those living in poverty all then become candidates for occupational therapy intervention. In all of these cases, significant impairments are obvious in the **occupational performance** areas of activities of daily living, work and play/leisure, and in numerous occupational performance components.

Fidler (1997) commends Baum and Christianson for moving the profession from the narrow focus on deficit and dysfunction to a more inclusive perspective on human performance. The profession's focus on occupational performance throughout the life span, in normal development as well as in health and illness, provides a unique framework for addressing society's critical needs and concerns.

In addition, occupational therapy must expand its focus on intervention to include health promotion and disability prevention. Why wait to intervene with occupational therapy principles after a disability has occurred? Occupational therapy's philosophy and principles are as applicable to health promotion and prevention as they are to rehabilitation. Occupational therapy has expertise and services to offer throughout the health-care continuum.

This broader perspective requires the profession to expand its notion of "holistic healing" to include a systems orientation to problem solving that incorporates the occupational therapy dedication to mind-body holism and person-environment interdependence. The focus on changing *individuals* with disabilities must give way to a

systems perspective on changing all elements—environmental, attitudinal, and sociopolitical—that perpetuate disability in society.

 # TRANSITIONS IN HEALTH CARE

A Pew Health Professions Commission report titled *Healthy America: Practitioners for 2005,* set forth an agenda for health professional schools in the United States (Shugars, O'Neil, and Bader, 1991). The report suggests a need for a new type of health-care practitioner with expanded capabilities and a broader perspective. The competencies for practitioners that the authors recommend include the ability to:

- Assess and use technology appropriately.
- Involve health-care consumers and families in the decision-making process.
- Incorporate prevention strategies in all areas of health-care practice.
- Promote healthy lifestyles.
- Implement measures to promote healthy environments for living.
- Care for the health of the community.

The current revolution in health care involves a fundamental shift in the way professionals and agencies relate to individuals and families who utilize their services, a shift from the medical model of service provision to a community model of service. The **community model** is dedicated to supporting individuals and communities and empowering them to make their own choices. It redefines the role of professionals as facilitators rather than decision makers.

This community revolution has generated much confusion, debate, concern, and controversy. Some professions have been quicker to respond and adapt than others. Occupational therapy, by virtue of its history and philosophy, can lead the way in this revolution. Within occupational therapy some practitioners have been advocating and supporting this **paradigm shift** for a number of years. Yet, as a whole, the field has been slow to respond to the call for a significant paradigm shift in service provision (Baum, 2000; Finn, 1972; Laukaran, 1977; West, 1969; Wiemer and West, 1970).

According to Wiemer and West (1970, p. 323), "the refinement of practice is a sensitive and appropriate response to societal needs, an enhancement of the utilization of the present body of knowledge, and an enrichment rather than violation of occupational therapy's traditional identification with medicine."

Occupational therapy must broaden its focus to include health promotion and prevention, as well as expand the unit of care from the individual to include the physical, social, and cultural milieu in which he or she lives.

Community health care is more than just a decentralization of services through outreach into the community. It also includes a focus on community health in addition to individual health. Functioning effectively in the community will require a range of new roles for the practitioner and a unique set of knowledge, skills, and attitudes (Wiemer and West, 1970).

A main difference between the model of community health espoused by Wiemer and West (1970) and the model that is currently being proposed is that Wiemer and West believed that community health was merely an extension of the medical model into community-based settings. The current belief is that community health requires a paradigm different from that of the medical model, a reductionist perspective, that is, a shift to a new way of thinking. This new paradigm is, however, consistent with the early foundations of occupational therapy and represents a return to the early principles of the profession.

The cornerstones of the emerging paradigm are "commitment to community, human relationships, functional teaching, individualization and flexibility" (Karan and Greenspan, 1995, p. 1). A focus on human dignity, preferences, and individuality is the mainstay of this model of service delivery.

At present, the medical model has serious limitations that can only be remedied by increased funding, research, and training of professionals. Clearly, in the era of health-care reform, these increases will not be forthcoming. A dramatic change in perspective and practice is needed.

 # COMMUNITY-BASED PRACTICE

DEFINITIONS OF TERMS

To conceptualize and operationalize community-based practice in occupational therapy, definitions of some terms have been adopted for the purposes of this textbook. These terms include health, community, community-based rehabilitation, community-based services, and community health promotion.

Health
Health is defined as "the extent to which an individual or group is able, on the one hand, to realize aspirations and satisfy needs, and on the other hand, to change or cope with the environment. Health is, therefore, seen as a resource for everyday life . . . a positive concept emphasizing social and personal resources, as well as physical capacities" (World Health Organization, 1986, p. 74).

Community
Community means different things to different people. Consider the following definitions of community. No single definition appears to capture the richness and diversity of the term. However, combining these definitions provides a perspective that is broad based and comprehensive.

The *American Heritage College Dictionary* (1997, p. 282) defines **community** as:

1. A group of people living in the same locality and under the same government.
2. A group of people having common interests.
3. Similarity or identity. Sharing, participation and fellowship.

Community refers to "noninstitutional aggregations of people linked together for common goals or other purposes" (Green and Raeburn, 1990, p. 41). Community is the same for everyone, disabled and non-disabled alike. It is the space where people think for themselves, dream their dreams, and come together to create and celebrate their common humanity (O'Connell, 1988). Community is "a social unit in which there is a transaction of common life among the people making up the unit" (Green and Anderson, 1982, p. 26). This social group has its own norms and through the regulation of resources organizes both the environment and individual and group behavior.

The community or neighborhood setting is a vital part of growing up, raising families, and meeting the many challenges and stresses of modern life (Warren and Warren, 1979). According to Nisbit (1972), people do not come together in community relationships merely to be together; they come together to do something that cannot easily be done in isolation.

Community-Based Rehabilitation
Community-based rehabilitation refers to "a strategy within community development for the rehabilitation, equalization of opportunities and social integration of all

people with disabilities" (International Labour Organization, United Nations, Educational, Scientific and Cultural Organization, World Health Organization, 1994). In the 1960s, the philosophy behind community-based occupational therapy services was the notion that in order to learn to function as independently as possible within the home and community—the ultimate goal of occupational therapy—the individual must have opportunities to practice utilizing community resources within his or her actual community setting (Howe and Dippy, 1968; Watanabe, 1967).

Community-Based Service

Community-based service is more comprehensive than community-based rehabilitation. Community-based service includes a broad range of health-related services: prevention and health promotion, acute and chronic medical care, habilitation and rehabilitation, direct and indirect service provision, all of which are provided in community settings. Community in this framework "means more than a geographic location for practice, but includes an orientation to collective health, social priorities, and different modes of service provision" (Kniepmann, 1997, p. 540). Community models are responsive to individual and family health needs in homes, workplaces, and community agencies. The goal in this type of community model is for the client and the practitioner to become integral parts of the community. Some hospitals and rehabilitation centers provide fieldtrips for patients/clients into the community and health fairs for community members, but these activities are not considered community-based services. They are more appropriately referred to as "community outreach" (Robnett, 1997).

Community Health Promotion

Community health promotion can be defined as "any combination of educational, social, and environmental supports for behavior conducive to health" (Green and Anderson, 1982, p. 3). Educational programs may be directed at individuals, families, groups, or communities through schools, worksites, organizations, and/or mass media. Social approaches focus on organizational, legal, political, and economic changes that support health and well-being. Environmental interventions are aimed at reducing environmental conditions that impair health while optimizing environmental factors that enhance well-being (Green and Anderson, 1982). "Organized community effort is the key to community health. There are some things the individual can do entirely alone, but many health benefits can be obtained only through united community effort" (Green and Anderson, 1982, p. 4).

HISTORICAL PERSPECTIVES

Community-based practice is not a new concept in occupational therapy (Table 1–1). Two founders of the profession, George Barton and Eleanor Clarke Slagle, developed community-based programs in the early 1900s. Barton, who was disabled by tuberculosis and a foot amputation, established "Consolation House" in New York in 1914. The program used occupations to enable convalescents to return to productive living (Punwar, 1994; Sabonis-Chafee, 1989). Eleanor Clarke Slagle was hired in 1915 to develop a program to provide persons with mental or physical disabilities an opportunity to work and become self-sufficient. The project was funded by philanthropic contributions and was located at Hull House, a settlement house in Chicago. In its first year of operation, the program served 77 persons who developed manual skills and received wages for their work. The goods produced in the workshop included: baskets, needlework, rugs, simple cabinets, and toys (Reed and Sanderson, 1999).

In the 1930s, Humphreys (1937) and Banyai (1938) wrote about community prac-

TABLE 1-1

HISTORICAL TIMELINE OF COMMUNITY PRACTICE IN OCCUPATIONAL THERAPY

Date	Event
1914	George Barton establishes Consolation House in New York.
1915	Eleanor Clarke Slagle establishes the work program at Hull House in Chicago.
1937	Humphreys advocates community treatment for persons with developmental disability.
1938	Banyai advocates following tuberculosis patients into the community after discharge from sanitariums.
1940	The American Occupational Therapy Association (AOTA) reports on roundtable discussions held at national conference on the role of occupational therapy in community health.
1968	Bockhoven suggests that occupational therapy take responsibility for community occupational development.
1969–1973	In the United States, West, Reilly, and Mosey describe the need for occupational therapy services in the community.
1972	Llorens describes a community-based program in San Francisco for pregnant teenagers.
1972	Finn argues that the profession move beyond the role of therapist to "health agent."
1973	In Canada, Opzoomer and McCordic describe the need for occupational therapy services in the community.
1973	Hasselkus and Kiernat describe an independent living program for the elderly.
1974	The AOTA Task Force on Target Populations expands the role of the profession to include health promotion and disability prevention.
1977	Laukaran describes the major obstacles to community-based practice.
1982	Kirchman, Reichenback, and Giambalvo describe a prevention program for the well elderly.

tice in an early journal titled *Occupational Therapy and Rehabilitation,* a precursor to the *American Journal of Occupational Therapy.* Humphreys (1937) describes occupational therapy services for persons with developmental disabilities. She proposes two broad functions for occupational therapy practitioners in the treatment of this population: orthopedic and socioeconomic. The orthopedic function is clearly focused on remediating any physical impairments. The socioeconomic function, according to Humphreys (1937), is focused on assisting a person with developmental disability to fit into the general social, economic, and political life of society. This socioeconomic function is best carried out in the actual community where the person lives (Humphreys, 1937). She believed that a lack of professional vision had prevented occupational therapists from moving outside of the traditional institutional settings into the community and acknowledging occupational therapy's responsibility to the larger social and economic needs of the nation (Humphreys, 1937).

Banyai (1938) wrote about treatment of tuberculosis in sanitariums. While acknowledging the importance of occupational therapy intervention in the institution, she emphasized the need to follow the patient into the community. The ultimate goal of treatment was to restore the individual to a satisfactory level of social and economic functioning. Banyai (1938) believed that this required the occupational therapist to work with the person in the community after discharge from the institution.

The American Occupational Therapy Association (1940) published a report of discussions that took place at the national convention. These roundtable discussions focused on the practice of occupational therapy in different settings. The topics considered included: occupational therapy in community health, the relationship between occupational therapy and vocational rehabilitation, recreation as a therapeutic agent, and the interpretation of occupational therapy to other professional groups.

The professional literature of the 1960s suggested that the field was on the verge of expanding its services outside of traditional medical settings (Laukaran, 1977). West (1969, p. 231) asserted that "the traditional role of the occupational therapist, that of the reintegration of social function, is not a hospital service but rather a function that can be best filled in the community." Reilly (1971) advocated that the future growth of the profession was predicated on the transition of occupational therapy services from the hospital to the community. The focus of occupational therapy, in her view, should be to develop experiences and programs in the individual's community environment that enhance adaptive competencies.

Mosey (1973) emphasized the profession's role in meeting the health needs of individuals. She defined "health needs" as those inherent human requirements that must be met for a person to achieve a sense of well-being. This perspective is much broader than the traditional view of occupational therapy. Mosey (1973) suggested that movement of practice out of institutional settings would be enhanced if therapists conceptualized their role as facilitating community members in meeting their health needs, instead of focusing solely on the remediation of individual dysfunction.

In Canada, Opzoomer and McCordic (1973) expressed a similar sentiment. These Canadian therapists believed that the traditional focus of occupational therapy was inadequate to respond to consumer demands to meet their health needs. They suggested that practitioners consider the family, community, and cultural framework of the individual in addition to the specific limitation imposed by the disability (Opzoomer and McCordic, 1973). This broader perspective requires the professional to provide therapeutic programming in the individual's milieu, including home, workplace, and community.

In spite of these early admonitions to focus on broader health needs and to provide services outside of institutional settings, the move to community-based practice was short-lived and very limited in scope. In the 1970s and 1980s, examples of outreach into the community included: an independent living project for the elderly, a project in San Francisco for pregnant teenage girls, and prevention services for the well elderly.

The independent living project for the elderly incorporated three basic components: adult education, transportation, and home consultation. An occupational therapist served as a consultant to the program and conducted the home evaluations. The government grant-funded project offered services free of charge to the participants (Hasselkus and Kiernat, 1973).

The program for pregnant teens focused on the developmental tasks of adolescence and preparation for motherhood. In addition, the children of these young mothers were screened routinely for developmental milestones. The mothers were trained in developmental stimulation and creative play activities (Llorens, 1972).

The prevention program for well elderly combined service provision and a research project (Kirchman, Reichenback, and Giambalvo, 1982). The goal of the program was to provide support services that enabled the elderly participants to remain in the community and resulted in improved life satisfaction. Interviews were conducted before and after the program was implemented. The results indicated improvement in four key areas, including general affect, life satisfaction, social resources, and economic resources (Kirchman et al., 1982).

According to Laukaran (1977), three major obstacles to community-based practice existed at that time. These barriers included practical constraints, historical factors within the discipline, and gaps in knowledge and theory related to community-based practice. The practical constraints were related to the limited number of opportunities that existed for community-based practice at that time and the public perception of occupational therapy as a medical discipline. Historically, occupational therapists' professional identity had been associated with work in medical institutions. In addition, professional education programs emphasized preparation for practice in medical rather than in the community-based settings. Laukaran (1977) noted that some theoretical frameworks of that era (occupational behavior, biopsychosocial, and developmental models) were compatible with community-based practice. However, these early models were inadequate in providing guidelines and rationales for services in community settings.

Some of these same obstacles exist today, however, in different forms. Opportunities for utilizing occupational therapy expertise in community settings are limitless, but typically not designated as occupational therapy positions. For the profession to move into these settings, practitioners must seek out positions, which although not labeled "occupational therapy" could benefit from the unique contributions of the discipline.

The perception of occupational therapy strictly as a medical discipline continues to exist both outside and within the profession. The identity of "medical professional" is an alluring one, as in the past it denoted an aura of legitimacy. Many occupational therapy practitioners today are still reluctant to "let go" of this restrictive image in favor of a more broadly defined role. In addition, professional preparation programs are slow to shift focus. However, many educators concur that the future of the profession will largely be determined by its ability to expand the scope of practice into community-based settings.

Many more theoretical frameworks exist today than in the 1960s. These newly emerging models, based on the work of previous theorists, are readily applicable to community-based practice. Some of these theories and models, including occupational science, the model of human occupation and occupational adaptation, are described in detail in a later chapter.

Interestingly, one of the boldest predictions and strongest support for the validity of occupational therapy services in the community came from a physician in 1968. Bockhoven (1968, p. 25) suggested a new role for occupational therapists, described as "taking responsibility for community occupational development, alongside the businessman, city planner and the economist . . . to support growth of respect for human individuality in occupation." The American Occupational Therapy Association (1974, p. 158) Task Force on Target Populations redefined occupational therapy as "the science of using occupation as a health determinant." This definition advanced the notion that occupational therapy was not limited to the seriously or chronically ill, but also could remediate mild to moderate impairments and contribute to health promotion and disability prevention. Finn, in the 1971 Eleanor Clarke Slagle Lecture, states (Finn, 1972, p. 59):

> In order for a profession to maintain its relevancy it must be responsive to the trends of the times. . . . Occupational therapists are being asked to move beyond the role of therapist to that of health agent. This expansion in role identity will require a reinterpretation of current knowledge, the addition of new knowledge and skills, and the revision of the educational process.

These words are still true today in the 21st century. The expanded role of **health agent** requires practitioners to move into the community and provide a continuum of services that includes health promotion and disability prevention in addition to the intervention services typically provided by the profession. Health agent is more than "therapist." Other roles, such as consultant, advocate, community organizer, program developer, and case manager, are also included.

TRENDS IN PRACTICE SETTINGS

According to the American Occupational Therapy Association (1997), a fairly dramatic shift in occupational therapist employment settings has occurred. Since 1973, the percentage of occupational therapists employed in hospital-based settings has significantly declined. In 1973, 13.8 percent of occupational therapists were employed in psychiatric hospitals. By 1996, this percentage had decreased to 1.7 percent. The data for occupational therapist employment in pediatric hospitals decreased from 2.9 percent in 1973 to 1.6 percent in 1996, and in rehabilitation hospitals employment decreased from 13.4 percent in 1973 to 9.5 percent in 1996.

Even in the six years between 1990 and 1996, dramatic changes are obvious in the percentage of occupational therapists employed in general hospitals. This data reflects all units of general hospitals, including specialized rehabilitation units, psychiatric units, and neonatal intensive care units. The percentage of occupational therapists employed in general hospitals declined from 25.4 percent in 1990 to 17.6 percent in 1996. This decrease reflects a national trend in managed care aimed at reducing the number of inpatient beds and decreasing the length of stay to minimize costs.

At the same time that the use of occupational therapists in general hospitals is declining, the percentage of therapists employed in community-based settings is increasing. This trend is most notable in home health agencies (0.9 percent in 1973 to 6.1 percent in 1996), outpatient clinics (2.5 percent in 1982 to 5.1 percent in 1996), private practice (1.3 percent in 1973 to 7.3 percent in 1996), and school systems (11.0 percent in 1973 to 17.9 percent in 1996). In addition, the percentage of occupational therapists employed in skilled nursing/intermediate care facilities has increased from 6.2 percent in 1973 to 18.2 percent in 1996. These data point to a shift from hospital-based services to services being provided in smaller, more cost-effective facilities in the community. The changes in employment settings for certified occupational therapy assistants mirror the trends in the employment of occupational therapists.

ROLES IN COMMUNITY-BASED PRACTICE

More than 30 years ago, West (1967) described her vision of the changing responsibility of occupational therapists to the community. This vision acknowledged the newly emerging focus on prevention and health promotion in medicine and the impact this new focus would have on practice settings, roles, and responsibilities. West (1967, p. 312) predicted that, as a result of the change in focus, practice would move into new settings, "namely, the communities in which our potential patients live, work and play." She described four emerging roles that at the time were adding new dimensions to the traditional role of the clinically based occupational therapist (West, 1967). These new roles included evaluator, consultant, supervisor, and researcher. West (1967) advocated that professional preparation programs respond to these changes in health-care delivery to produce practitioners able to meet these changing responsibilities in the community.

Other roles that community-based practitioners may fulfill include program planners and evaluators, staff trainers, community health advisors, policy makers, case managers, primary care providers, and advocates. As a community health advocate, practitioners can identify the social, physical, emotional, medical, educational, and occupational needs of community members for optimal functioning and advocate for services to meet those needs. In addition, practitioners can act as advocates and lobbyists by providing input and shaping legislation and government policies, thereby affecting local and national physical and mental health issues and changing environmental conditions to promote health.

OCCUPATIONAL THERAPY ROLES

The American Occupational Therapy Association (AOTA) (1993) roles document describes a variety of potential roles for occupational therapists and occupational therapy assistants. The more common and well known of these roles in the practice setting include practitioner, supervisor, administrator, and fieldwork educator. Other roles that are less obvious and may occur outside of the traditional practice setting include:

- Consultant
- Faculty member
- Researcher
- Private practice owner/entrepreneur

The roles document is not meant to be an exhaustive list. Rather, it represents roles within the occupational therapy profession only. The roles outlined in the document are not mutually exclusive. At any point in one's career, a person may fulfill a variety of occupational therapy roles.

Other potential roles outside of the profession include:

- Activity director
- Case manager
- Rehabilitation coordinator
- Program manager
- Hospital or skilled nursing facility administrator

According to the American Occupational Therapy Association (1993, p. 5), "career progression involves advancement within roles as well as transition to different roles. When transitioning occurs, practitioners need to have demonstrated performance potential and appropriate educational preparation for the new role. Preparation for new roles often involves self-reflection, continuing or advanced education, and acquisition of experience and skills required for the new role."

Occupational therapy practitioners have a significant role to play in supporting individuals in their homes and workplaces, facilitating their independence, and promoting their integration into the community (Stalker, Jones, and Ritchie, 1996). Broadening the role of occupational therapy requires learning to delegate and relinquish ownership of, and responsibility for, certain tasks. Practitioners in the community may function as consultants, case managers, program planners, and personnel trainers. It is important for community-based practitioners to develop networks for support and collaboration with other occupational therapists and occupational therapy assistants, health and social service professionals, and community leaders.

ROLE DESCRIPTIONS

The following role descriptions are based on official documents of the American Occupational Therapy Association (1993).

Consultant

An occupational therapy consultant provides consultative services to individuals, groups, programs, or organizations. The content of the consultation may relate to practice issues, program development, administrative concerns, and/or research protocols (American Occupational Therapy Association, 1993).

Occupational therapy practitioners, in the role of **consultant,** provide information and expert advice regarding program development and evaluation, supervisory models, organizational issues, and/or clinical concerns. Consultation services are most often utilized when new programs are being developed or undergoing significant change. Consultation services may be short term or long term, depending on the needs of the program. Within the community, occupational therapy practitioners can act as consultants to a variety of groups such as Scouts and Boys and Girls Clubs, adult education programs, adult day care, transitional living programs, independent living centers, community development and housing agencies, and worksite safety and health programs.

Case Manager

As a **case manager,** a practitioner would coordinate the provision of service; advise the consumer, family, or caregiver; evaluate financial resources; and advocate for needed services (American Occupational Therapy Association, 1993). Case management requires a professional who has ample clinical experience, understands reimbursement mechanisms, and has good organizational skills. Frequently, the qualifications and duties of case managers are dictated by state regulations. Occupational therapy practitioners are designated as case managers most frequently in mental health and pediatric practice. Case management may be a long-term process of coordinating service delivery for individuals and families coping with chronic disabilities.

Private Practice Owner/Entrepreneur

According to the roles document, an occupational therapy **entrepreneur** is someone who is partially or fully self-employed (American Occupational Therapy Association, 1993). The practitioner may own a private practice, provide services on a contractual basis, and/or function as a consultant. In order for entrepreneurs to be successful, they must be able to assess and respond to the unique needs of their communities.

 ## CHARACTERISTICS OF EFFECTIVE COMMUNITY-BASED OCCUPATIONAL THERAPY PRACTITIONERS

Linda Learnard has long been an advocate of occupational therapy service provision in community settings. She has spoken at numerous conferences about her unique philosophy and approach to community health. In an article published in *OT Practice,* Robnett (1997) interviews Learnard and writes about paradigms of community practice.

According to Learnard, "occupational therapy in community health is both an art and a science" (Robnett, 1997, p. 30). In addition to the typical occupational therapy skill of task analysis and understanding the impact of the environmental context and its relationship to function, occupational therapists in community-based practice need a variety of other skills and attributes. According to Robnett (1997), Learnard advocates several characteristics of effective community-based therapists. These include:

- A sense of positive hopefulness
- Understanding of individuals in their specific personal circumstances
- Creativity to envision a variety of possibilities
- Ability to set aside one's cultural, personal, and professional biases and respect individual choices rather than passing judgment

According to Learnard (Robnett, 1997), the focus of occupational therapy in the community should be on changing the environment, not on changing the individual. The goal is to create an accommodating and accepting environment for people with disabilities.

In addition, the following attributes and skills are recommended for those contemplating practice in community settings:

- Professional autonomy
- Flexibility
- Tolerance for ambiguity
- Attitude of collaboration
- Excellent interpersonal communication skills
- Strong organizational skills
- Networking skills
- Program planning and evaluation skills
- High-level problem-solving ability
- Good public relations skills
- Comfort with indirect service provision
- Grant-writing skills

 ## CONCLUSION

> It is time to start living out of our imagination,
> not out of our memory alone.

The lessons of the past have much to teach us. As the mentally ill were deinstitutionalized and moved into the community, occupational therapists failed to follow their lead. As a result, many jobs for occupational therapists were permanently lost while many other potential roles were filled by other professionals. As others with disabilities move out into the community to receive services, occupational therapy practitioners must be there to serve their needs.

Dasler (1984) contends that occupational therapists, regardless of their area of practice, should focus their attention on creating and filling more positions in community-based settings than in the traditional clinic environment. If occupational therapy professionals limit their job searches to positions labeled "occupational therapy," community-based practice gains will be few. Therapists must adapt their roles and skills to fit with the "outside" community environment. Dasler (1984, p. 31) refers to this as the "deinstitutionalization of the occupational therapist." If therapists continue to resist the move into community-based settings, where their services are most needed, in favor of clinic and hospital environments, then the future of the profession will surely be unnecessarily limited.

Occupational therapy philosophy and services are very compatible with community-based service provision. Now is the time for practitioners to move ahead with confidence and lead the way for others to follow. If the profession fails to assume the dynamic, new roles that are emerging in the community, other professionals will surely replace us.

In 1972, Finn suggested nine issues that need to be addressed as the profession moves from an emphasis on medical and clinical services to health promotion and community-based services. An updated interpretation of these issues follows. Occupational therapy practitioners need to:

1. Become knowledgeable about community organizations and institutions and how they operate.
2. Acquire a thorough understanding of the unique services they can offer in community settings and be able to communicate these services clearly.
3. Develop strategies to translate knowledge into actual programs that are responsive to community needs.

4. Be willing to take risks when faced with challenges in unfamiliar environments.
5. Learn to relate to and communicate effectively with nonmedical personnel and avoid the use of professional jargon.
6. Be willing to be proactive and go into the community offering services rather than waiting for their services to be solicited.
7. Be secure in their professional identity, develop the role of health agent, and appreciate the opportunities for personal and professional growth in the experience.

In addition, the profession must reinterpret and expand its knowledge base to support community-based initiatives as well as think creatively and develop new models of practice appropriate for community-based settings.

The time has come to make occupational therapy one of the grand and glorious concepts of the 21st century. It is our responsibility as a profession to respond to and help resolve the social problems of the 21st century, including poverty, homelessness, addiction, depression, and violence. With vision and creativity, the profession's potential contribution to the community and society is limitless.

 ## STUDY QUESTIONS

1. Is it appropriate for occupational therapy to broaden its definition of disability to include populations not typically served by OT? Why or why not?
2. What are the implications for the profession of making the paradigm shift from clinic-based practice to community-based practice?
3. What are the implications for the profession of *not* making the paradigm shift from clinic-based practice to community-based practice?
4. What are the characteristics of effective community-based practitioners?
5. What are the barriers to "deinstitutionalizing" the occupational practitioners?
6. Assess your own readiness to practice in community settings. What do you need to learn to be able to make this transition?

REFERENCES

American heritage college dictionary (3rd ed.). (1997). Boston: Houghton Mifflin.

American Occupational Therapy Association. (1940). Editorial: Reports of roundtables, AOTA convention. *Occupational Therapy and Rehabilitation, 19,* 387–411.

American Occupational Therapy Association. (1974). Task force on target populations: Report of the task force on target populations, report I. *American Journal of Occupational Therapy, 28,* 158–163.

American Occupational Therapy Association. (1993). Occupational therapy roles. *American Journal of Occupational Therapy, 47,* 1087–1099.

American Occupational Therapy Association. (1997). Percentage of registered occupational therapists and certified occupational therapy assistants by primary employment setting 1973–1996. Source: AOTA Member Surveys.

Banyai, A.L. (1938). Modern trends in the treatment of tuberculosis. *Occupational Therapy in Rehabilitation, 17,* 245–254.

Baum, C. (2000). Reinventing ourselves for the new millennium. *OT Practice, 5*(1), 12–15.

Bockhoven, J.S. (1968). Challenge of the new clinical approaches. *American Journal of Occupational Therapy, 22,* 23–25.

Christianson, C., and Baum, C. (1997). *Occupational therapy: Enabling function and well-being.* Thorofare, NJ: Slack.

Dasler, P.J. (1984). Deinstitutionalizing the occupational therapist. *Occupational Therapy in Health Care, 1*(1), 31–40.

Fidler, G.S. (1997). Foreword in C. Christianson and C. Baum (1997), *Occupational therapy: Enabling function and well-being*. Thorofare, NJ: Slack.

Finn, G.L. (1972). The occupational therapist in prevention programs. *American Journal of Occupational Therapy, 26*, 59–66.

Green, L.W., and Anderson, C.L. (1982). *Community health* (4th ed.). St. Louis: Mosby.

Green, L.W., and Raeburn, J. (1990). Contemporary developments in health promotion, definitions and challenges. In N. Bracht (Ed.), *Health promotion at the community level*. Newbury Park, CA: Sage.

Hasselkus, B.R., and Kiernat, J.M. (1973). Independent living for the elderly. *American Journal of Occupational Therapy, 27*(4), 181–188.

Howe, M., and Dippy, K. (1968). The role of occupational therapy in community mental health. *American Journal of Occupational Therapy, 22*, 521–524.

Humphreys, E.J. (1937). The value of occupational therapy to the developmentally deficient child. *Occupational Therapy and Rehabilitation, 16*, 1–13.

International Labour Organization, United Nations, Educational, Scientific and Cultural Organization, World Health Organization (1994). *Community-based rehabilitation for and with people with disabilities*. Geneva: WHO.

Karan, O.C., and Greenspan, S. (1995). *Community rehabilitation services for people with disabilities*. Boston: Butterworth-Heinemann.

Kirchman, M.M., Reichenback, V., and Giambalvo, B. (1982). Preventive activities and services for the well elderly. *American Journal of Occupational Therapy, 36*, 236–242.

Kneipmann, K. (1997). Prevention of disability and maintenance of health. In C. Christianson and C. Baum, *Occupational therapy: Enabling function and well-being* (pp. 531–555). Thorofare, N.J.: Slack.

Laukaran, V.H. (1977). Toward a model of occupational therapy for community health. *American Journal of Occupational Therapy, 31*(2), 71–74.

Llorens, L.A. (1972). Problem-solving the role of occupational therapy in a new environment. *American Journal of Occupational Therapy, 26*(5), 234–238.

Mosey, A.C. (1973). Meeting health needs. *American Journal of Occupational Therapy, 27*, 14–17.

Nisbit, R. (1972). *Quest for community*. New York: Oxford.

O'Connell, M. (1988). *The gift of hospitality*. Evanston, IL: Center for Urban Affairs and Policy Research.

Opzoomer, A., and McCordic, L. (1973). Occupational therapy—a change of focus. *Canadian Journal of Occupational Therapy, 40*, 125–129.

Punwar, A.J. (1994). *Occupational therapy: Principles and practice* (2nd ed.). Baltimore, MD: Williams and Wilkins.

Reed, K.L., and Sanderson, S.N. (1999). *Concepts of occupational therapy* (4th ed.). Philadelphia: Lippincott.

Reilly, M. (1962). Occupational therapy can be one of the great ideas of 20th century medicine. *American Journal of Occupational Therapy, 16*, 1–8.

Reilly, M. (1971). The modernization of occupational therapy. *American Journal of Occupational Therapy, 25*, 243–246.

Robnett, R. (1997). Paradigms of community practice. *OT Practice, 2*(5), 30–35.

Sabonis-Chafee, B. (1989). *Occupational therapy: Introductory concepts*. St. Louis: Mosby.

Shugars, D.A., O'Neil, E.H., and Bader, J.D. (Eds.). (1991). *Healthy America, practitioners for 2005: An agenda for U.S. health professional schools*. Durham, NC: The Pew Health Professions Commission.

Stalker, K., Jones, C., and Ritchie, P. (1996). All change? The role and tasks of community occupational therapists in Scotland. *British Journal of Occupational Therapy, 59*(3), 104–108.

Steib, P.A. (1997). A decade of change: 10 trends. *OT Week*, February 13, 1997, 18.

Warren, R., and Warren, D. (1979). *The neighborhood organizer's handbook*. Notre Dame, IN: University of Notre Dame.

Watanabe, S.G. (1967). The developing role of occupational therapy in psychiatric home service. *American Journal of Occupational Therapy, 21*, 353–356.

West, W.A. (1967). The occupational therapist's changing responsibility to the community. *American Journal of Occupational Therapy, 21*, 312–316.

West, W.A. (1969). The growing importance of prevention. *American Journal of Occupational Therapy, 23*, 226–231.

Wiemer, R.B., and West, W.A. (1970). Occupational therapy in community health care. *American Journal of Occupational Therapy, 24*, 323–328.

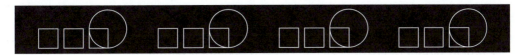

2 CHAPTER

Paradigm Shift: From the Medical Model to the Community Model

Marjorie E. Scaffa, PhD, OTR, FAOTA

■ OUTLINE

LEARNING OBJECTIVES

This chapter is designed to enable the reader to:
- Describe the characteristics and purposes of a paradigm.
- Illustrate the stages of a paradigm shift.
- Describe the history of paradigm shifts in occupational therapy.
- Identify the characteristics of the emerging paradigm in occupational therapy.
- Describe the basic concepts and principles of systems theory and explain its relevance to occupational therapy.
- Describe the history of paradigm shifts in public health and vocational rehabilitation and the implications for occupational therapy.
- Identify key characteristics of a community practice paradigm for occupational therapy.

> If you do not know where you are going, you are likely to end up someplace else.
>
> Lao Tsu

INTRODUCTION

The word **paradigm** comes from the Greek *paradeigma*, which means an example, pattern, or model (*American Heritage College Dictionary*, 1997). A paradigm is a conceptual framework that allows explanation and investigation of phenomena.

Thomas S. Kuhn (1970), in a classic text titled *The Structure of Scientific Revolutions*, described the concept of paradigm in detail. Kuhn (1970, p. viii) defined a paradigm as "universally recognized scientific achievements that for a time provide model problems and solutions to a community of practitioners." Paradigms have two essential characteristics: (1) a sufficiently unprecedented scientific achievement that draws a large number of constituents from competing areas of inquiry and (2) adequately open ended enough to allow for the exploration of solutions to a variety of problems.

A paradigm is a worldview that characterizes a particular group or discipline that has common interests. It is a "consensus-determined matrix of the most fundamental beliefs or assumptions of a field" (Kielhofner, 1983, p. 6). A profession or discipline-specific paradigm determines:

● How professionals view their phenomenon of interest

20

● What puzzles, problems, or questions practitioners will seek out in their work
● What solutions will emerge
● What goals will be set for the direction of the profession

A paradigm is the "cultural core of the discipline" and "provides professional identity" (Kielhofner, 1997, p. 17).

In short, according to Barker (1992, p. 32), a paradigm is a "set of rules and regulations (written or unwritten) that establishes or defines boundaries" and dictates the behaviors within those boundaries that are required for success. Every paradigm has a range of problems that it can successfully address. The more robust or powerful a paradigm, the greater the variety of problems to which it can be applied.

Paradigms act as filters of perception. Information or data that is contrary to one's paradigm is often filtered out of perception or its effect is minimized. This is referred to as the **paradigm effect** (Barker, 1992). What is obvious when perceived from one paradigm may be obscure when viewed from another paradigm. A paradigm can have both positive and negative effects on a profession. When utilized appropriately, a paradigm can distribute information into meaningful and useful categories and provide valuable guidelines for practice. The danger of paradigms is their potential for limiting problem solving and innovation by constraining thinking and perception. Typically, paradigms are not used deliberately to bias or deceive, but sometimes misrepresentation is a result of the inappropriate application of a paradigm. The worst-case scenario is the inability to perceive data that are clearly obvious and the resulting belief that change is impossible. Barker (1992, p. 92) states that "what is defined as 'impossible' today is impossible only in the context of present paradigms."

Paradigms are often not explicitly or consciously chosen by practitioners in a particular discipline but are internalized through the professional training process and modified in response to environmental demands. It is frequently difficult for individuals or groups to distance themselves enough from a discipline's prevailing paradigm to examine it dispassionately.

This chapter presents the major paradigm shifts in occupational therapy, highlighting the impact of systems theory. Paradigm shifts in other disciplines, such as public health and medicine and vocational rehabilitation, also are described. The chapter concludes with a discussion of the community practice paradigm as a client-centered approach to practice.

 ## PARADIGM SHIFTS

If one reviews the ontology of the development of professions and science, certain patterns become apparent. Kuhn (1970) asserts that paradigm acquisition, and the resultant research and inquiry permitted, is a reflection of maturity in a given discipline or scientific field. The history of physics and other well-developed disciplines suggests that the path to paradigm acquisition and research consensus is long and arduous.

According to Kuhn (1970, p. 15), "in the absence of a paradigm or some candidate for a paradigm, all of the facts that could possibly pertain to the development of a given science are likely to seem equally relevant." Fact gathering in such a discipline tends to be a random trial-and-error activity. This activity is essential for a paradigm to emerge, but it tends to produce a maze of information rather than a body of literature that could truly be labeled scientific.

Kuhn (1970) asserted that change within a discipline or profession does not occur gradually. Rather, it occurs very dramatically. When a discipline abandons one view of the world for another, it has undergone a revolution, a drastic conceptual restructuring, and a **paradigm shift**. Often, much resistance to paradigm shifts and to those initiating them is present. Paradigm shifts dramatically change the existing rules, create new trends, and trigger innovations. Paradigm shifts occur in four stages: pre-paradigm, paradigm, crisis, and return to paradigm (Figure 2–1).

The pre-paradigm stage represents the early preformalization phase of a discipline. Several groups may have a common interest in a set of phenomena, but perceive, define, and operationalize the phenomena differently. Eventually, one stream of thought prevails, becoming the dominant paradigm of the discipline. During the paradigm stage, this worldview becomes the filter through which the profession seeks out and solves

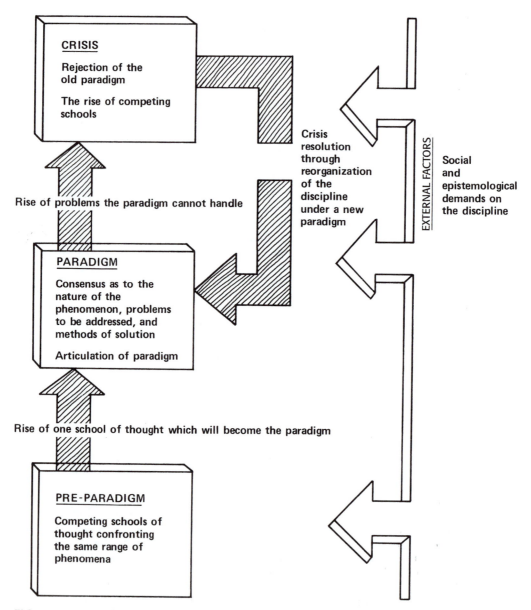

FIG. 2–1. Stages of a Paradigm Shift. *(From Kielhofner, G. [1983]*. Health through occupation: Theory and practice in occupational therapy. *Philadelphia: F. A. Davis. With permission.)*

problems. Over time, problems emerge that cannot be solved within the boundaries of the existing paradigm. As these "unsolvable" problems accumulate, the old paradigm is criticized and the discipline enters the crisis stage. During the crisis stage, alternative ways of thinking about the phenomenon appear and compete for prominence within the profession. Eventually, a new paradigm emerges that can successfully address the previously identified "unsolvable" problems. This return to paradigm requires significant reorganization of the discipline's knowledge base. However, information and technology generated by the old paradigm are typically retained (Kielhofner, 1983).

According to a model by Barker (1992), paradigms develop and paradigm shifts occur in a predictable manner (Figure 2–2). During the first phase, or phase A, a new way of solving problems emerges. A few interesting problems are solved using this new approach. Kuhn (1970) regards these special solutions as "exemplars." The boundaries of the new paradigm are explored, and the rules and regulations are discovered. As more is known about the emerging paradigm, more and more problems are solved and the trajectory or slope of the line in the B phase increases dramatically. Now, rapid problem solving is possible, new technologies emerge, and new approaches are developed.

At some point in phase C, the problem solving slows and the problems needing to be solved become increasingly more difficult. At this time, the paradigm begins to lose its usefulness as problems emerge that cannot be solved. Typically, a new paradigm has already taken root, usually somewhere in the B phase. However, when the new paradigm is introduced, it is usually rejected in favor of the old paradigm that has demonstrated success. Barker (1992, p. 52) states that "every paradigm will, in the process of finding new problems, uncover problems it cannot solve, and those unsolvable problems provide the catalyst for triggering the paradigm shift."

 ## PARADIGM SHIFTS IN OCCUPATIONAL THERAPY

Kielhofner conducted an historical examination of paradigm shifts in occupational therapy (Figure 2–3). According to Kielhofner (1983), the pre-paradigm stage in occupational therapy traces its roots to the moral treatment movement with its humanistic focus. Moral treatment proponents advocated that the treatment of persons with mental illness should emphasize a daily routine of occupations in a family-like atmosphere (Neidstadt and Crepeau, 1998). Participation in occupations was believed to normalize disorganized habits and behaviors (Kielhofner, 1997). During the 18th and 19th centuries, the moral treatment philosophy was competing with a pathology-oriented approach in the treatment of the mentally ill.

During the first four decades of the 20th century, a remarkable degree of consensus emerged among practitioners and in the literature regarding "occupation" as the central phenomenon of interest. Although the **paradigm of occupation** originated in the mental health arena, it was easily applicable to physical disabilities. Occupation referred to the balance of work, play, self-care, and rest. Occupational therapists of the time viewed the individual holistically, composed of both mind and body, participating in daily tasks in interactions with their environments. Occupations were graded according to the individual's capabilities. Persons progressed from simple activities that stimulated the senses to more demanding occupations requiring concentration and skill (Kielhofner, 1997).

The first paradigm crisis is evident in the professional literature of the late 1940s and early 1950s. Increasing pressure from medicine to be more scientific led to the questioning of the paradigm of occupation. The literature began to favor kinesiological, neurophysiological, and psychoanalytic approaches to occupational therapy

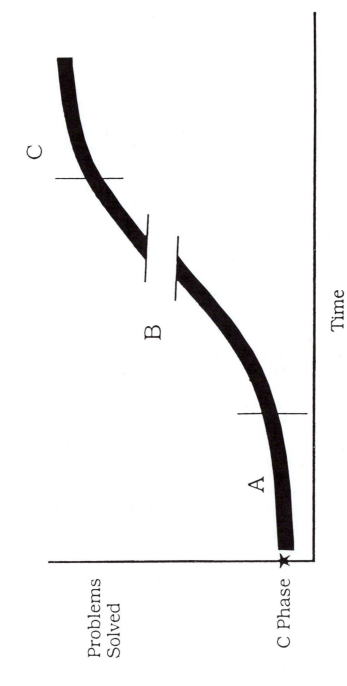

FIG. 2–2. The Paradigm Curve. *(From* Future Edge *by Joel Arthur Barker. Copyright © 1992 by Joel Arthur Barker. Reprinted by permission of HarperCollins Publishers, Inc.)*

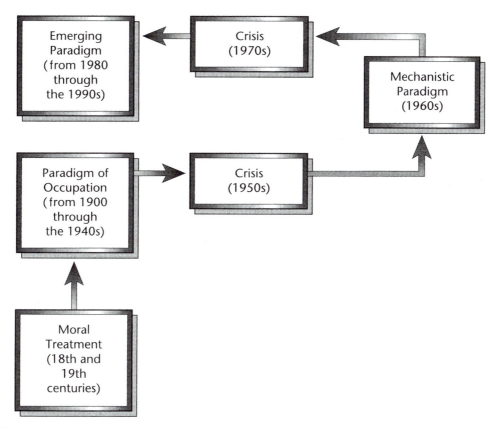

FIG. 2–3. Paradigm Shifts in Occupational Therapy. *(From Kielhofner, G. [1997, p. 48]. Conceptual foundations of occupational therapy [2nd ed.]. Philadelphia: F. A. Davis. With permission.)*

practice. The depression of the 1930s caused much job insecurity, compelling occupational therapy to develop a closer relationship with medicine. The American Medical Association began accrediting occupational therapy educational programs. Occupational therapy practice began to align itself more closely with the **medical model** and adopted the medical paradigm of reductionism with few modifications (Kielhofner, 1983).

The reductionist, or mechanistic, paradigm of the 1960s asserted that by focusing on the inner mechanisms of disease and disability (neurophysiology, anatomy, kinesiology, and psychoanalysis), occupational therapy could actually alter function and thereby gain professional respect as a scientific discipline. The early paradigm of occupation had a holistic appreciation of the occupational nature of human life. The new paradigm provided a more in-depth view and shifted professional thinking from the gestalt to a reductionist focus on parts. The medical model, or **reductionist paradigm,** was not simply added to the paradigm of occupation; it replaced it and, as a result, the focus of occupational therapy practice changed dramatically in the 1960s and 1970s. Practitioners dropped "occupations" from therapy in favor of exercise, talk groups, specialized treatment techniques, and modalities (Kielhofner, 1983).

The reductionist, or mechanistic, paradigm was not, and is not, altogether negative. New assistive devices and technology, new treatment techniques such as sensory integration and neurodevelopmental treatment, and greater respect from the medical community emerged from this approach. The major loss was the profession's commitment to the occupational nature of human beings and the importance of occupation as a therapeutic medium. Without this common theme of early practice, the specialty areas within the field began to drift apart, leading to a second paradigm crisis.

This paradigm crisis, which occurred in the 1970s, was precipitated by the recognition that reductionism was an inadequate framework for understanding the complexities of human occupational behavior. Awareness grew that the problems of the chronically disabled could not be solved by technology alone. In addition, occupational therapists expressed dissatisfaction over a loss of professional identity, a fragmented ideology, and a lack of professional unity (Kielhofner, 1983, 1997).

According to Kielhofner (1997), a new paradigm is emerging that recommits itself to the core construct of occupation and attempts to regain the profession's identity and its holistic orientation. The emerging paradigm is characterized by core constructs that "elucidate the occupational nature of humans, problems of occupational dysfunction, and occupation as a health determinant" (Kielhofner, 1997, p. 90). In addition, the emerging paradigm utilizes a systems perspective. A systems viewpoint emphasizes that occupational performance results from the dynamic interaction between the person, the environmental context, and the occupations in which the person engages. In addition, it allows for a more complex perspective on factors that impact occupational performance, and therefore a broader range of potential solutions to occupational performance problems (Kielhofner, 1997). The emerging paradigm also values a client-centered approach, active engagement and empowerment, and a balance of the art and science of practice.

BASIC PRINCIPLES OF SYSTEMS THEORY

General systems theory (GST) represents a major shift in scientific thinking from the prevailing paradigm of reductionism. This shift can be best understood as a transformation in the way in which science conceptualizes reality and in how it generates new knowledge. Von Bertalanffy (1969, p. 57) characterizes the paradigm shift from reductionism to GST as "a change in basic categories of knowledge . . . to deal with complexities, wholes, systems, organizations . . . a shift or re-orientation in scientific thinking."

In contrast to reductionism, which reduces phenomena into the smallest possible units that can be quantifiably measured, **systems theory** focuses on larger units, or systems, that are conceptualized as patterns and configurations. Explanations of phenomenon in reductionism are based on cause-and-effect relationships and linear models, whereas in systems theory, explanation is based on **laws of hierarchy** and circular or spiral models. In addition, reductionism is a mechanistic view of the world, while systems theory is more organismic in nature. GST acknowledges the importance of contextually appropriate human behavior in contrast to reductionism's emphasis on normative responses.

Historically, reductionism has been enormously successful in the basic sciences and has enhanced medical technology dramatically. However, as a paradigm for the behavioral and social sciences and as a means of explaining the behavior of human and social systems, it is incomplete, inadequate, and overly simplistic. Systems theory does not attempt to supplant reductionist approaches. Rather, it aims to enhance and expand the prior paradigm. Reductionism is genuinely appropriate and useful for particular classes of phenomena, but its application has been overextended and improperly utilized in the behavioral and social sciences, including occupational therapy.

According to Capra (1982, p. 43), systems theory "looks at the world in terms of the inter-relatedness and interdependence of all phenomenon, and in this framework an integrated whole whose properties cannot be reduced to those of its parts is called a system." A hierarchy of types of systems, based on levels of complexity, has been developed and includes from least complex to most complex: physical systems, biological systems, and social systems (von Bertalanffy, 1968).

All systems and components of systems are organized by levels and operate according to the laws of hierarchy. The laws of hierarchy state that lower levels of a system constrain higher levels and higher levels direct lower levels. This implies that open or living biological systems direct and organize lower-level physical systems which, in turn, limit and constrain the activities of higher-level biological systems. Two other laws of hierarchy concern change. Less time and effort are required for change to occur at higher levels than at lower levels, and a change at one level in a system resonates through all of the other levels, resulting in change in the system as a whole. At the level of biological systems, open systems represent the point at which living systems begin to be differentiated from closed, nonliving systems.

A recent reformulation of systems theory, referred to as *dynamical systems theory*, has replaced the concept of hierarchy with the concept of "self-organizing processes." Dynamical systems theory asserts that "states of order, including organized behavior, arise spontaneously in complex systems without any central agent or underlying causal mechanism" (Kielhofner, 1997, p. 75). In this view, hierarchies are functional entities engaged in a dynamical process, not rigid structures.

Open systems are those systems that interact with their environments and are self-maintaining through input, throughput, output, and feedback mechanisms (Kielhofner, 1978). An open system inputs information, material, and energy from the environment. It then transforms and manipulates the input in the throughput process and outputs some new action/behavior on the environment. The interaction of the system with its environment is further refined and guided by the feedback process. Feedback regarding the results and outcome of the new action or behavior that was initiated influences subsequent output (Kielhofner, 1978). Feedback also enables the system to modify its internal components in response to environmental demands.

The underlying themes and principles of systems theory have been incorporated, to varying degrees, in the research, practice, and theory development of a wide array of disciplines, including some health-related fields. Examining the uses of systems philosophy, approaches, and theory in these disciplines can provide a framework from which to develop and enhance systems applications in occupational therapy.

 PARADIGM SHIFTS IN OTHER DISCIPLINES

PUBLIC HEALTH AND MEDICINE

Public health can be defined as (Green and Anderson, 1982, p. 3):

> the science and art of preventing disease, prolonging life, and promoting health and well-being through organized community effort for the sanitation of the environment, the control of communicable infections, the organization of medical and nursing services for the early diagnosis and prevention of disease, the education of the individual in personal health, and the development of the social machinery to assure everyone a standard of living adequate for the maintenance or improvement of health.

In the United States, the "modern era" of public health can be traced back to the 1850s and represents an organized, rigorous assault on health problems and disease. According to Green and Anderson (1982), the "modern era" can be divided into *five* distinct phases as follows:

1. Miasma phase (1850–1880)
2. Disease control or health protection phase (1880–1920)
3. Health resources or medical phase (1920–1960)

4. Social engineering phase (1960–1975)
5. Health promotion phase (1975–present)

The Miasma Phase (1850–1880)

According to the *American Heritage College Dictionary* (1997, p. 860), miasma means "a noxious atmosphere or influence, a poisonous atmosphere once thought to rise from swamps and putrid matter and cause disease." The belief in the mid- to late 1800s was that noxious air, dirt, and lack of cleanliness caused illness. Disease prevention efforts focused on garbage collection, public sanitation, street cleaning, food handling, and personal hygiene education (Green and Anderson, 1982).

Disease Control or Health Protection Phase (1880–1920)

This phase of public health was initiated by the work of Louis Pasteur and was perpetuated by Robert Koch and Walter Reed. Pasteur demonstrated that organisms cause disease and the science of bacteriology was born. Disease control efforts focused on the development of inoculations against diseases such as rabies and typhoid fever, and an increased emphasis on quarantine to prevent the spread of communicable illnesses.

Health Resources or Medical Phase (1920–1960)

Health examinations of World War II Army recruits revealed that approximately one-third were unfit, either physically or mentally, to serve in the military. This finding refocused public health and medical efforts on the health of individual citizens. Financial resources were invested in the construction and expansion of hospitals, the development of health professionals, and the enhancement of biomedical research. At this time, the number of health professional schools, such as medicine, nursing, and dentistry, increased exponentially in order to staff the new hospitals. The National Institutes of Health was established. Additionally, voluntary health organizations assumed significant responsibility for bringing health concerns to the attention of the public (Green and Anderson, 1982). Occupational therapy services in the medical model expanded significantly during this time, but focused less on occupation and more on performance components (Kielhofner, 1983).

Social Engineering Phase (1960–1975)

In the early 1960s, it became evident that not all Americans were benefiting from the advancements of medical science. The economically disadvantaged had little access to mainstream health-care services. The passage of Medicare and Medicaid legislation in 1967 was an effort to make health-care services available to all citizens.

Other social concerns related to health were also addressed at the federal level, including housing, education, and poverty. Costs of medical care, technology, and biomedical research escalated at an unprecedented rate. Yet the overall health of the nation's citizens did not improve proportionately (Green and Anderson, 1982).

Health Promotion Phase (1975–Present)

By the late 1970s, a renewed interest in health promotion and disease prevention was evident due in large part to the recognition that a significant percentage of the remaining health problems were attributable to an individual's lifestyle and behavior. The leading causes of morbidity, mortality, and disability (heart disease, cancer, stroke, human immunodeficiency virus [HIV] infection, and accidents) are associated with significant lifestyle and behavioral etiologies.

Health promotion efforts combine social and environmental supports with strategies for health education and behavioral changes to prevent disease and disability and enhance health and well-being. In the mid- to late 1970s, the National Health Information and Health Promotion Act (1976) was enacted and the two-volume Surgeon General's report on the nation's health, *Healthy People* (1979) and *Promoting Health, Preventing Disease: Objectives for the Nation* (1980), was published. This set the federal disease prevention and health promotion agenda for the year 2000 (Green and Anderson, 1982), resulting in the publication of *Healthy People 2000* (U.S. Department of Health and Human Services, 1990). These documents are important to occupational therapy practice and are discussed in more detail in Chapter 3.

HEALTH-CARE DELIVERY FOR PERSONS WITH DISABILITIES

In the history of service provision to disabled populations, three distinct phases or paradigmatic shifts can be identified. The first phase was the era of **institutionalization,** which ended roughly in the mid-1970s. Individuals with cognitive, emotional, and/or physical disabilities were housed in large institutions and segregated from their families, friends, and the general public. The inadequacies and abuses in institutionalized care became glaringly obvious as class-action lawsuits were filed and people with disabilities became more vocal in their demands for autonomy (Bradley and Knoll, 1995).

The second era, **deinstitutionalization** and community development, focused on moving individuals with disabilities into the community, providing specialized housing and services in more "homelike" settings. The prevailing values of the time were individual rights, maximizing human potential, and placement in the "least restrictive environment." Professionals, however, were still the planners of service and retained authority.

One of the guiding principles of this era was referred to as "developmental theory." This theory posited that no matter what level of function a person had, he or she could develop skills and behaviors reflective of higher developmental levels. This assumption was responsible for the generation of the rehabilitation focus of the time. Generally, this model of service provision dominated from the mid-1970s to the late 1980s. One of the limitations of this approach has been the assumption that individuals could develop skills and behaviors in artificial contexts that would then generalize to the communities in which they lived (Bradley and Knoll, 1995).

The present phase could be referred to as the era of **community membership**. The current emphasis is on community supports to facilitate integration, autonomy, quality of life, and independence. The current focus is on providing services and supports in environments in which people live to allow them to function more effectively. The guiding principle is the adaptation of the environment to meet the individual's needs, rather than education of the individual to adapt to the environment. In reality, dysfunction is a dynamic interplay between an individual's limitations and resources and the demands and constraints of the environment.

The philosophical underpinnings of this model are derived from Kurt Lewin's (1935) classic formulation that behavior is a function of the interaction between the person and the environment. Subsequent research by Dembo, Leviton, and Wright (1956), which focused on people with physical disabilities, found that the limitations experienced by persons with disabilities were more often the result of societal and environmental constraints than inherent in the physical disability.

In this community membership perspective, three potential areas for change exist: (1) the individual, (2) the environment, and (3) societal expectations and attitudes. In the past, most of the focus has been on changing the individual, with some attention to modifying specific environments for accessibility. The emerging paradigm calls for a greater emphasis on modifying environments and dramatically changing societal attitudes. It is a systems approach to change that recognizes and appreciates the dynamic interplay among individuals, families, communities, health-care services, public policy, and societal norms.

Although earlier perspectives have diminished in intensity, the medical model of institutional care and segregation of the sick and disabled continues to persist. Deinstitutionalized care in specialized housing and segregated "treatment" programs has become more of the norm, while *full* community membership for individuals with disabilities remains mainly a dream pursued.

VOCATIONAL REHABILITATION

In the 1980s, Stubbins and Albee wrote about changing ideologies or paradigms in the practice of vocational rehabilitation. They described two models of practice, the clinical model and the ecological model, asserting that these models "are more than alternative scientific models but encompass different value attitudes and moral perspectives concerning how to deal with the employment problems of disabled persons" (Stubbins and Albee, 1984, p. 350).

In the **clinical model of vocational rehabilitation,** the disabled individual is presumed to be unemployed because of some personal deficit that may or may not be remediable. Therefore, the person with a disability must be assessed, counseled, and treated to make him or her more employable. The model's primary focus of vocational rehabilitation is to modify or restructure the individual's psychological and vocational skills and behaviors (Stubbins and Albee, 1984). This approach has a tendency to "blame the victim." Very little attention, if any, is paid to the fact that segregated housing and education, architectural barriers, and societal attitudes developmentally disadvantage disabled individuals. The clinical model has not been generally successful in meeting the vocational needs of persons with disabilities, particularly those who are severely physically disabled or mentally ill.

An alternative to the clinical model of vocational rehabilitation is the **ecological or environmental model of vocational rehabilitation**. The underlying premise of this paradigm is that numerous environmental, social, and economic forces affect the person with a disability (Stubbins and Albee, 1984). These forces have the potential to limit or expand the individual's capacity to function in his or her own best interest and are therefore targets of intervention. The focus is on modifying all aspects of the environment (physical, social, and political) to support optimal vocational function. Stubbins and Albee (1984) believe that expanding vocational rehabilitation to include these domains of concern is a significant professional advancement over the more limited focus on the individual's capacity for change through clinical intervention.

 # COMMUNITY PRACTICE PARADIGM

Though it is easy to critique the limitations of medical models of health-care delivery, it is far more difficult to describe the essential components of a new, more community-oriented paradigm. Clearly, the role of the professional and the therapeutic relationship between provider and "patient" is different in the two paradigms (Table 2–1). In addition, some basic terminology from the medical model, such as "patient," is clearly inappropriate in community settings.

Occupational therapy practitioners must make a conscious effort to modify their use of terminology from patient to *client,* from treatment to *intervention,* and from reimbursement to *funding*. Use of medical language can limit one's perspective, unnecessarily narrow professional focus, and decrease the ability to perceive options.

TABLE 2–1

CONTRASTING PARADIGMS

Medical Model	*Community Model*
Professional is responsible.	Community member is responsible.
Professional has power.	Community member has power.
Professional makes decisions.	Community member makes decisions.
Professional is the "expert."	Community member is the "expert."
Professional answers to the agency.	Professional answers to the consumer.
Planning is fragmented.	Planning is coordinated.
Culture is denied.	Culture is appreciated.

The community paradigm requires a **client-centered approach** to practice. A client-centered approach "promotes participation, exchange of information, client decision-making, and respect for choice" and "focuses on the issues which are most important to the person and his or her family" (Law, 1998, preface). The collaborative process is designed to enable the client to identify occupational performance problems, engage in problem solving and propose solutions that meet their unique individual needs and circumstances. The occupational therapist is a facilitator, educator, and mentor in the process (Law, 1998). Use of the term "client" in the community paradigm may refer to an individual, a family, an organization, or an entire community. Regardless of the type of client identified, the principles of client-centered practice are still relevant.

In the transition from a medical model paradigm to a **community practice paradigm,** professionals need to relinquish responsibility, power, and control to the recipient of services, client, or community member. The client is the expert regarding his or her situation, needs, and desires. Therefore, the client is the person who makes the decisions regarding the services utilized. For community practice to be successful, planning must be coordinated with and through a variety of agencies, organizations, and individuals in the community. The impact of culture also must be recognized, appreciated, and incorporated into service delivery. Ultimately, the professional reports to the client who is both the recipient and evaluator of the services provided.

In the community practice paradigm, professionals function as facilitators whose role is to build and reinforce capacity and develop leadership in others. This requires humility, the ability to share successes with others, and patience. Successful practice in the community requires more time than in the typical clinical setting, as consensus must be developed and resources identified and obtained to support individuals in maintaining a satisfying lifestyle in the community of their choice.

A systems perspective is extremely useful in conceptualizing community practice. Throughout history (Green and Anderson, 1982, p. 22),

> people have organized themselves into families, institutions, communities, and societies to exercise more control over the environment and over the behavior of each other. Rules of behavior become community norms that are transmitted from one generation to another as culture. Culture defines acceptable social organization (family interaction patterns, roles and responsibilities of institutions and leaders, and the functions of government) as well as individual behavior. The influence of all these cultural, economic, organizational, and institutional forces on the environment, on individual behavior, and on health may be referred to as the social history of health.

A systems approach recognizes the complexity of the social history of health and provides a framework for assessment and intervention at various levels of systems, including individual, interpersonal, organizational, community, and public policy levels. The focus of intervention in community practice might be the individual recipient of service. However, just as frequently, if not more frequently, the focus of intervention is the family or the community as a whole. Impacting one level of the systems hierarchy will indirectly affect other levels. Individuals are embedded in a number of systems that must be addressed even when the focus of intervention is at the individual level. An individual's level of self-fulfillment and independence in the community may well be more a function of environmental, institutional, and social barriers than the individual's disability itself. Therefore, intervention may focus on several levels of systems simultaneously.

Assessment of individuals in the community paradigm may include the traditional components of occupational therapy evaluation based upon performance areas and performance components. However, this type of evaluation is usually insufficient in the community setting. Performance components are often the primary focus in the medical model. In the community paradigm, the performance areas of activities of daily living, work and productive activities, play/leisure activities, and performance contexts take on much more significance. If the focus of intervention is not the individual, but rather a collection of individuals—for example, a family, a community, or some subpopulation of a community such as members of a senior center—then assessment must be much broader in scope. Assessment in community settings requires attention to the population to be served and the context in which the services will be delivered (Box 2-1). Intervention planning utilizes the information generated from the comprehensive assessment, and potential programs of services are identified with input from the intended service recipients and community organizations. Community

---

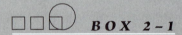 **BOX 2-1**

Assessment of Population and Context

I. **Assessment of the population:**
   A. General demographics (age, gender, diagnoses, etc.)
   B. Current and anticipated living and working environments and role expectations
   C. Current performance in areas of activities of daily living, work and productive activities, and play/leisure activities
   D. General performance component assets and deficits
   E. Significance of these factors with respect to community members' goals and needs
II. **Assessment of the context:**
   A. General characteristics of the agency/program (mission, goals, etc.)
   B. Characteristics of the physical environment
   C. Characteristics of the social environment/milieu (norms, emotional and cultural climate, etc.)
   D. Availability of resources (space, materials, staff, etc.)
   E. Significance of these factors with respect to community members' goals and needs

institutions, such as schools, churches and synagogues, social organizations, health-care providers, and political entities, are all part of the context of service and therefore are integral components of assessment and intervention. Chapter 6 describes the process of program development in community settings in detail.

 ## CONCLUSION

As occupational therapy services in the community increase and as practitioners become more comfortable with indirect service provision and designing interventions for populations, the paradigm of community practice will evolve. Currently, the paradigm of direct-service provision to individuals in clinical settings is inadequate for these emerging areas of practice in the community. The old paradigms are insufficient for identifying relevant issues and solving the problems associated with community practice. The emerging paradigm, as described by Kielhofner (1997), has the potential to fill this void. Learning from other disciplines, which have had a community focus for all or most of their existence (for example, sociology, social psychology, public health, and community health education), can be a powerful tool in facilitating occupational therapy's transition into the community. All occupational therapy practitioners, educators, and students are critical links in this monumental paradigm shift in the profession.

 ## STUDY QUESTIONS

1. Describe the positive and negative aspects of having a well-developed paradigm for the profession.
2. Identify the characteristics of the emerging paradigm in occupational therapy.
3. Compare and contrast the paradigm shifts in occupational therapy with those of public health and vocational rehabilitation.
4. Discuss the usefulness of systems theory to community practice.
5. Describe what you believe should be the basic components and/or characteristics of a community practice paradigm in occupational therapy.
6. Describe a situation in your personal or professional life that required a significant change in perspective or paradigm shift in your thinking.

REFERENCES

American heritage college dictionary (3rd ed.). (1997). Boston: Houghton Mifflin.

Barker, J.A. (1992). *Future edge*. New York: William Morrow.

Bradley, V.J., and Knoll, J. (1995). Shifting paradigms in services to people with disabilities. In O.C. Karan and S. Greenspan, *Community rehabilitation services for people with disabilities*. Boston: Butterworth-Heinemann.

Capra, F. (1982). *The turning point*. New York: Bantam.

Dembo, T., Leviton, G.L., and Wright, B.A. (1956). Adjustment to misfortune—a problem of social psychological rehabilitation. *Artificial Limbs, 3,* 4–62.

Green, L.W., and Anderson, C.L. (1982). *Community health*. St. Louis: Mosby.

Kielhofner, G. (1978). General systems theory: Implications for theory and action in occupational therapy. *American Journal of Occupational Therapy, 32*(10), 637–645.

Kielhofner, G. (1983). *Health through occupation: Theory and practice in occupational therapy*. Philadelphia: F. A. Davis.

Kielhofner, G. (1997). *Conceptual foundations of occupational therapy*. Philadelphia: F. A. Davis.

Kuhn, T.S. (1970). *The structure of scientific revolutions* (2nd ed.). Chicago: The University of Chicago Press.

Law, M. (1998). *Client-centered occupational therapy*. Thorofare, NJ: Slack.

Lewin, K. (1935). *A dynamic theory of personality*. New York: McGraw-Hill.

Neidstadt, M.E., and Crepeau, E.B. (1998). *Willard and Spackman's occupational therapy*. Philadelphia: Lippincott.

Stubbins, J., and Albee, G.W. (1984). Ideologies of clinical and ecological models. *Rehabilitation Literature, 45*(11–12), 349–353.

U.S. Department of Health and Human Services. (1980). *Promoting health/preventing disease: Objectives for the nation*. Washington, DC: U.S. Government Printing Office.

U.S. Department of Health and Human Services. (1990). *Healthy people 2000: National health promotion and disease prevention objectives* (Publication No. 017-001-00474–0). Washington, DC: U.S. Government Printing Office.

U.S. Department of Health, Education and Welfare. (1979). *Healthy people: Surgeon General's report on health promotion/disease prevention* (Publication No. 79–55071). Washington, DC: U.S. Government Printing Office.

von Bertalanffy, L. (1968). General systems theory—the skeleton of science. In W. Buckley (Ed.), *Modern systems research for the behavioral scientist*. Chicago: Aldine.

von Bertalanffy, L. (1969). Chance or law. In A. Koestler and J.R. Smythies (Eds.), *Beyond reductionism*. Boston: Beacon.

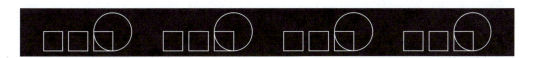

3

CHAPTER

Public Health, Community Health, and Occupational Therapy

Marjorie E. Scaffa, PhD, OTR, FAOTA
Sharon Desmond, PhD
Carol A. Brownson, MSPH

■ OUTLINE

Activity limitation	Occupational alienation
Community	Occupational deprivation
Community health	Occupational imbalance
Community health interventions	Prevalence
Determinants of health	Prevention
Functional limitation	Preventive occupation
Epidemiology	Primary prevention
Health	Public health
Health promotion	Resiliency factors
Healthy People	Risk factors
Healthy People 2010	Secondary prevention
Incidence	Tertiary prevention

LEARNING OBJECTIVES

This chapter is designed to enable the reader to:
- Define the terms public health, community health, epidemiology, and risk factors.
- Discuss the major concepts associated with public health.
- Differentiate between public health and medicine.
- Discuss strategies for primary, secondary, and tertiary prevention.
- Compare the development of the national health goals and objectives from the 1979 *Healthy People* document with those in the *Healthy People 2010* report.
- Explain occupational therapy's role within the context of health promotion, community, and public health.

 INTRODUCTION

Although a sound knowledge base in occupational therapy (OT) is likely, the reader may be less familiar with the areas of public health and community health. This chapter presents the underlying concepts and principles of public health and community health as a foundation for providing OT from a community perspective. The chapter discusses key public and community health concepts such as health promotion, prevention, national health goals, and disability. It also addresses the roles that may be assumed by OT and measures that may be implemented to improve the health of the community.

 PUBLIC HEALTH

Public health is concerned with optimizing the health status of populations. Detels and Breslow (1997, p. 3) stated that public health is "the process of mobilizing local, state, national, and international resources to ensure the conditions in which people can be healthy." To achieve these healthy conditions, four public health strategies are used: (1) promoting health and preventing disease, (2) improving medical care, (3) promoting health-enhancing behaviors, and (4) controlling the environment (Detels and Breslow, 1997). These authors also identified three principles of public health that must be considered before any action can be taken to alleviate health concerns: (1) the specific problems affecting the community's health must be assessed, (2) any strategies implemented must be based on scientific knowledge and available resources, and (3) the level of social and political commitment that currently exists must be determined.

A comprehensive definition of public health was put forth by Winslow in 1920 (p. 30):

> Public health is the science and art of preventing disease, prolonging life, and promoting physical health and efficiency through organized community efforts for the sanitation of the environment, the control of communicable infections, the education of the individual in principles of personal hygiene, the organization of medical and nursing service for the early diagnosis and preventive treatment of disease, and the development of the social machinery which will ensure to every individual in the community a standard of living adequate for the maintenance of health.

Public health is often defined in terms of its aims and goals, rather than grounded in a specific body of knowledge (Fee, 1997; Detels, Holland, McEwen, and Omenn, 1997). Winslow's broad definition accurately implies that many disciplines contribute to the field of public health, including epidemiology, the biological and clinical sciences, biostatistics, nursing, health education, sanitation, industrial hygiene, sociology, psychology, economics, law, and engineering. However, the fundamental scientific basis of public health is **epidemiology,** the study of the distribution, frequencies, and determinants of disease, injury, and disability in human populations (MacMahon and Trichopoulos, 1996).

Epidemiology uses health statistics, including measures of incidence and prevalence, to estimate disease, injury, and disability in a variety of population groups; analyze health trends; plan and evaluate public health initiatives; and make informed health policy decisions. **Incidence** refers to the number of new cases of disease, injury, or disability within a specified time frame, typically a year. **Prevalence** refers to the total number of cases of disease, injury, or disability in a community, city, state, or nation existing at one point in time (Pickett and Hanlon, 1990).

According to Pickett and Hanlon (1990), preventive interventions attempt to reduce the incidence rate of a disease or an injury, and early detection procedures and rapid treatment attempt to reduce the duration of illness. Either strategy would result in a decreased prevalence rate. Combining the two strategies of prevention and early detection is the most effective approach to reducing overall prevalence.

Public health practitioners also are very interested in risk factors, both modifiable and nonmodifiable, that compromise health. **Risk factors** are those precursors that increase an individual's or population's vulnerability to developing a disease or disability or sustaining an injury (Scaffa, 1998). Often when people hear or use the term "risk factor," they are thinking of a physical condition that contributes to a disease. For example, high cholesterol, hypertension, and obesity are risk factors that can contribute to cardiovascular disease. However, risk factors are not just physical, behavioral, or genetic. They can also be social, economic, political, and environmental. Some risk factors are considered causal because the health problem cannot occur in the absence of the risk factor. Other risk factors are considered contributory because they interact with other risk factors leading to the development, exacerbation, or maintenance of disease, injury, or disability (Scaffa, 1998).

In addition to risk factors, public health professionals attempt to increase resiliency or protective factors that contribute to improved health and well-being. **Resiliency factors** are those precursors that appear to increase an individual's or population's resistance to developing a disease or disability or sustaining an injury (Scaffa, 1998). Resiliency factors may include the individual's genetic composition, personality, and health behavior patterns and social factors such as peer and family relationships and environmental and institutional supports for health. Public health interventions attempt to modify all types of risk factors and strengthen resiliency or protective factors to enhance the overall health and well-being of populations.

HEALTH PROMOTION

Health promotion, a key public health strategy, is defined as any planned combination of educational, political, regulatory, environmental, and organizational supports for actions and conditions of living conducive to the health of individuals, groups, or communities (American Hospital Association, 1985; Green and Kreuter, 1991). More simply, it is "the process of enabling people to increase control over and to improve their health" (World Health Organization, 1986, p. iii). Health promotion encompasses strategies impacting all societal levels, including individuals, groups, organizations, communities, and government policy makers. A key purpose of health promotion is the prevention of disease and disability in individuals and populations.

PREVENTION

Prevention refers to "anticipatory action taken to reduce the possibility of an event or condition from occurring or developing, or to minimize the damage that may result from the event or condition if it does occur" (Pickett and Hanlon, 1990, p. 81). When applying the term to public health, prevention refers to reducing the likelihood of the occurrence of disease/disability or inhibiting its progression to enhance optimal health and quality of life. Specifically, there are three levels of prevention—primary, secondary, and tertiary. Each level focuses on preventing or stopping disease at a particular point along the natural continuum of the disease process.

Primary prevention focuses on healthy individuals who potentially could be at risk for a particular health problem. The goal is to prevent the disease from ever occurring by taking steps to maintain one's current healthy status and reduce susceptibility. For example, an already healthy person could continue to eat nutritious foods in the proper quantities and exercise regularly. Doing so could potentially avert obesity, diabetes, or cardiovascular disease. Another primary prevention strategy is to always wear a seat belt while in a motor vehicle, possibly avoiding injury if a crash occurred.

Secondary prevention focuses on the detection and treatment of disease early on in its preclinical or clinical stages. The goal is to slow the disease process, attempt to cure or control it as soon as possible, and prevent complications and disability. Arresting or reversing disease communicability is also a focus because early treatment of an infectious disease will limit exposure to others. An example of secondary prevention is an individual with hypertension exercising and maintaining an optimal weight so he or she can achieve normal blood pressure readings, and thus reduce the risk of myocardial infarction (MI) and cerebrovascular accident (CVA).

Tertiary prevention, the third level, refers to measures used in the advanced stages of disease, to limit disability and other complications. Tertiary prevention is implemented when a person is already ill and the initial damage has already occurred. The goal is to restore as much functionality as possible, rehabilitate the individual, and attempt to prevent further damage. This level of prevention is the most familiar to OT practitioners. For example, OT practitioners routinely teach joint protection techniques to individuals with rheumatoid arthritis to prevent deformity. Energy-conservation techniques are taught to individuals with cardiac conditions to prevent myocardial infarction.

DIFFERENTIATION FROM MEDICINE

Examination of the unique qualities of medicine and public health may provide a better understanding of the three types of prevention and further clarify the two professions. Public health is primarily concerned with the health of entire populations. Health is thought of as a tool for achieving human well-being and optimal potential, not merely the absence of disease (Pickett and Hanlon, 1990). A strong sense of social responsibility and justice is present. Attention is paid to health-care costs and cost-benefit analyses, and the government is involved in disseminating services and identifying priorities (Pickett and Hanlon, 1990). The impact of social and environmental factors and their contribution to health and disease is emphasized (Pickett and Hanlon, 1990).

Medicine, on the other hand, is primarily concerned with the health of the individual and benefiting the individual, with or without regard to cost. The focus is on clinical medicine, that is, curing disease and tertiary prevention, rather than on primary prevention (Pickett and Hanlon, 1990). Technological, pharmaceutical, and surgical interventions are emphasized. The mind-body dichotomy is present. The central concern is fixing the physical body (Pickett and Hanlon, 1990).

Ideally, public health professionals focus on primary and secondary prevention—working with healthy and at-risk populations to prevent disease and illness from occurring in the first place, rather than waiting for people to be sick or disabled before taking action (tertiary prevention). This orientation reflects a move away from the traditional medical model in which physicians direct priorities and technology and patients are passive recipients of care. Today, clients are encouraged to be active health-care consumers. Prevention and quality of life are emphasized.

In reality, all three levels of prevention (primary, secondary, and tertiary) are necessary for optimal health. Historically, though, the United States has focused its energies, resources, and efforts almost exclusively on tertiary prevention. However, recently, with the rising cost of health care, limited resources, the chronic nature of the leading causes of death, and the aging of the population, researchers have suggested concentrating on primary prevention. Such an orientation may improve the health status of all individuals and may ultimately be more cost effective.

Currently, Americans are in the midst of a transition in terms of how they obtain health-care services. Increasingly, outpatient centers and clinics are being used for services. As a result, community-based health care is thriving while inpatient hospital-based care is declining. Managed care also has become the norm. Thus, how OT practitioners and other allied health professionals provide services and work with clients is becoming more community-based with an orientation toward primary and secondary prevention.

 ## COMMUNITY HEALTH

Typically, when people use the terms "community" and "health," they assume others define the words in the same manner. In reality, definitions can vary widely. To avoid misunderstandings, these two words are defined here for this discussion. **Community** refers to "noninstitutional aggregations of people linked together for common goals or other purposes" (Green and Raeburn, 1990, p. 41). Inherent is the idea that a community does not have to be comprised of individuals within a particular geographical region. **Health** is defined as the blending of a person's physical, emotional, social, intellectual, and spiritual resources so that he or she can master the developmental tasks necessary to enjoy a satisfying and productive life (Dintiman and Greenberg, 1980). Thus, **community health** refers to the physical, emotional, social, and spiritual well-being of a group of people who are linked together in some way, possibly through geographical proximity or shared interests.

Using a community-based approach can be optimal when providing prevention and health-care services to individuals. Social support, the ability to reach many consumers, targeted interventions that meet specific community needs, active community involvement, community-driven priorities, and the potential for a systems approach where problems can be addressed at multiple levels are included. Using a systems-oriented approach allows all involved to see the big picture and better understand relationships, connections, and dependencies. Because consequences and interactions are integral components, employing a systems view is helpful when trying to prioritize community needs and determine solutions to problems.

Community health interventions can be defined as "any combination of educational, social, and environmental supports for behavior conducive to health" (Green and Anderson, 1982, p. 3). Also, according to Green and Anderson (1982, pp. 3–4):

> The educational interventions may be directed at high-risk individuals, families, or groups or at whole communities through mass media, schools, worksites, and organizations. Social interventions may include economic, political, legal and organizational changes designed to support actions conducive to health. Environmental supports include the structure and distribution of physical, chemical and biological resources, and facilities and substances required for people to protect their health. The health behavior of a community includes the actions of the people whose health is in question and the actions of community decision makers, professionals, peers, teachers, employers, parents and others who may influence health behaviors, resources or services in the community.

The goal of community health promotion is that every member of the community experience a level of well-being and vitality, enabling him or her to choose, participate in, and enjoy the activities of the community.

 ## NATIONAL HEALTH GOALS AND OBJECTIVES FOR THE UNITED STATES

In 1979, the Surgeon General's office, in the Department of Health, Education and Welfare (now the Department of Health and Human Services [DHHS]), published a document titled *Healthy People*. This document was designed to identify national health goals and discuss health promotion and disease prevention in the United States, so increasingly scarce health-care resources could be used most efficiently and effectively. The concept underlying *Healthy People* came from Canada's LaLonde Report, a document published in 1974 describing the health status of Canadians. This framework proposed that all morbidity and mortality can be attributed to four primary elements: (1) inadequacies in the existing health-care system, (2) behavioral factors or unhealthy lifestyles, (3) environmental hazards, and (4) human biological factors (LaLonde, 1974).

The *Healthy People* document (U.S. Department of Health, Education and Welfare, 1979) emphasized the importance of lifestyle changes in reducing morbidity and mortality rates, primarily because identified unhealthy behavioral and lifestyle factors contributed to almost 50 percent of all deaths. Then, and still currently, the leading causes of death for adults included chronic diseases such as cardiovascular disease and cancer. Lifestyle factors also contributed to the leading cause of death for adolescents and young adults—unintentional and intentional injuries.

Five major health goals for the nation were identified and categorized according to life span. That is, one major goal was identified for each age group (infants, children, adolescents and young adults, adults, and older adults). Goals, several subgoals, and other problems experienced by that particular age group also were presented for each major age group. For example, the national health goal for adults was to improve the health of adults and, by 1990, to reduce deaths among people ages 25 to 64 by at least 25 percent (U.S. Department of Health, Education and Welfare, 1979). Subgoals included reducing the number of persons experiencing heart attacks, strokes, and cancer. Additionally, alcohol abuse, mental health problems, and periodontal disease were identified as necessary problems to address.

In 1980, the Surgeon General's office published *Promoting Health/Preventing Disease Objectives for the Nation* (U.S. Department of Health and Human Services, 1980), a companion report to *Healthy People*. The purpose of this document was to identify specific objectives that would enable achievement of the five national health goals. Fifteen subject areas were recognized and categorized under three main headings. Five areas were identified for preventive health services, for example, family planning and immunizations; five areas for health protection, such as occupational safety and health and fluoridation of community water supplies; and five areas for health promotion, for example, smoking cessation and improved nutrition. A total of 226 specific health objectives were written and included in the report.

A special issue of *Public Health Reports*, published in 1983, described the implementation plans and various strategies that agencies could use to help achieve the national health objectives. The document, *A Midcourse Review*, came out in 1986 and updated readers on progress toward achieving the objectives. Some objectives were already met, or were certain to be met by 1990, while some others were not likely to be reached, and still others had backtracked. A major problem recognized via *A Midcourse Review* was that available data were insufficient to measure some of the objectives.

Based on experience with *Healthy People* and the previously mentioned subsequent related documents, the Surgeon General's office in the Department of Health and Human Services made some changes to the new document, *Healthy People 2000*, released in 1990. With this document, the focus became the improvement in quality of life and people's sense of well-being, rather than only the reduction of mortality rates. The new health goals for the nation were to:

1. Increase the span of healthy life for Americans.
2. Reduce health disparities among Americans.
3. Achieve access to preventive health services for all Americans (U.S. Department of Health and Human Services, 1990).

In *Healthy People 2000*, 22 priority areas were identified for the focus of the nation's health promotion and disease prevention efforts. These areas were listed under the same three broad categories used in the 1979 document (health promotion, health protection, and preventive health services) with the addition of another category, surveillance and data systems. The purpose of this last category was to improve data collection methods.

The 1990 document also targeted another important area, the needs of several population subgroups. Previously and currently, serious disparities in health status and access to health care between the majority of the population and specific subgroups exist. These subgroups include people with low income, people with disabilities, and people in minority groups (including African Americans, Hispanic Americans, Asian and Pacific Islander Americans, Native Americans, and Alaska Natives). Two of the three national health goals identified by the 1990 document specifically address these gaps. Additionally, to achieve the goals, social and environmental factors must be addressed and emphasized because focusing on individual behaviors is insufficient. Other helpful strategies might include adopting new policies, regulations, and laws, or instituting organizational change.

The latest document, *Healthy People 2010*, was released in January 2000. Due to advances in preventive therapies, vaccines and pharmaceuticals, assistive technologies, and computerized systems, the context in which *Healthy People 2010* was developed differed from that in which *Healthy People 2000* was framed (U.S. Department of Health and Human Services, 1998). *Healthy People 2010* has two comprehensive goals: (1) to increase the quality and years of healthy life and (2) to eliminate health disparities. Progress toward these goals will be measured by 467 objectives that are organized into 28 focus areas (see Box 3–1). According to the U.S. Department of Health and Human Services (1998, Goals 3):

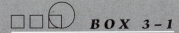 **BOX 3–1**

Healthy People 2010 **Focus Areas**

Access to quality health services
Arthritis, osteoporosis, and chronic back conditions
Cancer
Chronic kidney disease
Diabetes
Disability and secondary conditions
Educational and community-based programs
Environmental health
Family planning
Food safety
Health communication
Heart disease and stroke
HIV
Immunization and infectious diseases
Injury and violence prevention
Maternal, infant, and child health
Medical product safety
Mental health and mental disorders
Nutrition and overweight
Occupational safety and health
Oral health
Physical activity and fitness
Public health infrastructure
Respiratory diseases
Sexually transmitted diseases
Substance abuse
Tobacco use
Vision and hearing

Source: U.S. Department of Health and Human Services. (2000). *Healthy people 2010* (Conference ed., p. 17). Washington, DC: U.S. Government Printing Office.

> The first goal of Healthy People 2010 is to increase the quality as well as the years of healthy life. Here the emphasis is on the health status and nature of life, not just longevity. . . . People have become increasingly interested in other health goals such as preventing disability, improving functioning, and relieving pain and the distress caused by physical and emotional symptoms. . . . From an individual perspective, healthy life means a full range of functional capacity at each life stage, from infancy through old age, allowing one the ability to enter into satisfying relationships with others, to work and to play. From a national perspective, healthy life means a vital, creative, and productive citizenry contributing to thriving communities and a thriving nation.

Healthy People 2010 acknowledges the relationship between individual and community health and the complex interaction among six **determinants of health,** including "individual biology and behavior, the physical and social environments, policies and interventions, and access to quality health care" (U.S. Department of Health and Human Services, 2000, p. 20). "Healthy People in Healthy Communities" is the underlying premise of *Healthy People 2010*. Individual health is dependent, to some degree, on the physical and social environments that exist in the community. Likewise, community health is affected by the collective attitudes and behaviors of community members.

   Healthy People 2010 provides a framework for interdisciplinary collaboration in prevention and health promotion activities. The objectives require systematic intervention and are therefore not the purview of any one segment of society. OT practitioners need to be aware of these national priorities and participate in accomplishing these objectives.

 ## DEMOGRAPHICS OF DISABILITY AND THE NEED FOR PREVENTION

Overall, the prevalence of disability is increasing due to decreasing mortality rates for a number of disabling conditions and the aging of the population of the United States. For example, in 1980, less than 10 percent of Americans who sustained severe traumatic brain injury survived more than two years after the injury. However, in 1997, due to advances in trauma care, the survival rate improved to greater than 90 percent. In addition, while the mortality rate after CVA has declined, the incidence of CVA has not decreased (Jones, Sanford, and Bell, 1997).

   According to Jones et al. (1997, p. 36),

> advances in emergency medical care, a focus on comprehensive rehabilitation teams, continued research to develop new capabilities in assistive technology and the growth of wellness programs are contributing to the increasing numbers of people with long-term disabilities. The aging baby boomers will only add to these numbers, and the power of this growing minority.

   The term "disability" is defined in a variety of ways. Some federal agencies define disability in terms of activity limitations, while others relate disability to functional limitations. The National Center for Health Statistics estimates that 14 percent of the U.S. population have activity limitations. An **activity limitation** is defined as any "long-term reduction in a person's capacity to perform the usual kind or amount of activities associated with his or her age group" (U.S. Department of Health and Human Services, 1997, p. 317). About 38 percent of individuals with activity limitations report mobility impairments. The causes of activity limitation vary with age. Among children and adolescents, activity limitations are most often associated with cognitive limitations, asthma, deafness, speech impairment, and mental illness. Among the elderly, activity limitations are most often associated with degenerative diseases, particularly arthritis and cardiovascular disorders (U.S. Department of Health and Human Services, 1990).

The U.S. Bureau of the Census estimates that about 20 percent of Americans over age 15 have functional limitations. A **functional limitation** is defined in terms of a person's ability to perform a list of nine specified sensory and physical tasks. The prevalence of activity limitations, functional limitations, and disability increases with age. Estimations reveal that, by the year 2040, as the population of baby boomers ages, the number of Americans with disabilities will have increased threefold from what it was in 1997 (Jones et al., 1997).

A significant number of the health objectives for the nation outlined in *Healthy People 2010* address the disabled population specifically. Box 3–2 contains examples of these objectives, many of which are directly relevant for OT intervention.

 ## IMPROVING THE HEALTH OF THE COMMUNITY THROUGH OCCUPATION

The Guide to Occupational Therapy Practice (Moyers, 1999) affirms the profession's participation in health promotion and disability prevention. Health promotion services provided by OT practitioners typically involve "lifestyle redesign," or the development of supports for healthy engagement in occupations as a means of preventing the unhealthy effects of inactivity.

Wilcock (1998, p. 110) defines health from an occupational perspective as

> the absence of illness, but not necessarily disability; a balance of physical, mental and social well being attained through socially valued and individually meaningful occupation; enhancement of capacities and opportunity to strive for individual potential; community cohesion and opportunity; and social integration, support and justice, all within and as part of a sustainable ecology.

A variety of risk factors to health can result from less than optimal use, choice, opportunity, or balance in occupation. Risk factors for occupational dysfunction include occupational imbalance, deprivation, and alienation (Wilcock, 1998).

Occupational imbalance is a lack of balance between self-care, work, rest, and play/leisure that fails to meet an individual's physical or psychosocial needs, thereby resulting in decreased health and well-being. **Occupational deprivation** includes circumstances or limitations that prevent a person from acquiring, using, or enjoying an occupation. Conditions that lead to occupational deprivation may include poor health, disability, lack of transportation, isolation, homelessness, etc. **Occupational alienation** is a lack of satisfaction in one's occupations. Tasks that are perceived as stressful, meaningless, or boring may result in an experience of occupational alienation (Wilcock, 1998).

OT practice is based on the premise that participation in meaningful occupations can improve occupational performance and overall health. Therefore, **preventive occupation** can be characterized as the application of occupational science in the prevention of disease and disability and the promotion of health and well-being of individuals and communities through meaningful engagement in occupations.

THE WELL ELDERLY STUDY

An excellent example of the power of preventive occupation was demonstrated in a comprehensive research project commonly referred to as the "Well Elderly Study" conducted at the University of Southern California (Clark et al., 1997). This randomized, controlled trial, involving 361 men and women aged 60 years or older, living independently in the community, was designed to evaluate the effectiveness of a preventive OT program.

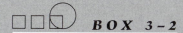 **BOX 3-2**

Objectives Targeting People with Disabilities

The overall goal in this focus area is to "promote the health of people with disabilities, prevent secondary conditions, and eliminate disparities between people with and without disabilities in the U.S."

- Include in the core of all relevant *Healthy People 2010* surveillance instruments a standardized set of questions that identify "people with disabilities."
- Reduce the proportion of children and adolescents with disabilities who are reported to be sad, unhappy, or depressed.
- Reduce the proportion of adults with disabilities who report feelings such as sadness, unhappiness, or depression that prevent them from being active.
- Increase the proportion of adults with disabilities who participate in social activities.
- Increase the proportion of adults with disabilities reporting sufficient emotional support.
- Increase the proportion of adults with disabilities reporting satisfaction with life.
- Reduce the number of people with disabilities in congregate care facilities, consistent with permanency planning principles.
- Eliminate disparities in employment rates between working-aged adults with and without disabilities.
- Increase the proportion of children and youth with disabilities who spend at least 80 percent of their time in regular education programs.
- Increase the proportion of health and wellness and treatment programs and facilities that provide full access for people with disabilities.
- Reduce the proportion of people with disabilities who report not having the assistive devices and technology needed.
- Reduce the proportion of people with disabilities reporting environmental barriers to participation in home, school, work, or community activities.
- Increase the number of tribes, states, and the District of Columbia that have public health surveillance and health promotion programs for people with disabilities and caregivers.

Source: U.S. Department of Health and Human Services. (2000). *Healthy People 2010* (Conference ed., pp. 6-2–6-22). Washington, DC: U.S. Government Printing Office.

The experimental design consisted of pre- and posttesting of three distinct groups: (1) a group that received OT services, (2) a group that participated in social activities, and (3) a control group that received no treatment. The intervention lasted nine months and occurred in two government-subsidized apartment complexes for the elderly. The pre- and posttest measurement tools included the following:

- Functional Status Questionnaire
- Life Satisfaction Index-Z
- Center for Epidemiologic Studies (CES) Depression Scale

- Medical Outcomes Study (MOS) Short Form General Health Survey
- RAND 36-Item Health Status Survey, Short Form-36

The main outcome measures of interest were "physical and social function, self-rated health, life satisfaction and depressive symptoms" (Clark et al., 1997, p. 1321).

Subjects who were randomly assigned to the OT group received OT services two hours each week in a group setting and a total of nine hours of individual OT services. Topics covered in these sessions included:

- The importance of activity to health and well-being
- Principles of joint protection and energy conservation
- Use of adaptive equipment
- Use of public transportation
- Home and community safety

Statistically significant ($p > .05$) health benefits were found among the subjects who received OT services when compared to those subjects who participated in social activities and those who received no treatment. Those receiving OT services demonstrated improved vitality, physical and social functioning, life satisfaction, and general mental health. They also demonstrated decreased bodily pain and fewer role limitations as a result of emotional or physical health problems.

Demonstration by the OT group of significant benefits when compared with the social activity group debunks any misconceptions that "activity simply for activity's sake" is health enhancing. The results of this study indicated that professionally provided services, based on OT theoretical principles, were far superior to participation in social activity programs. In fact, social activity appeared to be no more effective than no treatment at all in maintaining and improving the health and well-being of elderly persons living in the community.

PRACTITIONER ROLES IN COMMUNITY HEALTH

Changes in demographics, including the rapid growth in the number of elderly who are at risk for injuries, illnesses, and disabilities, provide an opportunity for OT practitioners to expand their role in health promotion and disease/disability prevention.

OT practitioners assume three major roles in health promotion and disease/disability prevention:

1. The promotion of healthy lifestyles for all clients and their families regardless of disability status. Lifestyle risk factors, such as tobacco use, unhealthy diet, physical inactivity, and substance abuse, are often overlooked among persons with disabilities. Standard health promotion programs and services may be inappropriate for persons with disabilities. OT practitioners are capable of adapting these programs to meet the special needs of individuals living with disabling conditions.
2. Complementing existing health promotion efforts by adding the unique perspective of occupation to programs developed by experts in areas such as health education, nutrition, and exercise. For example, in working with a person with a lower-extremity amputation due to diabetes, the OT practitioner may focus on the occupation of meal preparation using foods and preparation methods recommended in the nutritionist's health promotion program. This enables the achievement of the OT goal of functional independence in the kitchen while reinforcing the importance of proper nutrition for the prevention of further disability.
3. Development of occupation-based health promotion programs, targeting a variety of constituencies and levels of society, including individuals (both with and without disabilities), groups, organizations, communities, and governmental policies.

A variety of examples of occupation-focused health promotion interventions are listed in Box 3–3.

Injury Prevention

Injury prevention is an area rich in potential for OT intervention. According to the National Academy of Sciences, injury is probably the most underrecognized major public health problem facing the nation today. Injuries are the result of "acute exposure to physical agents such as mechanical energy, heat, electricity, chemicals and ionizing ra-

---

 BOX 3 – 3

Occupation-Based Health Promotion Interventions

Occupation-focused health promotion interventions at each level may include but are not limited to:

Individual-level interventions
- Adaptation of physical activities/exercises for people with disabilities
- Education of caregivers about proper body mechanics for lifting to prevent back injuries
- Driving evaluation and training for persons with physical or cognitive impairments

Group-level interventions
- Repetitive strain injury education and prevention and management programs for workers
- Parenting skills training for adolescent mothers
- Education of day-care providers regarding normal growth and development, handling behavioral problems, and identifying children at risk for developmental delay

Organizational-level interventions
- Consultation with industrial managers regarding the benefits of ergonomic workspace design and worksite injury prevention strategies
- Disability awareness training for service-industry personnel such as airlines, hotels, restaurants, etc.

Community-level interventions
- Modification of community recreational facilities to increase accessibility for persons with disabilities
- Consultation with contractors, architects, and city planners regarding accessibility and universal design

Governmental-policy interventions
- Promotion of full inclusion of children with disabilities in schools and day-care programs
- Lobbying for public funds to support programs to improve the quality of life for at-risk populations

diation interacting with the body in amounts or at rates that exceed the threshold of human tolerance" (U.S. Department of Health and Human Services, 1997, p. 15).

Unlike accidents, injuries typically do not happen by chance. Scientific study of injuries has demonstrated that injuries are not random occurrences. Like disease, injuries follow an identifiable pattern. Death rates due to injury vary depending on age, showing "relatively higher (rates) in infancy than for young children, rising through the early to mid-twenties, then declining through middle age, and rising again among the elderly" (U.S. Department of Health and Human Services, 1997, p. 20). Unintentional injury, including transportation-related incidents, exposure to harmful substances or environments, contact with objects and equipment, falls, and fires and explosions, accounts for the largest proportion of deaths due to injury. Suicide and homicide account for the majority of the remainder of injury-related deaths. Understanding causes and patterns of injuries makes it possible to predict and prevent a significant percentage of injuries.

OT practitioners can play a major role in a variety of injury-prevention initiatives. A few examples of programs appropriate for OT involvement are briefly described here.

ELDERLY FALL PREVENTION. Fall-prevention programs typically impact three major areas that interact to cause falls. The three assessment and intervention domains are: (1) the individual, (2) the environment, and (3) society. Attributes of the individual, which may predispose a person to fall, include sensory and perceptual deficits, musculoskeletal limitations, balance problems, and cardiovascular impairments. Fall-prevention efforts are often directed at improving aerobic fitness, muscle strength, and balance. Environmental targets for intervention may include improving lighting, modifying floor surfaces, removal of safety hazards, and installing assistive devices. Fall-prevention programs may also include education of the general public in an effort to increase acceptance and use of ambulatory aids and other safety devices (Holliday, Cott, and Torresin, 1992).

In one randomized, controlled trial conducted in seven pairs of nursing homes, investigators found that simple interventions, such as repairing wheelchairs, ensuring properly fitted shoes, removing room clutter, monitoring psychotropic medication, assisting patients more frequently, and reminding patients about safety issues, helped reduce the number of recurrent falls in the elderly by 19 percent. In addition, these interventions resulted in 50 percent fewer injurious falls by elderly residents who previously had experienced three or more falls (Ray et al., 1997).

RECREATIONAL INJURY PREVENTION. Sports and recreational injuries are a frequent cause of visits to hospital emergency rooms. Most of these injuries are associated with basketball, football, baseball, bicycles, and playground equipment (U.S. Department of Health and Human Services, 1997). In one prospective cohort study, the use of break-away bases among "high-performance" baseball players decreased the number and severity of baseball sliding injuries by 80 percent. Break-away bases are cost effective and safer than standard stationary bases in both recreational and sports settings (Janda et al., 1993). Occupational therapists can provide services to recreational facilities and programs to evaluate safety hazards and propose strategies to reduce the risk of injury in these settings.

WORK INJURY PREVENTION. In the United States, work-related injuries are expensive, costing billions of dollars in lost wages, decreased productivity, and health-care expenses. OT practitioners have the expertise to develop and implement programs to prevent back and cumulative trauma injuries, promote on-the-job safety, and design ergonomically efficient workspaces. In addition, OT practitioners can evaluate the nature and extent of work-related injuries, assess job demands, and facilitate the employee's return to work safely (Rothman and Levine, 1992).

CONCLUSION

Philosophically, OT and public health are quite compatible and even complementary. OT practitioners can learn much from collaboration with public health, health promotion, and health education professionals in terms of primary and secondary prevention strategies and community health initiatives. Public health programs can benefit from the unique contribution of occupation and occupational science perspective that OT professionals can provide. The focus of *Healthy People 2010* on quality of life, satisfying relationships, and functional capacity to work and play invites the participation and inclusion of the OT profession in public health, health promotion, prevention, and community health initiatives.

 STUDY QUESTIONS

1. Identify and describe similarities, differences, and relationships among the following concepts/terms: public health, prevention, health promotion, and community health.
2. Describe the differences between public health and medical approaches to health and disease. Discuss the implications of these two approaches with respect to OT practice.
3. Identify potential OT strategies at primary, secondary, and tertiary levels of prevention.
4. Describe the history of the development of national health goals and objectives and potential roles for OT practitioners within the *Healthy People* framework.

REFERENCES

American Hospital Association. (1985). *Health promotion for older adults: Planning for action.* Chicago: Center for Health Promotion.

Clark, F., Azen, S.P., Zemke, R., Jackson, J., Carlson, M., Mandel, D., Hay, J., Josephson, K., Cherry, B., Hessel, C., Palmer, J., and Lipson, L. (1997). Occupational therapy for independent living older adults: A randomized controlled trial. *Journal of the American Medical Association, 278,* 1321–1326.

Detels, R., and Breslow, L. (1997). Current scope and concerns in public health. In R. Detels, W.W. Holland, J. McEwen, and G.S. Omenn (Eds.), *Oxford textbook of public health.* New York: Oxford.

Detels, R., Holland, W.W., McEwen, J., and Omenn, G.S. (1997). *Oxford textbook of public health.* New York: Oxford.

Dintiman, G.B., and Greenberg, J.S. (1980). *Health through discovery.* Menlo Park, CA: Addison Wesley Longman.

Fee, E. (1997). The origins and development of public health in the United States (Chap. 3, pp. 35–54). In R. Detels, W.W. Holland, J. McEwen, and G.S. Omenn (Eds.), *Oxford textbook of public health.* New York: Oxford Univerity Press.

Green, L.W., and Anderson, C.L. (1982). *Community health.* St. Louis: Mosby.

Green, L.W., and Kreuter, M.W. (1991). *Health promotion planning: An educational and environmental approach* (2nd ed.). Mountainview, CA: Mayfield.

Green, L.W., and Raeburn, J. (1990). Contemporary developments in health promotion, definitions and challenges. In N. Bracht (Ed.), *Health promotion at the community level.* Newbury Park, CA: Sage.

Holliday, P.J., Cott, C.A., and Torresin, W.D. (1992). Preventing accidental falls by the elderly. In J. Rothman and R. Levine (Eds.), *Prevention practice: Strategies for physical therapy and occupational therapy.* Philadelphia: Saunders.

Janda, D.H., Maguire, R., Mackesy, D., Hawkins, R., Fowler, P., and Boyd, J. (1993). Sliding injuries in college and professional baseball—a prospective study comparing standard and break-away bases. *Clinical Journal of Sports Medicine, 3,* 78–81.

Jones, M., Sanford, J., and Bell, R.B. (1997). Disability demographics: How are they changing? *Team Rehab Report, 8*(10), 36–44.

LaLonde, M. (1974). *A new perspective on the health of Canadians: A working document.* Ottawa: Ministry of National Health and Welfare.

MacMahon, B., and Trichopoulos, D. (1996). *Epidemiology principles and methods.* Boston: Little, Brown.

Moyers, P.A. (1999). *The guide to occupational therapy practice.* Bethesda, MD: American Occupational Therapy Association.

Pickett, G., and Hanlon, J.J. (1990). *Public health: Administration and practice.* St. Louis: Times Mirror/Mosby.

Ray, W., Taylor, J., Meador, K., Thapa, P., Brown, A., Kajihara, H., David, C., Giddeon, P., and Griffin, M. (1997). A randomized trial of a consultation service to reduce falls in nursing homes. *Journal of the American Medical Association, 278*(7), 557–562.

Rothman, J., and Levine, R. (1992). *Prevention practice: Strategies for physical therapy and occupational therapy.* Philadelphia: Saunders.

Scaffa, M.E. (1998). Adolescents and alcohol use. In A. Henderson, S. Champlin, and W. Evashwick (Eds.), *Promoting teen health: Linking schools, health organizations and community.* Thousand Oaks, CA: Sage.

U.S. Department of Health and Human Services. (1980). *Promoting health/preventing disease: Objectives for the nation.* Washington, DC: U.S. Government Printing Office.

U.S. Department of Health and Human Services. (1986). *The 1990 health objectives for the nation: A midcourse review.* Washington, DC: U.S. Government Printing Office.

U.S. Department of Health and Human Services. (1990). *Healthy people 2000: National health promotion and disease prevention objectives* (Publication No. 017-001-00474-0). Washington, DC: U.S. Government Printing Office.

U.S. Department of Health and Human Services. (1997). *Health, United States, 1996–97 and injury chartbook.* Hyattsville, MD: National Center for Health Statistics.

U.S. Department of Health and Human Services. (1998). *Healthy people 2010 objectives: Draft for public comment.* Washington, DC: U.S. Department of Health and Human Services.

U.S. Department of Health and Human Services. (2000). *Healthy people 2010* (Conference ed.). Washington, DC: U.S. Department of Health and Human Services.

U.S. Department of Health, Education and Welfare. (1979). *Healthy people: Surgeon General's report on health promotion/disease prevention* (Publication No. 79-55071). Washington, DC: U.S. Government Printing Office.

Wilcock, A.A. (1998). *An occupational perspective of health.* Thorofare, NJ: Slack.

Winslow, C-E.A. (1920). The untilled fields of public health. *Science, 51,* 23–33.

World Health Organization. (1947). Constitution of the World Health Organization. *Chronicle of the World Health Organization, 1.*

World Health Organization. (1986). The Ottawa charter for health promotion. *Health Promotion, 1,* iii–v.

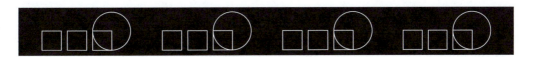

4 CHAPTER

Theoretical Frameworks for Community-Based Practice

S. Maggie Reitz, PhD, OTR, FAOTA
Marjorie E. Scaffa, PhD, OTR, FAOTA

■ OUTLINE

Community organization
Concept
Conceptual model of practice
Construct
Ecology of human performance
Frame of reference
Health belief model
Model
Model of human occupation
Occupational adaptation
Occupational science

Paradigm
Person-environment-
    occupational performance
    model
PRECEDE-PROCEED model
Principle
Social learning theory
Theory
Transtheoretical model of health
    behavior change

This chapter is designed to enable the reader to:
- Appreciate the need for practitioners to be knowledgeable and competent in the use of theory.
- Identify and define terms related to theory and the relationships among these terms.
- Describe the general characteristics and principles of some occupational therapy theories that could be used in community-based practice.
- Critique the appropriateness of these occupational therapy theories for community practice and research.
- Describe the general characteristics and principles of some health education and public health theories that could be used in community-based practice.
- Critique the appropriateness of these health education and public health theories for community practice and research.
- Define the term "community organization," describing strategies for organizing communities to meet health needs.
- Identify several reasons for the limited growth of community-based occupational therapy services.

 INTRODUCTION

This chapter explores the importance of theory and its application to community-based occupational therapy (OT) practice, with an emphasis on health promotion planning and implementation. A brief review of the terminology used is provided to help establish a common basis of understanding for the theoretical discussion. This review is followed by a description of theoretical frameworks from OT and other health disciplines. These theoretical frameworks can be used to support greater involvement in assisting communities in their efforts to improve their residents' health and quality of life.

THEORY AND THE ORGANIZATION OF KNOWLEDGE

IMPORTANCE OF THEORY TO COMMUNITY-BASED PRACTICE

One of the fundamental characteristics of a true profession is the existence of a theoretical base underlying its practice, defining the parameters within which the profession operates (Shireffs, 1984). Typically, in the development of the sciences, theory precedes application. A well-developed theoretical foundation for community-based practice is essential for a variety of reasons. Theories and models provide the foundation and context for basic and applied research, program design, implementation, and evaluation (Scaffa, 1992). Therefore, up-to-date knowledge of theories in OT and related disciplines is imperative for comprehensive community-based programming.

Experienced OT practitioners frequently have limited opportunity to keep abreast of new and evolving conceptual models of practice and theories (Reitz, 1998a). Workplace demands often inhibit practitioners' knowledge of current theory. When OT professionals are unfamiliar with current developments in theory, they may neglect an area of potential benefit for the development or refinement of ongoing or new community-based programs.

Many reasons exist for the limited use of theory in program planning (Reitz, 1998a). Two of the most prominent are today's rapid pace of change and the current sense of uncertainty in professional practice. In addition, an explosion of knowledge has taken place in this area subsequent to many practitioners' graduation from school. In the past, few students had the opportunity to observe theory application during their field-work experiences. Once a practitioner has graduated, limited emphasis is placed on theory in continuing education. Inconsistent and conflicting terminology use is also problematic, possibly creating confusion for the student of theory. Miller (1993b) has identified five reasons why OT professionals should be knowledgeable of and competent in the use of theory (Box 4–1). Both students and practitioners must feel comfortable articulating the theory base of OT and applying theory to treatment and program planning.

This chapter provides an overview of four conceptual models of OT practice and

---

 ### *B O X   4 – 1*

Miller's Reasons for Advocating Knowledge and Competency in Theory

- To validate and guide practice
- To justify reimbursement
- To clarify specialization issues
- To enhance the growth of the profession and the professionalism of its members
- To educate competent practitioners

Source: Miller, R.J. (1993b). What is theory, and why does it matter? In R.J. Miller and K.F. Walker (Eds.), *Perspectives on theory for the practice of occupational therapy* (2nd ed., pp. 8–11). Gaithersburg, MD: Aspen.

introduces models from other disciplines that can add to the body of knowledge. In the current climate of rapid change and the need to justify and substantiate the role of OT, knowledge of theory is essential. New and evolving models are well suited to support OT's role in health-care institutions and the community. However, before these models can be fully understood and implemented, it is important to clarify the terminology used in the application of theory, as well as to understand the broader structures that organize and support the various levels of knowledge.

REVIEW OF TERMINOLOGY

The following terms will be defined and described: concept, construct, principle, model, theory, paradigm, frame of reference, and conceptual model of practice. These terms are presented in sequence beginning with those used to describe the basic building blocks of theory to terms that describe higher levels of conceptualization. However, the placement of the terms "frame of reference" and "conceptual model of practice" are two exceptions to this progression.

Concepts and Constructs

A **concept** "describes some regularity or relationship within a group of facts and is designated by some sign or symbol" (Payton, 1988, p. 12). At times the term "concept" is divided into two distinct terms—concept and construct. When this distinction is utilized, the term "concept" is employed to describe images based on tangible objects such as a splint or ball, while the term **construct** is used to refer to images of intangible ideas, such as intelligence (Miller, 1993b).

Fidler (1981) used the term "concept" to identify and refer to both tangible and intangible ideas. "Competence, mastery, achievement, self-esteem, self-value, and worth are interrelated concepts" (Fidler, 1981, p. 568). Fidler lamented that these concepts are "difficult to quantify," which "explains to some extent the infrequent use of these concepts in the areas of physical disabilities as compared to psychiatry" (Fidler, 1981, p. 568). This statement was based on Fidler's review of "concepts" in OT literature from 1917 to 1977, reported by Gillette and Kielhofner (1979). It is essential that these very concepts be examined, defined, and explained in terms of their potential contribution to community-based practice.

Principle

A **principle** describes the relationship between two or more concepts, constructs, or a combination of constructs and concepts. Related principles are then organized into theories (Miller, 1993b; Payton, 1988). Examples of principles from Nelson's Conceptual Framework of Therapeutic Occupation (Nelson, 1997, p. 13) include:

- Occupation influences the world around the person
- The person can affect his or her own future occupational forms
- A person can literally change his or her own nature by engaging in occupation
- Brief occupations are nested within higher-level occupations

Model

A **model** can be defined as a semantic or diagrammatic representation of concepts and their interrelationships. This representation allows for operationalization, experimental assessment, and application of a theory (Parcel, 1984). Models can be viewed as a subclass of theories (McKenzie and Smeltzer, 1997). However, not all theories possess corresponding models and not all models are founded on specific, well-defined theories.

Theory

A scientific **theory** can be defined as a model of a specific phenomenon and a set of rules or laws that accurately describes and predicts a large class of observations related to that phenomenon (Hawking, 1988). Theory, grounded in reality, is a powerful tool for both understanding the world around us and for exerting some control over it. A robust theory describes a set of concepts in detail, dimensionalizes these concepts, systematizes the relationships among the concepts, identifies the process of change over time, and withstands strong attempts to refute it (Strauss and Corbin, 1990). The explanatory power of a theory is increased if it includes (Strauss and Corbin, 1990):

- A description of the causal, or antecedent, conditions that led to the development or occurrence of the phenomenon
- The context, or set of conditions, within which the phenomenon takes place
- The intervening conditions that facilitate and/or constrain the phenomenon
- The action/interaction strategies that can be used to manage and/or respond to the phenomenon
- The consequences, outcomes, or results of action and interaction

A well-constructed theory satisfies four basic criteria: (1) fit, (2) understanding, (3) generality, and (4) control. For a theory to have a good *fit*, it must reflect the everyday reality of the phenomenon it is designed to represent. *Understanding* refers to the need for the theory to be rational, logical, and make sense both to the researcher/theorist and to the individuals who were studied. *Generality* means that a well-developed theory is comprehensive and includes sufficient variation to provide applicability to a diversity of contexts. Lastly, it should allow for a degree of *control* over the phenomenon in question (Strauss and Corbin, 1990).

Paradigm

A paradigm guides the thinking and development of new knowledge for the use of a discipline. It is used in a variety of disciplines to address both the overall vision of the discipline as well as the practical knowledge employed in daily activities of the discipline. In the nursing literature, Marriner (1986, p. 22) presented the following description of paradigm. A **paradigm** is

> used to denote the prevailing network of science, philosophy, and theory accepted by a discipline.... The prevailing paradigm directs the activities of a discipline. As such, it is accepted by the majority of individuals within the discipline and suggests the areas of study of interest to the discipline and the means to study them.

The term paradigm has been used to describe the overall conceptualization of knowledge in a profession. In OT, however, complete agreement regarding the use of the term is lacking (Kielhofner, 1997; Miller, 1993b). Kielhofner has been influenced by Kuhn, the originator of the term paradigm, and refers to Kuhn's discussion of paradigm in writings concerning the organization of OT knowledge (Kielhofner, 1985, 1997). Kielhofner's descriptions of paradigm have evolved over time. In 1985, Kielhofner described the concept of paradigm and its relationship to OT as follows (Kielhofner, 1985, p. xvii):

> ... it is useful to think of theory as divided into two levels. The highest level is the gestalt knowledge of the field that incorporates *all* the field's concerns, concepts and technical expertise. This highest level of knowledge also defines the field, sets boundaries on its activities and specifies its values and goals. This gestalt level of knowledge in occupational therapy has been referred to as the *paradigm* of the field.

More recently, Kielhofner identified three elements of the OT paradigm: (1) core constructs, (2) focal viewpoint, and (3) integrating values (Kielhofner, 1997). These elements are represented in Figure 4–1.

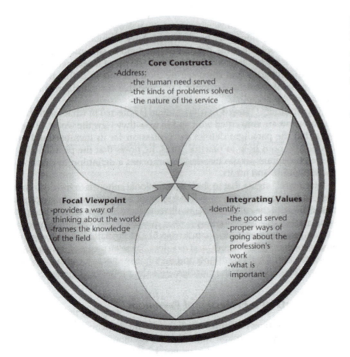

FIG. 4–1. Kielhofner's Three Elements of a Paradigm. (*From Kielhofner, G. [1997]*. Conceptual foundations of occupational therapy *[2nd ed., p. 18]. Philadelphia: F. A. Davis. With permission.*)

Frame of Reference

This term was "occasionally used in the OT literature prior to 1968" (Mosey, 1981, p. 129). Mosey defined **frame of reference** as a "set of interrelated internally consistent concepts, definitions, and postulates that provide a systematic description of and prescription for a practitioner's interaction within a particular aspect of the profession's domain of concern." Examples of commonly used frames of reference identified by Dutton, Levy, and Simon (1993) include behavioral, biomechanical, cognitive disability, developmental, neurodevelopmental, sensory integration, model of human occupation, rehabilitation, psychodynamic, spatiotemporal adaptation, and occupational adaptation.

Conceptual Model of Practice

A **conceptual model of practice** "presents and organizes a number of theoretical concepts used by therapists in their work. Each model explains an area of functioning and specifies the interventions pertaining to particular kinds of problems" (Kielhofner, 1997, p. 22). Examples of conceptual models of practice identified by Kielhofner include biomechanical model, cognitive disabilities model, cognitive-perceptual model, group work model, model of human occupation, motor control model, sensory integration model, and spatiotemporal adaptation model.

There are several "models" that also appear on the preceding list as frames of reference, which would lead one to make the assumption that conceptual models of practice and frames of reference describe the same level of knowledge. Although Kielhofner (1997) agrees that they share "attributes," he sees a distinct difference in the two entities. Namely, a frame of reference often "borrows a theory from another discipline and applies it to occupational therapy without formulating unique occupational therapy theory" (Kielhofner, 1997, p. 24). In addition, "a mature conceptual model of practice organizes concepts from within and outside the field into *unique theoretical arguments* that reflect the paradigm of the profession" (Kielhofner, 1997, p. 24).

ORGANIZATION OF KNOWLEDGE

Knowledge has been organized into systems to facilitate discussion of ideas and foster development of thought. These systems seek to explain the relationships between philosophy, theory, research, and practice and have been visualized and described in different ways. Disciplines organize knowledge for practical use into theories, models, and frames of reference. These organizational structures can be viewed as parts of larger, more complex organizational systems that contain and support the knowledge used by a profession. Figures 4–2 through 4–5 display four different schemes for organizing OT knowledge. These organizational schemes are presented to provide a high-level view and act as helpful tools in showing the links between the "science" of occupation and health, the core values and beliefs of the profession, and the historical ideals of community-based practice.

Although many similarities exist among these five viewpoints for organizing knowledge, fundamental differences also are present. Kielhofner (1997) views the paradigm of the profession as its core with conceptual practice models drawing from, and using, related knowledge under the guidance of the values and focal viewpoint provided by the paradigm. Christiansen (1991) offers a different viewpoint. He focuses on the relationships between paradigms, theories, and frames of reference.

Reitz (1998b) adds the recipient of service, possibly including an individual, a family, or a community, as an important entity to include in examining the organization of knowledge for the profession. This paradigm is visualized as being similar to a comet moving in time. The comet has a history, a present, and a trajectory or future path. The comet also changes over time but its core remains stable. An additional aspect of this method of organizing knowledge is that the comet's configuration and future travels are influenced significantly by its preceding journey through history.

Levy (1993) shows a hierarchical relationship between theory, philosophy, and practice. Mosey (1981), however, depicts philosophy as influencing science, ethics, and the arts, which, in turn, are the primary catalysts of the profession's model and continued development. This perspective is very different from Levy's view that as-

FIG. 4–2. The Relationship between Related Knowledge, Conceptual Practice Models, and Paradigms. *(From Kielhofner, G. [1997]. Conceptual foundations of occupational therapy [2nd ed., p. 15]. Philadelphia: F. A. Davis. With permission.)*

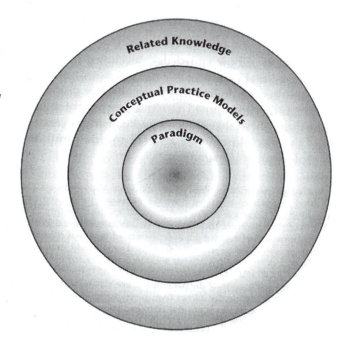

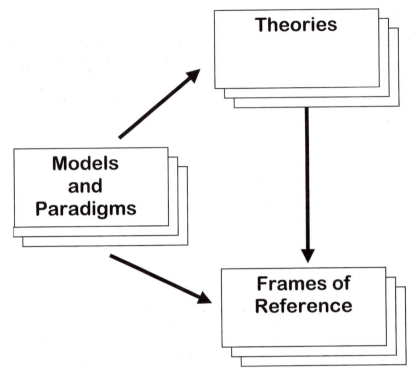

FIG. 4–3. The Relationship between Theories, Frames of Reference, and Models and Paradigms. *(Reprinted from Christiansen, C., and Baum, C. [Eds.], Occupational Therapy: Enabling Function and Well-Being [p. 41], 1997, with permission from SLACK Incorporated.)*

serts theories "from the scientific bases" (Levy, 1993, p. 61) of other fields are the beginning point for the organization of knowledge for practical use by the profession. Levy believes that theories need to be transformed before they can be of use in practice and thus begins the hierarchy with theory. An additional difference between Levy's view and the other methods presented is the inclusion of occupational science. **Occupational science** is clearly represented as the academic discipline primarily responsible for providing the profession of "occupational therapy with its own theory base" (Hopkins, 1993, p. 59). Reitz (2000) also has recently incorporated the role of occupational science when depicting the organization of OT knowledge. Occupational science is viewed as the academic discipline that supports the practice of OT. In addition, occupational science assists OT practitioners in filtering knowledge from other disciplines and simultaneously feeds other disciplines' knowledge systems.

 ## THEORIES RELATED TO COMMUNITY-BASED PRACTICE

The following is a description of popular constructs, concepts, theories, and models found in the professional literature and a critique of their appropriateness for community-based practice and research. This description is not meant to be an exhaustive account of relevant theoretical approaches, but rather a sampling to illustrate theories related to OT community-based practice. Occupational science has not been included

Comet Analogy Explained

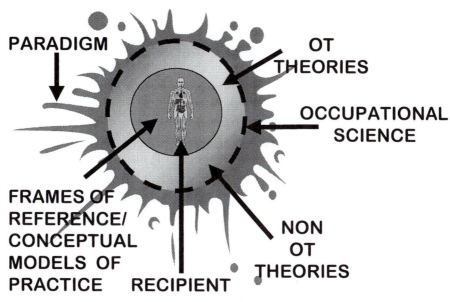

FIG. 4–4. The Relationship between the Terms of Paradigm, Theory, Frames of Reference/Conceptual Models of Practice, and Recipient of Service. *(From Reitz, S.M. [2000]. Ways to organize OT knowledge. Course Packet [OCTH 611]. Towson, MD: Towson University. With permission.)*

since it is viewed as an academic discipline (Hopkins, 1993; Levy, 1993; Zemke and Clark, 1996). The purpose of occupational science "is to generate knowledge about the form, the function, and the meaning of human occupation" (Zemke and Clark, 1996, p. vii). This is not to say that occupational science is not relevant for the practitioner when developing community-based programs. In fact, the community was the context for a very exciting study conducted by the Department of Occupational Therapy and Occupational Science at the University of Southern California (Clark et al., 1997; Jackson, Carlson, Mandel, Zemke, and Clark, 1998). The results of this research provide essential data regarding the efficacy of OT and community-based practice.

SELECTED OT CONCEPTUAL MODELS OF PRACTICE

In the past decade, a surge has occurred in the development of conceptual models of practice and frames of reference in the profession. Some models, such as the model of human occupation, continue to evolve (Kielhofner, 1997) while others, such as the ecology of human performance (Dunn, Brown, and McGuigan, 1994) and the conceptual framework of therapeutic occupation (Nelson, 1997), are more recent additions to the profession's theory base. In addition, some models such as occupational adaptation (Schkade and Schultz, 1992; Schultz and Schkade, 1992), which was developed for application in practice, can also be used for education and research. This is similar to occupational genesis (Breines, 1995), which can be used to assist in curriculum design, teaching, and clinical practice (E. Breines, personal communication, June 3, 1998).

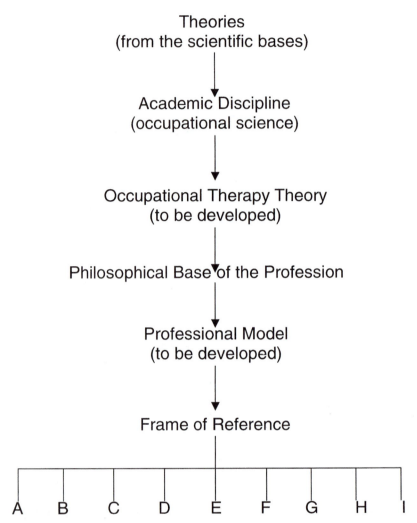

FIG. 4–5. Levy's View of the Relationship of Theory, Philosophy, and Practice. *(From Levy, L.L. [1993]. Current basis for theory and philosophy of occupational therapy, section 2—theory base. In H.L. Hopkins and H.D. Smith (Eds.),* Willard and Spackman's occupational therapy *[8th ed., p. 61]. Philadelphia: Lippincott. With permission.)*

Of the many OT models used to assist in community health program planning, four have been selected for analysis in this chapter. However, various other models are also useful in community-based practice. It is hoped that the reader will explore other models and conduct an independent analysis to determine the most appropriate model to address the health needs of their unique community. The four models discussed in this chapter were selected due to their applicability for use either individually or in conjunction with models and approaches from other disciplines presented later in this chapter.

Model of Human Occupation

The **model of human occupation (MOHO)** was developed by Kielhofner and Burke to provide a link between practice and Reilly's theory of occupational behavior (Miller,

1993a). In 1980, a four-part article describing the MOHO was published in the *American Journal of Occupational Therapy*. Kielhofner either authored or coauthored each of these articles and has been the catalyst for the model's further development. However, "scholars and clinicians worldwide now contribute to its development and application" (Kielhofner, 1997, p. 187). According to the original articles on the model, the human system interacts with the environment via a cycle of input, throughput, output, and feedback (Kielhofner and Burke, 1980). The traditional application of this model views the individual as receiving input from the environment as well as being the site of the throughput process. *Throughput* is a process composed of three subsystems: (1) volitional, (2) habituation, and (3) performance. This process was originally portrayed as being hierarchical in nature, where the higher subsystems "command lower ones and . . . lower ones constrain the higher" (Kielhofner, 1985, p. 504). More recently, it has been described as a heterarchy, where each of the subsystems works in unison to perform occupational behaviors "according to the demands of the situations in which they are performing, not according to a preordained or fixed structure" (Kielhofner, 1995, p. 34).

The output of the system is occupational behavior (Kielhofner, 1997), or purposeful interaction with the environment. This interaction, which is termed *feedback*, produces additional information to the individual regarding his or her performance. A thorough understanding of the role of the three hierarchical subsystems of throughput is necessary before applying or adapting this model. These subsystems, when working in unison, serve to organize the individual's response to the environment.

Through the years the description of the components of the environment has been modified to reflect both the continued development of the model and the influence of other theorists. In the current language of the MOHO (Kielhofner, 1997), the environment consists of physical aspects (i.e., objects and spaces) as well as social aspects (i.e., occupational forms and groups). The environment both "affords" and "presses" the individual (Kielhofner, 1997), meaning it simultaneously facilitates and constrains the human system. Figure 4–6 provides a visual picture of the relationships between these components and subsystems.

The throughput subsystems play important roles. The performance subsystem has been modified and renamed the *mind-brain-body performance subsystem* (Kielhofner, 1995, 1997). This subsystem involves the "interplay of the musculoskeletal, neurological, perceptual, and cognitive phenomena" (Kielhofner, 1997, p. 194) that allows the individual to meet the demands of both the environment and the remaining two subsystems. The primary function of this subsystem is to produce "the actions required to accomplish occupation" (Kielhofner, 1997, p. 194).

The *habituation subsystem* functions to maintain the organism by providing "everyday patterns of behaviors without ongoing conscious choices" (Kielhofner and Burke, 1985, p. 24). This maintenance is done through the development and refinement of habits and internalized roles (e.g., worker, student, mother, and spouse). Habits and internalized roles provide humans with a sense of order and predictability. In addition, they allow humans to be energy and time efficient.

The *volitional subsystem*, the final component of the throughput system, causes the individual to "enact" or "motivate" the individual to action. This subsystem, which originally was viewed as the subsystem that governed the other subsystems, is composed of three "structural components": (1) personal causation, (2) values, and (3) interests (Kielhofner and Burke, 1980, p. 576). Kielhofner and Burke (1985) defined *personal causation* as "a collection of beliefs and expectations which a person holds about his or her effectiveness in the environment" (p. 15). These beliefs include "belief in skill, belief in efficacy of skill, expectancy of success/failure, and internal/external control" (Kielhofner and Burke, 1985, p. 16). In addition, Kielhofner and Burke view values as "images of what is good, right and/or important" (p. 17), whereas interests concern the self-knowledge of activities or occupations that provide pleasure to the

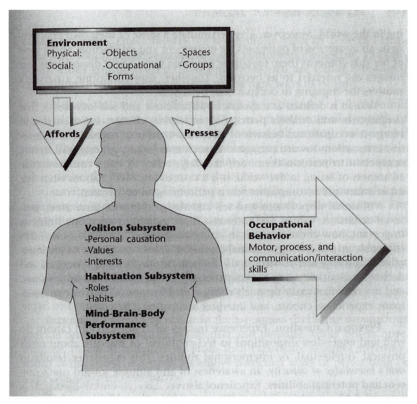

FIG. 4–6. The Major Components of the MOHO. *(From Kielhofner, G. [1997]. Conceptual foundations of occupational therapy [2nd ed., p. 189]. Philadelphia: F. A. Davis. With permission.)*

individual. This self-knowledge includes the ability to recognize patterns of like activities and an understanding of which activities have more "potency" than others.

Two related constructs that explain how the human system changes within and in response to the environment over time are also important to understand when using this model. These constructs are "the trajectory of change" and "adaptive and maladaptive cycles." The *trajectory of change* is the self-transformation of the system over time. An *adaptive cycle* supports the individual in satisfying internal demands as well as the demands of the environment (Kielhofner and Burke, 1980; Miller, 1993a). Kielhofner described a *maladaptive cycle* as failing "to meet one or both" of the internal or environmental demands just mentioned (1980, p. 737). It is possible, however, to "reverse" a maladaptive cycle and encourage the development of an adaptive cycle.

The MOHO has been applied to the treatment of individuals with a variety of disorders. This model also has potential use for well individuals in an OT community-based program. In addition, it is believed that it can be used in community-based health promotion programming where the recipient of services is the community rather than an individual or family. Figure 4–7 illustrates a simplified adaptation of the MOHO for use as a community empowerment model (Reitz, 1990). Although the latest texts (Kielhofner, 1995, 1997) describe the reworked performance subsystem, it is believed that earlier versions of the model (Kielhofner, 1985, 1992) provide a more useful framework for community-based practice. Hence, different representations of the performance subsystem are shown in Figures 4–6 and 4–7.

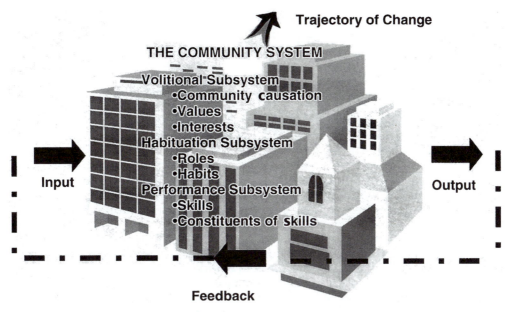

FIG. 4–7. The Model of Human Occupation as a Framework for Use in Community-Based Practice. *(From Reitz, S.M. [1990]. Community development model: An application of the model of human occupation. Unpublished paper for HEALTH 688—P, Community Health Issues for Minority Populations, University of Maryland, College Park. Adapted from Kielhofner, Burke, and Igi [1980] and Kielhofner [1985, 1992]. With permission.)*

The following fictional example illustrates the possible use of the adapted MOHO depicted in Figure 4–7 to community-based practice. In this scenario, an OT practitioner employed by a school system has been asked by the Parent-Teacher-Student Association (PTSA) to assist with the development of a violence prevention program in the county's only high school. In this example, the community's volitional subsystem has already enacted the community to make the decision to seek assistance. Thus, the community is already exhibiting "community causation" by identifying the problem and believing it has the power to take steps to make its school safer.

The actual steps the community or PTSA decides to take will be greatly influenced by the community's cultural norms (e.g., values and interests) as well as the habits and roles of its members. The practitioner can assist the community in identifying values and interests that will influence decision making relative to changes in the physical structure of the school and community habits. The community may need to collectively determine the relative priorities of potentially conflicting values. For example, the community will need to weigh the value it places on personal freedom against the value it places on student safety and comfort when deciding whether to require students to wear identification or to install security cameras.

In addressing the habituation level of this model, the practitioner would identify potentially dangerous habits (e.g., propping open exterior doors on balmy days) and roles (e.g., identification of "disengaged" students with no apparent role in the school community). In addition, the community's skills and skill constituents would be identified. This analysis would then be used to facilitate the community's current skills to maximize habit and role performance as well as identify necessary skills requiring development.

Ecology of Human Performance

The **ecology of human performance (EHP)** model was developed by the faculty at the University of Kansas to address their concerns regarding the "lack of consideration for the complexities of context" in both evaluation and intervention (Dunn et al., 1994, p. 595). Figure 4–8 depicts the major components of this conceptual model of practice—the person and his or her skills, abilities, tasks, and performance range.

A human's skills and abilities, in combination with a perception of his or her context, support the selection and performance of specific tasks, defined in the model as "objective sets of behaviors necessary to accomplish a goal" (Dunn et al., 1994, p. 599). Each individual's performance range depends on both past experience and current resources. Limited resources, possibly due to a temporary state of affairs or a more permanent situation, may impact a human's performance range even if he or she has a variety of skills and abilities. For example, a competent parent of a toddler may find his or her parenting repertoire (i.e., performance range) significantly hindered by a change of context brought about by the cramped confines of an airplane seat. If the same competent parent were sentenced to serve a 10-year prison term, the change in resources for parenting would obviously be of longer duration. However, even though the parent had a variety of skills and abilities, he or she would not have access to resources to support a broad performance range.

The EHP model provides "five alternatives for therapeutic intervention" (Dunn et al., 1994, p. 603). The first of these five levels is identified as the *establish/restore* level. This level includes traditional interventions that seek to restore function via the improvement of skills and abilities. Another traditional level of treatment is that of *adapt*. At this level, the therapist adapts "the contextual features and task demands to support performance in context" (p. 604). Yet another treatment level is the *alter* level. At this level, the therapist changes the actual context versus adapting the current one. An

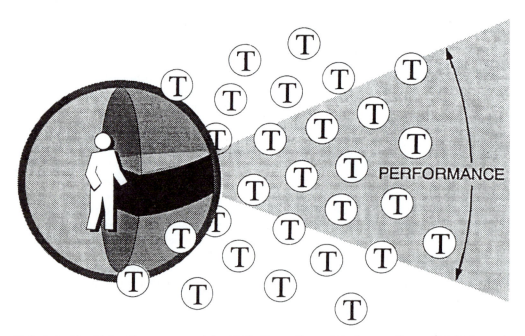

FIG. 4–8. The Major Components of the EHP. *(From Dunn, W., Brown, C., and McGuigan, A. [1994]. The ecology of human performance: A framework for considering the effect of context.* American Journal of Occupational Therapy, 48, *p. 600. With permission.)*

example of such an intervention would be moving an individual who uses a walker to a street-level apartment so the individual would not be forced to climb stairs. The *prevent* level of intervention seeks to "prevent the occurrence or evolution of maladaptive performance in context" (p. 604). The last level of intervention in the EHP is the *create* level. This level has great potential for community-based practice since its goal is to create "circumstances that promote more adaptable or complex performance in context" (p. 604). Policy initiatives, program development, community development, and community empowerment are all activities at this level of intervention.

In the EHP model, treatment, regardless of the level of intervention, is always guided by the culture of the individual or the community. Tasks that an individual or community select to pursue are guided by skills and abilities as well as personal choices, priorities, and values that are often guided by both life experience and cultural values. For example, a child's choice to play soccer may, at first, be influenced by his or her family's cultural background, which highly values the sport. Continued interest may be influenced by natural aptitude and early skill development, coupled with pride for a grandfather's past achievements as a semiprofessional player overseas.

This flexible model can also be highly effective in meeting the changing demands of OT practice. For example, it has been identified as an appropriate framework for health promotion, as described here (Lutz, 1998, p. 17):

> Interventions are intended to assist individuals in recognizing their health needs, acting, and gaining competence in the performance of these behaviors. Two of the EHP's intervention alternatives relate directly to preventive health behaviors. The "Prevent" and "Create" alternatives address how therapists assess an individual's context and take steps to avoid the occurrence of negative outcomes, or formulate a new set of circumstances to encourage the individual's success.

These levels of intervention can be readily adapted to facilitate the development of community-based health promotion activities. An intervention at the prevent level may, for example, include the development of an interdisciplinary program to educate seniors with diabetes in healthy eating habits and cooking techniques to avoid complications of an uncontrolled disease process (Lutz, 1998). Forming a daily walking group at a senior center to promote exercise, leisure skills, and a healthy lifestyle is an example of a create level intervention.

This model is still fairly new and has yet to be substantiated by a solid base of published research. However, it shows promise for use in both institutions and community-based practice. It is one of several models that are taught to fieldwork students and applied in treatment at Springfield Psychiatric Hospital Center in Maryland (C. Hays, personal communication, July 8, 1998). As stated earlier, the fifth alternative treatment level, create, appears to be particularly well suited for community-based program development since it "does not assume a disability is present" and it focuses on "providing enriched contextual and task experiences that will enhance performance" (Dunn et al., 1994, p. 606).

Occupational Adaptation

This model was developed by Schkade and Schultz and adopted by Texas Woman's University as a tool for research. **Occupational adaptation (OA)** was described by Schkade and Schultz (1993, p. 87) as "an integrative frame of reference . . . [that] provides an additional dimension to the understanding of occupation and adaptation and their relationship to health." According to OA, these two constructs (i.e., occupation and adaptation) are woven together into "an integrated phenomenon that describes an innate human process" (Schkade and Schultz, 1993, p. 87). The schematic representation of the model (Figure 4–9) appears extremely complex and can be overwhelming at first. However, the organization of this holistic model becomes readily apparent on closer examination by utilizing the flowchart format.

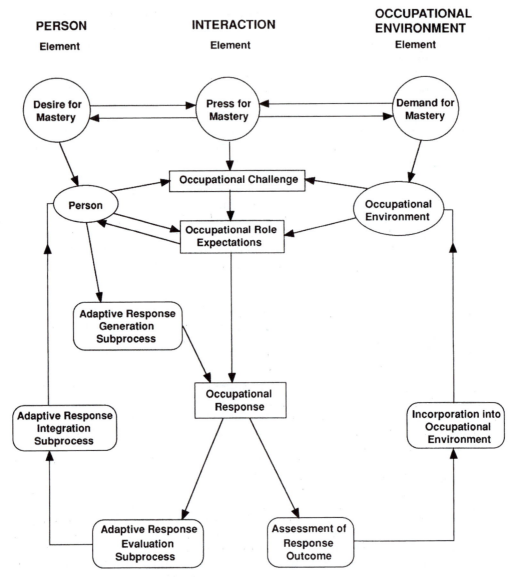

FIG. 4–9. Occupational Adaptation Model. *(From Schkade, J.K., and Schultz, S. [1992]. Occupational adaptation: Toward a holistic approach for contemporary practice, part 1.* American Journal of Occupational Therapy, 46, *p. 832. With permission.)*

The first segment of the original two-part article that was published in the *American Journal of Occupational Therapy* (Schkade and Schultz, 1992) describes the conceptual framework of the OA model. The second portion of this article (Schultz and Schkade, 1992) applies the OA model to a variety of OT practice examples. These examples include:

● A working mother recovering from carpal tunnel surgery receiving treatment on an outpatient basis
● An individual receiving inpatient therapy following a traumatic brain injury

- A husband receiving therapy in an inpatient setting following a CVA with secondary depression and aphasia
- An adolescent receiving treatment in the public school system for a behavior disorder and fine motor-control problems

Although this model has been identified as appropriate for both basic and applied research, little research either on the model or its use as a theoretical framework has been published to date. One exception is a research study on the effects of skiing on adolescents' relative mastery (Pasek and Schkade, 1996). This study investigated the impact of a six-day ski trip on 14 adolescents with limb deficiencies. The OA model was selected as the theoretical framework for this qualitative research project. However, the true potential of this model to guide research was not realized in this study since its focus was limited to one primary construct of the model (i.e., relative mastery) and its relationship to self-esteem. Attention to additional constructs (e.g., changes in self-initiation and generalization) may have been unrealistic for this study due to its short duration (i.e., six days) and the impetus for the research (i.e., graduate school project), but expanding the study's scope may have provided improved structure and more definitive results. Although little research has been published thus far, the authors of the OA model report that research is under way using both qualitative and quantitative methods, including a study examining community integration following cardiovascular accidents (Schkade and Schultz, 1992).

Towson University graduate students, under the direction of Stevens-Ratchford, have conducted unpublished research using this model (Barthel, Brzuszek, and Weaver, 1998; Bekker and Deijkers, 1998; Meyer and Ray, 1998). The students conducted a series of qualitative research studies using data collected on adaptive reminiscence from 30 older-adult stroke-survivor volunteers. One group investigated adaptive reminiscence patterns of stroke survivors with regard to changes in life autonomy (Bekker and Deijkers, 1998). Another group explored the reminiscences of poststroke life-role changes (Meyer and Ray, 1998), and a third group "examined coping mechanisms as an adaptive reminiscence factor" (Barthel et al., 1998, p. iii). Students reported that the OA model was a useful tool to organize theory for research purposes (Barthel et al., 1998). The OA model could be used to establish a successful community-based aging program using reminiscence, as well as a tool to conduct research on the impact of such an intervention.

Law et al. (1997) identified the model's dependence on a "close therapeutic relationship with the patient. This may not always be possible, particularly in some acute, community or consultation situations where patients are seen only once or twice" (Law et al., 1997, p. 95). While a close therapeutic relationship would be unlikely in current community-based or consultative practice, this may not be the case if the community is the "client" or the intervention point of service. The development of a close relationship that is maintained on a regular basis by a consistent therapist may not be a weakness but rather a strength in facilitating changes in the community's occupational performance.

Person-Environment-Occupational Performance Model

The **person-environment-occupational performance model (PEOPM)** was developed by Christiansen and Baum and first published in 1991. This model has since been revised and appears in its current form in Figure 4–10 (Law et al., 1997). The PEOPM was "developed to emphasize a view of the performance as an interaction between a person and his or her environment" (Law et al., 1997, p. 87).

The principles of this model, identified as concepts and assumptions by Law et al. (1997, p. 87), include:

- Performance results from complex interactions between the person and the environments in which he or she carries out tasks and roles.

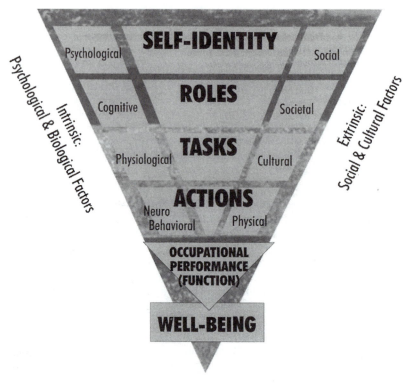

FIG. 4–10. Person-Environment-Occupational Performance Model. *(Reprinted from Law, M., Cooper, B.A., Strong, S., Stewart, D., Rigby, P., and Letts, L., Theoretical Context for the Practice of Occupational Therapy. In Christiansen, C., and Baum, C. [Eds.],* Occupational Therapy: Enabling Function and Well-Being *[2nd ed., p. 88], 1997, with permission from SLACK Incorporated.*

- Developmental stage influences performance.
- Intrinsic enablers (in person), environmental factors, and the meaning of the occupation facilitate performance.
- OT intervention can facilitate a person's adaptation when he or she encounters problems in performance.
- A personal sense of competence influences performance.

This model is new and still evolving and has yet to be substantiated with a body of research. However, its focus on the interactions between humans and the environment would make it a candidate for possible adaptation to community-based practice. The therapist's role in this model is portrayed as that of a "teacher-facilitator." The structure of the PEOPM suggests that it would be an appropriate tool to use with individuals in a community-based practice. One such example might be an OT practitioner working on an interdisciplinary team to facilitate the development of vocational skills, life skills (e.g., money management, apartment searching), and healthy development of leisure activities in individuals scheduled to be released from correctional facilities.

In addition, it is proposed that the PEOPM can be easily modified, as the MOHO was done earlier in this chapter, to examine a community as the recipient of service. The model's principles related to development stage and sense of competence can be modified to examine how occupation can be used to facilitate the development and competence of a community. If these principles were used in this manner, the term self-identity modified to community-identity, and additional principles from related disciplines incorporated, this model could be a useful framework for community development and empowerment.

SELECTED HEALTH EDUCATION AND PUBLIC HEALTH MODELS AND THEORIES

Many theories have been referred to in the health education and public health literature, but one of the most frequently cited is the social learning theory (Bandura, 1977a; Rotter, 1954). This theory will be examined in moderate detail, while three additional models will be described briefly. Since the 1950s, the fields of health education, public health, and health psychology have been developing and employing models to explain why people do or do not engage in health behaviors. The health belief model (Rosenstock, Strecher, and Becker, 1994) and newer models, such as Prochaska and DiClemente's transtheoretical model of health behavior change (1983, 1992), have been widely researched (DiClemente et al., 1994). Both of these models, as well as the precede-proceed model, are very popular in the professional literature and are frequently used in community-based health education. The health belief model (HBM) is a model of the precursors of health behavior, while the transtheoretical model of health behavior change explains the stages people experience as they seek to change their health behavior (McKenzie and Smeltzer, 1997). The precede-proceed model is a program planning and evaluation tool.

Social Learning Theory

Rotter (1954) established the foundation for **social learning theory (SLT),** which was renamed social cognitive theory (Bandura, 1986). Rotter postulated that an individual's expectations of the consequences of a particular action determined whether or not that behavior was performed.

Bandura (1977b) expanded on Rotter's work and developed an integral component of SLT—the concept of self-efficacy. *Self-efficacy* is defined as the individual's perception that he or she will be able to successfully perform a specific behavior (Bandura, 1977b). It is the belief in one's own competence to execute an action that will achieve the desired outcome. The most basic postulate of SLT is that individuals perform behaviors that result in certain outcomes. However, both the behavior and the outcomes are mediated by expectancies. An *expectancy* is the value an individual places on a particular outcome (Bandura, 1977b). There are three types of expectancies: (1) efficacy expectations, (2) outcome expectations, and (3) environmental expectations. Expectancies, sometimes referred to as incentives, possess a positive or negative value as well as a magnitude (Parcel and Baranowski, 1981).

Efficacy expectations, whether or not an individual believes in his or her ability to perform a given behavior, are derived from personal performance attainments, vicarious experiences, verbal persuasion, and emotional arousal. Successful accomplishment of a behavior enhances one's expectation for future endeavors. The more similar the current task to ones performed successfully in the past, the greater the efficacy expectations will be. Observations of others, who are perceived as similar to oneself, engaging in activities and achieving the desired outcome, can also increase one's expectations for accomplishment. According to this theory, verbal encouragement, receipt of permission to attempt a specific behavior, and a perceived physiological and emotional state that is conducive to successful execution of the task will also enhance an individual's confidence and self-efficacy relative to that behavior.

According to Bandura (1977a), *outcome expectations* are the individual's belief that a given behavior will lead to specific outcomes. Bandura (1977a) and others (Eiser, 1985;

Rosenstock et al., 1988; Wodarski, 1987) consider the locus of control construct an element of outcome expectations. The interaction of the constructs of self-efficacy and locus of control forms the foundation for SLT and is the basis on which behavior can be predicted (Bandura, 1977a). According to this theory, the expectation is that individuals who have high levels of self-efficacy for a behavior and an internal locus of control will be more likely to attempt to execute that particular behavior. These individuals would have a high level of confidence in their ability to successfully accomplish the task and tend to believe that performance of the behavior would directly affect the outcome (Rosenstock et al.). Individuals with low levels of self-efficacy for a behavior and an external locus of control would be less likely to attempt the given behavior. Typically, they have low levels of confidence in their ability to perform the behavior and believe their actions would not produce the desired outcome (Rosenstock et al.).

Environmental expectations are beliefs about how events are related to each other and what one may expect from any given environment (Bandura, 1977a). The SLT relies on the postulate of *reciprocal determinism,* which states that there is a continuous reciprocal, interdependent interaction of the person, the person's behavior, and the environment. The relative contribution of each of these factors in the determination of an outcome differs according to the setting and the behavior in question (Bandura, 1977a).

Behavior change, in the SLT paradigm, can be achieved in the following ways: (1) directly, by reinforcement of particular behaviors; (2) indirectly, through social modeling or observing someone else being reinforced for the behavior; and (3) through self-management or by having the individual monitor and self-reward (Parcel and Baranowski, 1981). According to Rosenstock et al. (1988), lifestyle changes will occur if the individual believes:

● Current behaviors pose a threat to a personally valued outcome, for example, health or appearance (environmental cue).
● Specific behavioral change will be likely to reduce these threats (outcome efficacy).
● Their own personal competence will allow them to perform the desired behavior (efficacy expectation).

In general, SLT provides a unique perspective for community-based practice. The constructs of self-efficacy, outcome expectancy, behavioral capability, modeling, reciprocal determinism, and self-control appear to be particularly relevant for the development of OT interventions. However, there are some significant limitations to the usefulness of SLT in health education. These include:

● The limited number of reliable and valid instruments designed to measure the constructs
● The lack of delineation of appropriate sources of modeling
● An insufficient description of the relationship of one construct to another and the nature of change over time

The absence of research that measures all constructs at once and evaluates the relationship among constructs limits the degree of variance that can be predicted by the theory. This research is the essential next step if SLT is to be considered a comprehensive and appropriate framework for health behavior change.

Health Belief Model

The health belief model (HBM) is one of many models of health-related behavior. Cummings, Becker, and Maile (1980), in a review of 14 models used in health education research, concluded that there is considerable overlap in the constructs or variables that make up these frameworks. Cummings et al. (1980) attempted to develop a unified framework for explaining health behavior by involving the authors of the various models in categorizing over 100 variables derived from the models. Six factors emerged from the multidimensional scaling analysis: (1) access to health-care services; (2) attitudes toward health care; (3) perception of threat of illness; (4) characteristics of the social network, interactions, norms, and structure; (5) knowledge about disease; and (6) demographic characteristics (Cummings et al., 1980).

Of all of the models studied by Cummings et al. (1980), the HBM is, by far, the most extensively used. The HBM was originally developed by Hochbaum, Kegeles, Leventhal, and Rosenstock to explain preventive health behaviors, but was quickly adapted to study sick role and illness behavior (Becker, 1974; Kirscht, 1974). The model is based on theories from social psychology, most notably, Lewin's aspiration theory (Maiman and Becker, 1974). Two underlying premises of the model, borrowed from Lewinian tradition, are the phenomenological orientation and the ahistorical perspective. The *phenomenological orientation* states that the individual's perceptions determine behavior, not the environment. An *ahistorical perspective* mandates a focus on the current dynamics affecting an individual's behavior, not on past history or prior experiences (Rosenstock, 1974).

The **health belief model** describes the relationships between a person's beliefs about health and his or her health-specific behaviors. The beliefs that mediate health behavior are, according to the model, perceived susceptibility, severity, benefits, and barriers. In addition to the beliefs just mentioned, cues to action are viewed as necessary triggers of behavior. *Perceived susceptibility* is the individual's subjective impression of the risk of contracting a disease or illness. *Perceived severity* refers to the convictions a person holds regarding the degree of seriousness of a given health problem. *Perceived benefits* are the beliefs a person has regarding the availability and effectiveness of a variety of possible actions in reducing the threat of illness. *Perceived barriers* are the costs or negative aspects associated with engaging in a specific health behavior. Cues to action are defined as instigating events that stimulate the initiation of behavior. These cues may be internal, such as perceptions of pain, or external, such as feedback from a health-care provider (Rosenstock, 1974).

According to the model, in order for a person to take action to avoid illness, the positive forces need to outweigh the negative forces. If an individual believes that: (1) he or she is personally susceptible to the disease or illness, (2) the occurrence of the health problem is severe enough to negatively impact his or her life, (3) taking specific actions would have beneficial effects, (4) the barriers to such action do not overwhelm the benefits, and (5) the individual is exposed to cues for action, then it is likely that the health behavior will occur (Rosenstock, 1974).

The HBM has been applied to a variety of populations and a diversity of health issues, including:

● Alcoholism (Bardsley and Beckman, 1988)
● Compliance with a diabetes regimen (Becker and Janz, 1985)
● Breast self-examination (Champion, 1985)
● Contraceptive behavior (Herold, 1983; Hester and Macrina, 1985)
● Medication compliance among psychiatric outpatients (Kelly, Mamon, and Scott, 1987)

The majority of studies are retrospective in nature, however, and the predictive value of the model is in question (Kegeles and Lund, 1982). Although the constructs of the model are fairly well defined, the causal associations among the variables and an explanation of why particular factors are more important in one population than in another are not addressed.

Perceived threat, which encompasses perceived susceptibility, has been suggested to be an important first cognitive step in the health-action link described by this model. In 1994, Rosenstock, Strecher, and Becker provided an updated schema of the HBM. They modified the schema by incorporating the construct of self-efficacy and by reordering the components of the model to more clearly elucidate the belief-action link. Figure 4–11 presents an adapted schematic representation of the updated HBM as applied to the goal of increasing physical activity.

PRECEDE-PROCEED Model

The precede model, developed by Green, Kreuter, Deeds, and Partridge (1980) with financial support from the National Institutes of Health, is a planning model for health education based on principles, both theoretical and applied, from epidemiology, education, administration, and the social/behavioral sciences. The acronym PRECEDE stands for predisposing, reinforcing, and enabling causes in educational diagnosis and evaluation (Green et al., 1980). In 1991, the model was revised to accommodate the evolving nature and broader perspective of health promotion. The addition of a new set of steps called PROCEED (policy, regulatory, and organizational constructions in educational and environmental development) has been superimposed on the original model in Figure 4–12 to illustrate the complete **PRECEDE-PROCEED model** (Green and Kreuter, 1991).

The PRECEDE model was to be readily applicable across a variety of settings, providing structure and organization to health education program planning and evaluation. Application of this approach occurs in several phases and involves the diagnoses of variables in five domains: (1) social, (2) epidemiological, (3) behavioral, (4) educational, and (5) administrative (Green et al., 1980). It is unique in that it begins

THE HEALTH BELIEF MODEL

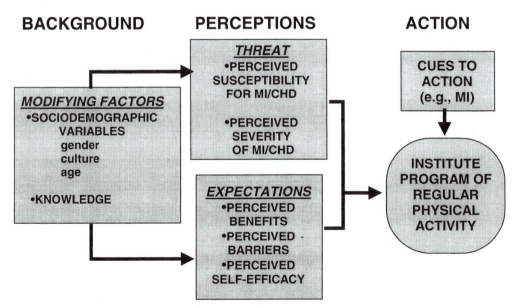

FIG. 4–11. The Revised Health Belief Model as a Framework to Investigate Compliance with Required Physical Activity. *(From Rosenstock, I.M., Strecher, V.J., and Becker, M.H. [1994]. The health belief model and HIV risk behavior change. In R.J. DiClemente and J.L. Peterson [Eds.], Preventing AIDS: Theories and methods for behavioral interventions [p. 11]. New York: Plenum. With permission.)*

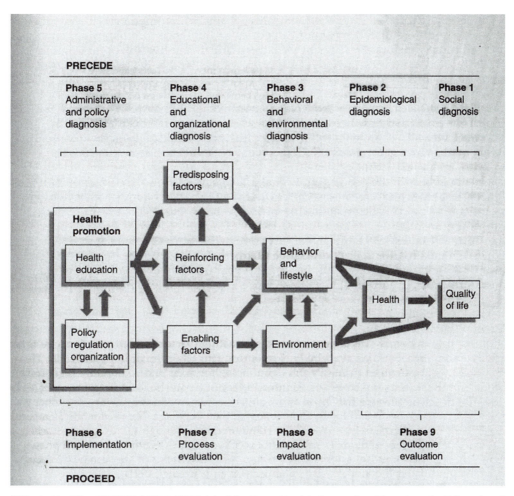

FIG. 4–12. The PRECEDE-PROCEED Model. *(From* Health Promotion Planning: An Educational and Ecological Approach, Third Edition, *by Lawrence W. Green and Marshall W. Kreuter. Copyright © 1999 by Mayfield Publishing Company. Reprinted by permission of the publisher.)*

with the desired final outcome and works backward, taking into account factors that must precede a certain result.

Phase 1 of the model is *social diagnosis.* An analysis of the social problems that exist in a community is a necessary prerequisite in assessing the quality of life of the target population. The purpose of this phase is to ascertain the relationship between a given health problem and the social problems of the population. Phase 2, *epidemiological diagnosis,* is an evaluation of the health problems associated with the community's quality of life. Morbidity, mortality, fertility, and disability are the primary indicators of the health of a population (Green et al., 1980).

Behavioral diagnosis, phase 3, attempts to identify the health-related behaviors that impact on the health problems isolated in the epidemiological diagnosis. It is important at this stage to also acknowledge the nonbehavioral factors, such as age, gender, and environment, which may contribute to the health problem of interest. Behavioral factors are then rated on a scale of importance and changeability. Factors rated high in importance and changeability are usually selected as targets for intervention (Green et al., 1980).

In phase 4, *educational diagnosis,* the health behaviors identified in the behavioral diagnosis are differentiated by three categories of influence: predisposing, enabling, and reinforcing factors. *Predisposing factors* provide the motivation or rationale for the behavior; for example, knowledge, attitudes, values, and beliefs. *Enabling factors* include personal skills and assets as well as community resources. Predisposing and enabling factors are antecedent to the health behavior and allow for the behavior to occur. *Reinforcing factors* supply the reward, incentive, or punishment of a behavior that contributes to its maintenance or extinction. Each group of factors is analyzed in terms of importance and changeability, and priorities are established for the intervention. Based on the nature of the targets for intervention, educational methodologies are selected (Green et al., 1980).

The final phase of the process is *administrative diagnosis.* It assesses budgetary implications, identifies and allocates resources, defines the nature of any cooperative agreements, and sets a realistic timetable for the intervention. Neglect of this important step can doom an otherwise viable intervention to failure. The proceed modifications (Green and Kreuter, 1991), utilized at this point in the model, include an assessment of policies, regulations, and organizational factors that impact on the implementation of health promotion programs and the development of strategies to effectively manage these influences. In addition, the revised precede-proceed model includes a discussion of implementation issues as well as process, outcome, and impact evaluation.

The PRECEDE model has been used in a variety of settings with a number of different populations, including planning an adolescent school-based sexuality program (Rubinson and Baillie, 1981), analysis of school health education programs (Green and Iverson, 1982), and educational interventions for hypertension control (Levine et al., 1982). Its application to injury prevention is shown in Figure 4–13. Although the model is robust in its possible applications, it is not by itself a theoretical model as it does not describe the relationships among the factors or variables (Parcel, 1984).

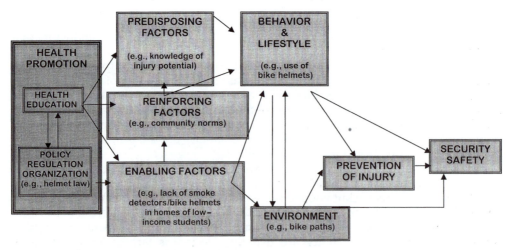

FIG. 4–13. The PRECEDE Model Applied to Injury Prevention.

Transtheoretical Model of Health Behavior Change

This model also is often more simply referred to as the stages of change model (McKenzie and Smeltzer, 1997). The **transtheoretical model of health behavior change (TMHBC),** which originated in the late 1970s and early 1980s, is a complex model consisting of stages and processes of change (Prochaska and DiClemente, 1983, 1992). Figure 4–14 shows the relationship between the stages and processes. The relationship of these stages to selected constructs of the HBM and SCT is displayed in Figure 4–15. This diagram depicts the various relationships between the theoretical components and will be described later.

As can be seen from the diagram, for a woman to engage in breast self-examination (BSE) or mammography, she must first feel threatened by being at risk for, or susceptible to, breast cancer and believe that it would be a serious matter to be diagnosed with breast cancer. Once this realization occurs, she moves from the stage of precontemplation of action to contemplation. Cues to action can be instrumental in increasing perceived susceptibility by consciousness-raising. Examples of such cues to action would be receiving information on the prevalence of breast cancer and shower cards that depict BSE.

Continued presence of a cue to action, for example, a shower card, will encourage self-re-evaluation and facilitate movement from contemplation to preparation. In addition, increased knowledge regarding the facts about the early diagnosis of breast cancer through these targeted behaviors would impact on the woman's beliefs regarding outcome expectations. More positive beliefs regarding these practices may, in turn, act as a stimulus to move from contemplation to preparation.

Continued movement toward engagement in the behavior will be influenced by continued presence of cues to action, self-efficacy (e.g., beliefs about the ability to perform BSE), and ability to perform self-liberation by confronting any remaining interpersonal barriers to performing BSE (e.g., dislike of touching one's breasts). As an in-

THE TRANSTHEORETICAL MODEL
OF BEHAVIOR CHANGE

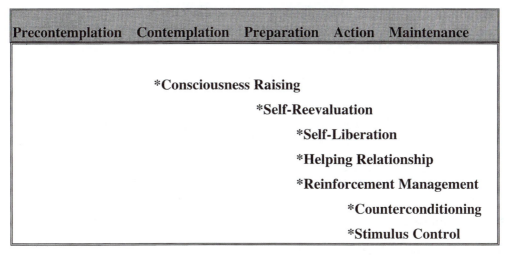

Fig. 4–14. The Transtheoretical Model of Behavior Change. *(From Prochaska, J.O., and DiClemente, C.C. [1983]. Stages and processes of self-change of smoking: Toward an integrative model of change.* Journal of Consulting and Clinical Psychology, 51 *[3], 394. Copyright © 1983 by the American Psychological Association. Reprinted with permission.)*

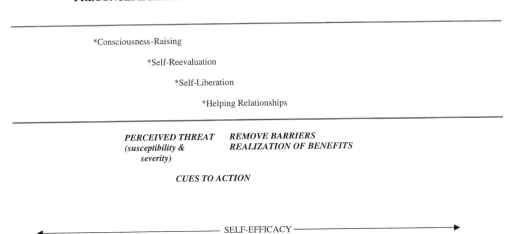

FIG. 4–15. The Relationship between Related Constructs of the HBM, SLT, and THBC.

dividual moves from the preparation stage to action, barriers can have a significant impact on further progress. If these barriers are removed, then the individual can proceed to engagement in the behavior and the realization of the benefits of the behavior (e.g., feeling of relief resulting from an absence of breast lumps and increased self-esteem for taking care of health needs). Continued exposure to social support, shower cards, and mass media campaigns will facilitate the maintenance of this behavior.

COMMUNITY ORGANIZATION THEORIES AND MODELS

Community organization has been defined as "the process by which community groups are helped to identify common problems or goals, mobilize resources, and in other ways develop and implement strategies for reaching goals they have set" (Minkler, 1990, p. 257). Before initiating a community organization effort, familiarity with the community, as well as the language of community development and the values and assumptions of community organization, is important. Terms associated with community organization are listed and defined in Box 4–2 (McKenzie and Smeltzer, 1997). Ross (1967) describes several assumptions underlying community organization. These include:

● Communities can develop strategies to respond to their specific needs and problems.
● Individuals have the ability to change and want to change.
● Community members should be involved in the change-making process.
● Changes that are internally motivated have more meaning and are more lasting than changes imposed from the outside.
● A "holistic" approach to change is more effective than a "fragmented" approach.

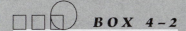 **BOX 4–2**

Terms Associated with Community Organization

Citizen participation:	The bottom-up, grassroots mobilization of citizens for the purpose of undertaking activities to improve the condition of something in the community.
Community development:	A process designed to create conditions for economic and social progress for the whole community with its active participation and the fullest possible reliance on the community's initiative (United Nations, 1955, p. 6).
Community organization:	The method of intervention whereby individuals, groups, and organizations engage in planned action to influence social problems. It is concerned with the enrichment, development, and/or change of social institutions (Brager, Specht, and Torczyner, 1987, p. 55).
Community participation:	A process of involving people in the institutions or decisions that affect their lives (Checkoway, 1989, p. 18).
Empowered community:	One in which individuals and organizations apply their skills and resources in collective efforts to meet their respective needs (Israel, Checkoway, Schulz, and Zimmerman, 1994).
Grassroots participation:	Bottom-up efforts of people taking collective actions on their own behalf, which involves the use of a sophisticated blend of confrontation and cooperation in order to achieve their ends (Perlman, 1978, p. 65).
Macro practice:	The methods of professional change that deal with issues beyond the individual, family, and small group level.

Source: From McKenzie, J.F., and Smeltzer, J.L., *Planning, Implementing, and Evaluating Health Promotion Programs: A Primer* (2nd ed.). Copyright © 1997 by Allyn & Bacon. Reprinted by permission.

● Democracy requires the "cooperative participation and action" of community members and the requisite skills that make this possible.
● Communities may need assistance to effectively organize to meet their needs.

The professional literature regarding community organization focuses more on methods than structured theoretical models. These methods have been classified into different systems. One frequently cited classification method, developed by Rothman (Minkler, 1990), separates the models into three categories: (1) locality development, (2) social planning, and (3) social action (McKenzie and Smeltzer, 1997; Minkler, 1990). McKenzie and Smeltzer (1997, p. 160) provide examples of each type of model; the Peace Corps is an example of locality development, the United Way is an example of social planning, and the social action model "was most useful during the civil rights and gay rights movements." In addition, they furnish a generic approach to community organization that combines the three types of models, with social planning being the most heavily used (Figure 4–16).

Regardless of the model chosen to facilitate the empowerment of a community, potential conflict must be anticipated and managed. Flick, Reese, Rogers, Fletcher, and Sonn (1994) stressed the importance of combining conflict management knowledge along with empowerment education theory for successful community organization to occur. Flick et al. (1994) described a long-term partnership between a community and a university that had as its goal the improvement of overall health for those most disadvantaged in the community. Their approach was based on Freire's theory of adult education. The use of Freire's theory in health education is described well by Marsick (1987). The seven-year partnership was successful, but conflict arose on at least two oc-

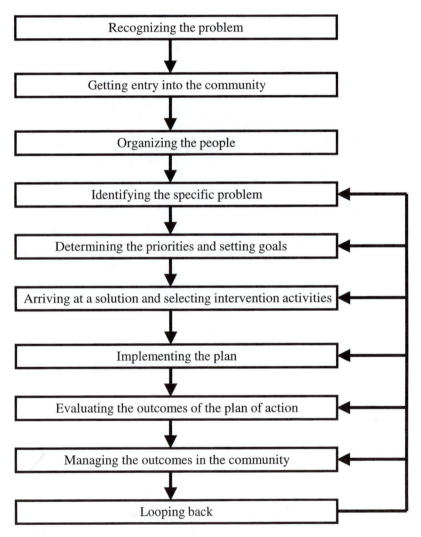

FIG. 4–16. Steps of Community Organization. *(From McKenzie, James F., and Smeltzer, Jan L., Planning, Implementing, and Evaluating Health Promotion Programs: A Primer [2nd ed.]. Copyright © 1997 by Allyn & Bacon. Reprinted by permission.)*

casions. These conflicts, presented as case studies by Flick et al. (1994), are helpful resources prior to engaging in community organization. The case studies illustrate the importance of university representatives (i.e., faculty and students) having both a variety of skills and an appropriate skill level in order to best serve a community. Critical skills include early recognition of conflict, conflict analysis, and conflict management.

OT practitioners, who are trained in group dynamics and psychosocial development and behavior, possess the prerequisite knowledge to become skilled in the early detection and resolution of conflict in community organization. However, additional benefit can be gained through the use of a structured format to focus the application of these skills. The steps, described by McKenzie and Smeltzer (1997), can serve as useful guides for OT practitioners who are new to working with the community as the point of service. These steps provide the basic roadmap of tasks that are required to enter and organize a community. However, they do not provide sufficient guidance to develop and evaluate an intervention. These principles, combined with one or more of the models discussed in this chapter, provide an excellent framework for the development of an empowered community.

An example of a community that may request assistance from an OT practitioner might be a homeless shelter (i.e., a community of individuals). In this example, the community has acted based on concern for the healthy development of its children. The community has already taken the first two necessary steps by recognizing the problem and inviting the OT professional into the community. The practitioner can use the EHP to define the scope of the problem but then will need to follow the remaining steps shown in Figure 4–16. Therefore, the next step would be to report the findings in lay terms to the community and then work with the community to determine priorities and set goals. Interventions are then selected, according to the EHP, from the five alternative treatment levels. The OT practitioner and the community will jointly implement activities and evaluate the outcomes. The community would then take responsibility for continued monitoring, consulting the professional for assistance in re-evaluation as needed.

As with all areas of OT practice, outcomes research is needed to evaluate the efficacy of interventions. This is particularly true in community-based practice. The profession can draw on the expertise of individuals conducting research on community empowerment initiatives in the fields of public health and health education. One such resource is a description of a "research model developed to study community organization influence on local public health care policy" (Brown, 1984, p. 205). Both the research methodology and the study's results are helpful to the potential researcher in this area. For example, one of the study's findings was that the group that used "political leverage" was more successful than those that used factual, educational testimony at public hearings. Another finding of this study's results was that lobbying and the presence of "other groups and leaders" help encourage support within the community (Brown, 1984, p. 229).

As OT practitioners seek to assist communities in reaching their potential, they need to be simultaneously collecting data to determine the efficacy of the interventions. Research is less effective and more costly if attempted in retrospect. Research by other professionals in community development and empowerment can be used to facilitate the development of research projects to study the efficacy of OT in community-based practice.

 ## CONCLUSION

OT practitioners are increasingly being encouraged to enter community-based practice, identified as the practice area of the future (Baum and Law, 1998). The January 1998 *American Journal of Occupational Therapy* special issue on this topic indicates the

American Occupational Therapy Association's projection of growth in this practice area. The authors recognize that the community has historically been a practice area of OT (Brownson, 1998; Reitz, 1992) and wish to facilitate its continued development. Community-based practice has not realized its full potential. To do so, both theorists and practitioners must reflect on past work of this nature, the close relationship between this type of practice and the core values and beliefs of the profession (American Occupational Therapy Association, 1993; Townsend, 1991), as well as the beliefs of the profession's founders. The authors believe the outcome of the preceding reflection will provide support for the profession's continued development of its potential to meet the health and occupation needs of individuals in their communities.

One reason for the minimal growth of community-based practice may be the limited number of theoretical models that can be easily applied to the community (McColl, 1998). It is hoped that this chapter has provided several alternatives and resources for investigating potential theoretical models to use in the development of community-based practice. There are also many sociopolitical reasons for the limited development of this practice area (e.g., limited reimbursement, lower salaries, and shortage of community-based OT practitioners).

Another reason for the minimal growth of community-based practice is that OT students generally lack the necessary preparation to enter this area of practice. McColl (1998) stressed academia's responsibility to provide students with knowledge about communities and their function as well as the tools and methods to promote healthy change in communities and society. Recently, new academic programs have been developed with health promotion and community development viewed as core content. Other educational programs have added courses that include both content and fieldwork experiences in community-based practice. A new course titled "Occupational Therapy Health Promotion Initiatives in the Community," offered at Towson University, is an example.

Yet another barrier to the widespread establishment of community-based practice may be the lack of common terminology in this area. Community-based practice often involves a team approach wherein the membership of the team does not conform to the familiar traditional hospital-based interdisciplinary team. Public health experts, health educators, community developers and organizers, and politicians are all examples of potential community-based team members who may work together on a community initiative. Many of these professionals share a common language that is represented in the nonoccupational therapy models presented in this chapter. It is hoped that exposure to these models will facilitate interdisciplinary work in the community by practitioners. For OT to reach its potential in the community, its practitioners must possess the knowledge and skill to join together with a varied group of stakeholders, gatekeepers, community members, and other health professionals to creatively and cost effectively facilitate the achievement of the health goals of diverse communities.

 STUDY QUESTIONS

1. Identify five reasons why OT professionals need to be knowledgeable and competent in the use of theory.
2. Identify and define the following terms: concept, construct, principle, model, theory, paradigm, frame of reference, and conceptual model of practice. Describe how these terms are related.
3. Describe the general characteristics and principles of the model of human occupation, ecology of human performance, occupational adaptation, and the person-environment-occupational performance model.

4. Compare and contrast these OT theories in terms of their appropriateness for community practice and research.

5. Describe the general characteristics and principles of social learning theory, the health belief model, PRECEDE-PROCEED model, and the transtheoretical model of health behavior change.

6. Compare and contrast these health education and public health theories in terms of their appropriateness for community practice and research.

7. Describe the potential roles of OT practitioners in community organization to meet health needs.

8. Describe ways to overcome the barriers to community-based practice and increase the viability of OT in community settings.

REFERENCES

American Occupational Therapy Association. (1993). Core values and attitudes of occupational therapy practice. *American Journal of Occupational Therapy, 47,* 1085–1086.

Bandura, A. (1977a). *Social learning theory.* Upper Saddle River, NJ: Prentice Hall.

Bandura, A. (1977b). Self-efficacy: Toward a unifying theory of behavioral change. *Psychological Review, 84,* 191.

Bandura, A. (1986). The explanatory and predictive scope of self-efficacy theory. *Journal of Social and Clinical Psychology, 4,* 359–373.

Bardsley, P., and Beckman, L. (1988). The health belief model and entry into alcoholism treatment. *International Journal of the Addictions, 23,* 19–28.

Barthel, J., Brzuszek, K.L., and Weaver, C. (1998). Adaptive reminiscence: Coping mechanisms of stroke survivors. Unpublished master's project, Towson University, Towson, MD.

Baum, C., and Law, M. (1998). Community health: A responsibility, an opportunity, and a fit for occupational therapy. *American Journal of Occupational Therapy, 52,* 7–10.

Becker, M. (Ed.). (1974). *The health belief model and personal health behavior.* Thorofare, NJ: Slack.

Bekker, S., and Deijkers, L.C.P. (1998). Adaptive reminiscence: Occupational responses of stroke survivors to changes in life autonomy. Unpublished master's project, Towson University, Towson, Maryland.

Becker, M., and Janz, N. (1985). The health belief model applied to understanding diabetes regimen compliance. *Diabetes Educator, 11,* 41–47.

Brager, G., Specht, H., and Torczyner, J.L. (1987). *Community organizing.* New York: Columbia University Press.

Breines, E.B. (1995). *Occupational therapy: Activities from clay to computers.* Philadelphia: F. A. Davis.

Brown, E.R. (1984). Community organization influences on local public health policy: A general research comparative study. *Health Education Quarterly, 10*(3/4), 205–233.

Brownson, C.A. (1998). Funding community practice. *American Journal of Occupational Therapy, 52,* 60–64.

Champion, V. (1985). Use of the health belief model in determining frequency of breast self-examination. *Research in Nursing and Health, 8,* 373–379.

Checkoway, B. (1989). Community participation for health promotion: Prescription for public policy. *Wellness Perspectives: Research, Theory and Practice, 6*(1), 18–26.

Christiansen, C. (1991). Occupational therapy: Intervention for life performance. In C. Christiansen and C. Baum (Eds.), *Occupational therapy: Overcoming performance deficits* (pp. 2–43). Thorofare, NJ: Slack.

Clark, F., Azen, S.P., Zemke, R., Jackson, J., Carlson, M., Mandel, D., Hay, J., Josephson, K., Cherry, B., Hessel, C., Palmer, J., and Lipson, L. (1997). Occupational therapy for independent-living older adults. *Journal of the American Medical Association, 278,* 1321–1326.

Cummings, K.M., Becker, M.H., and Maile, M.C. (1980). Bringing the models together: An empirical approach to combining variables used to explain health outcomes. *Journal of Behavioral Medicine, 3,* 123–145.

DiClemente, C.C., Prochaska, J.O., Fairhurst, S.K., Velcier, W.F., Velasquez, M.M., and Rossi, J.S. (1991). The process of smoking cessation: An analysis of precontemplation, contemplation, and preparation stages of change. *Journal of Consulting and Clinical Psychology, 59,* 295–304.

Dunn, W., Brown, C., and McGuigan, A. (1994). The ecology of human performance: A framework for considering the effect of context. *American Journal of Occupational Therapy, 48,* 595–607.

Dutton, R., Levy, L.L., and Simon, C.J. (1993). Current basis for theory and philosophy of occupational therapy, section 3—frames of reference in occupational therapy: Introduction. In H.L. Hopkins and H.D. Smith (Eds.), *Willard and Spackman's occupational therapy* (8th ed., pp. 62–63). Philadelphia: Lippincott.

Eiser, J.R. (1985). Smoking: The social learning of addiction. *Journal of Social and Clinical Psychology, 3,* 357–446.

Fidler, G.S. (1981). From crafts to competence. *American Journal of Occupational Therapy, 35,* 567–573.

Flick, L.H., Reese, C.G., Rogers, G., Fletcher, P., and Sonn, J. (1994). Building community for health: Lessons from a seven-year-old neighborhood/university partnership. *Health Education Quarterly, 21* (3), 369–380.

Gillette, N., and Kielhofner, G. (1979). The impact of specialization on the professionalization and survival of occupational therapy. *American Journal of Occupational Therapy, 33,* 20–28.

Green, L.W., and Iverson, D. (1982). School health education. *Annual Review of Public Health, 3,* 321–328.

Green, L.W., and Kreuter, M.W. (1991). *Health promotion planning: An educational and environmental approach* (2nd ed.). Mountainview, CA: Mayfield.

Green, L.W., Kreuter, M.W., Deeds, S.G., and Partridge, K.B. (1980). *Health education planning: A diagnostic approach.* Palo Alto, CA: Mayfield.

Hawking, S. (1988). *A brief history of time.* New York: Bantam.

Herold, E. (1983). The health belief model: Can it help us understand contraceptive use among adolescents? *Journal of School Health, 53,* 19–21.

Hester, N., and Macrina, D. (1985). The health belief model and the contraceptive behavior of college women: Implications for health education. *Journal of American College Health, 33,* 245–252.

Hopkins, H.L. (1993). Current basis for theory and philosophy of occupational therapy, section 1—philosophical base of occupational therapy. In H.L. Hopkins and H.D. Smith (Eds.), *Willard and Spackman's occupational therapy* (8th ed., pp. 58–59). Philadelphia: Lippincott.

Israel, B.A., Checkoway, B., Schulz, A., and Zimmerman, M. (1994). Health education and community empowerment: Conceptualizing and measuring perceptions of individual, organizational, and community control. *Health Education Quarterly, 21*(2), 149–170.

Jackson, J., Carlson, M., Mandel, D., Zemke, R., and Clark, F. (1998). Occupation in lifestyle redesign: The well elderly study occupational therapy program. *American Journal of Occupational Therapy, 52,* 326–336.

Kegeles, S., and Lund, A. (1982). Adolescents' health beliefs and acceptance of a novel preventive dental activity: Replication and extension. *Health Education Quarterly, 9,* 96–112.

Kelly, G., Mamon, J., and Scott, J. (1987). Utility of the health belief model in examining medication compliance among psychiatric outpatients. *Social Science Medicine, 25,* 1205–1211.

Kielhofner, G. (Ed.). (1985). *A model of human occupation: Theory and application.* Baltimore: Williams and Wilkins.

Kielhofner, G. (1992). *Conceptual foundations of occupational therapy.* Philadelphia: F. A. Davis.

Kielhofner, G. (Ed.). (1995). *A model of human occupation: Theory and application* (2nd ed.). Baltimore: Williams and Wilkins.

Kielhofner, G. (1997). *Conceptual foundations of occupational therapy* (2nd ed.). Philadelphia: F. A. Davis.

Kielhofner, G., and Burke, J. (1980). A model of human occupation, part 1: Conceptual framework and content. *American Journal of Occupational Therapy, 34,* 572–581.

Kielhofner, G., and Burke, J. (1985). Components and determinants of human occupation. In G. Kielhofner (Ed.), *A model of human occupation: Theory and application* (pp. 12–36). Baltimore: Williams and Wilkins.

Kirscht, J. (1974). The health belief model and illness behavior. In M. Becker (Ed.), *The health belief model and personal health behavior.* Thorofare, NJ: Slack.

Law, M., Cooper, B.A., Strong, S., Stewart, D., Rigby, P., and Letts, L. (1997). Theoretical context for the practice of occupational therapy. In C. Christiansen and C. Baum (Eds.), *Occupational therapy: Enabling function and well-being* (2nd ed., pp. 72–102). Thorofare, NJ: Slack.

Levine, D.M., Morisky, D.E., Bone, L.R., Lewis, C., Ward, K.B., and Green, L.W. (1982). Data-based planning for educational interventions through hypertension control programs for urban and rural populations in Maryland. *Public Health Reports, 97,* 107–112.

Levy, L.L. (1993). Current basis for theory and philosophy of occupational therapy, section 2—theory base. In H.L. Hopkins and H.D. Smith (Eds.), *Willard and Spackman's occupational therapy* (8th ed., pp. 59–62). Philadelphia: Lippincott.

Lutz, C. (1998). Interdisciplinary prevention in rural communities: Outcome evaluation of the *Strides for Life* walking program for older adults. Gerontology graduate research project. Unpublished master's project, Towson University, Towson, MD.

Maiman, L., and Becker, M. (1974). The health belief model: Origins and correlates in psychological theory. In M. Becker (Ed.), *The health belief model and personal health behavior.* Thorofare, NJ: Slack.

Marriner, A. (Ed.). (1986). *Nursing theorists and their works.* St. Louis: Mosby.

Marsick, V.J. (1987). Designing health education programs. In P.M. Lazes, L.H. Kaplan, and K.A. Gordon, *The handbook of health education* (2nd ed., pp. 3–30). Rockville, MD: Aspen.

McColl, M.A. (1998). What do we need to know to practice occupational therapy in the community? *American Journal of Occupational Therapy, 52,* 11–18.

McKenzie, J.F., and Smeltzer, J.L. (1997). *Planning, implementing, and evaluating health promotion programs: A primer* (2nd ed.). Boston: Allyn and Bacon.

Meyer, M.B., and Ray, H.M. (1998). Adaptive reminiscence of stroke survivors: Life role changes. Unpublished master's project, Towson University, Towson, MD.

Miller, R.J. (1993a). Gary Kielhofner. In R.J. Miller and K.F. Walker (Eds.), *Perspectives on theory for the practice of occupational therapy* (2nd ed., pp. 179–218). Gaithersburg, MD: Aspen.

Miller, R.J. (1993b). What is theory, and why does it matter? In R.J. Miller and K.F. Walker (Eds.), *Perspectives on theory for the practice of occupational therapy* (2nd ed., pp. 1–16). Gaithersburg, MD: Aspen.

Minkler, M. (1990). Improving health through community organization. In K. Glanz, F.M. Lewis, and B.K. Rimer (Eds.), *Health behavior and health education* (pp. 257–287). San Francisco: Josey-Bass.

Mosey, A.C. (1981). *Occupational therapy: Configuration of a profession.* New York: Raven.

Nelson, D.L. (1997). Why the profession of occupational therapy will flourish in the 21st century. *American Journal of Occupational Therapy, 51*(1), 11–24.

Parcel, G.S. (1984). Theoretical models for application in school health education research. Special combined issue of *Journal of School Health, 54* and *Health Education, 15,* 39–49.

Parcel, G., and Baranowski, T. (1981). Social learning theory and health education. *Health Education, 12,* 14–18.

Pasek, P.B., and Schkade, J.K. (1996). Effects of a skiing experience on adolescents with limb deficiencies: An occupational adaptation perspective. *American Journal of Occupational Therapy, 50*(1), 24–31.

Payton, O.D. (1988). *Research: The validation of clinical practice* (2nd ed.). Philadelphia: F. A. Davis.

Perlman, J. (1978). Grassroots participation from neighborhood to nation. In S. Langton (Ed.), *Citizen participation in America* (pp. 65–79). Lexington, MA: Lexington Books.

Prochaska, J.O., and DiClemente, C.C. (1983). Stages and processes of self-change of smoking: Toward an integrative model of change. *Journal of Counseling and Clinical Psychology, 51*(3), 390–395.

Prochaska, J.O., and DiClemente, C.C. (1992). Stages of change in the modification of behavior problems. In M. Hersen, R.M. Eisler, and P.M. Miller (Eds.), *Progress in behavior modification* (pp. 184–214). Sycamore, IL: Sycamore Press.

Reitz, S.M. (1990, Fall). Community development model: An application of the model of human occupation. Unpublished paper for HEALTH 688—P, Community Health Issues for Minority Populations, University of Maryland, College Park.

Reitz, S.M. (1992). A historical review of occupational therapy's role in preventive health and wellness. *American Journal of Occupational Therapy, 46,* 50–55.

Reitz, S.M. (1998a). Bridging the gulf between theory and practice. Poster session presented at the 12th International Congress of the World Federation of Occupational Therapists, Montreal.

Reitz, S.M. (1998b). Ways to organize OT knowledge. Course packet (OCTH 211). Towson, MD: Towson University.

Reitz, S.M. (2000). Ways to organize OT knowledge. Course packet (OCTH 611). Towson, MD: Towson University.

Rosenstock, I. (1974). Historical origins of the health belief model. In M. Becker (Ed.), *The health belief model and personal behavior*. Thorofare, NJ: Slack.

Rosenstock, I.M., Strecher, V.J., and Becker, M. (1988). Social learning theory and the health belief model. *Health Education Quarterly, 15,* 175–183.

Rosenstock, I.M., Strecher, V.J., and Becker, M.H. (1994). The health belief model and HIV risk behavior change. In R.J. DiClemente and J.L. Peterson (Eds.), *Preventing AIDS: Theories and methods for behavioral interventions* (pp. 5–24). New York: Plenum.

Ross, M.G. (1967). *Community organization: Theory, principles and practice.* New York: Harper and Row.

Rotter, J.B. (1954). *Social learning and clinical psychology.* Upper Saddle River, NJ: Prentice Hall.

Rubinson, L., and Baillie, L. (1981). Planning school based sexuality programs using the PRECEDE model. *Journal of School Health, 51,* 282–287.

Scaffa, M. (1992). *The development of comprehensive theory in health education: A feasibility study.* Dissertation Abstracts International.

Schkade, J.K., and Schultz, S. (1992). Occupational adaptation: Toward a holistic approach for contemporary practice, part 1. *American Journal of Occupational Therapy, 46,* 829–837.

Schkade, J.K., and Schultz, S. (1993). Current basis for theory and philosophy of occupational therapy, section 3K—occupational adaptation: An integrative frame of reference. In H.L. Hopkins and H.D. Smith (Eds.), *Willard and Spackman's occupational therapy* (8th ed., pp. 87–91). Philadelphia: Lippincott.

Schultz, S., and Schkade, J.K. (1992). Occupational adaptation: Toward a holistic approach for contemporary practice, part 2. *American Journal of Occupational Therapy, 46,* 917–925.

Shireffs, J.A. (1984). The nature and meaning of health education. In L. Rubinson and W.F. Alles (Eds.), *Health education: Foundations for the future.* St. Louis: Times Mirror/Mosby.

Strauss, A., and Corbin, J. (1990). *Basics of qualitative research: Grounded theory procedures and techniques.* London: Sage.

Townsend, B. (1991). Beyond our clinics: A vision of the future. *American Journal of Occupational Therapy, 45,* 871–873.

United Nations (1955). *Social progress through community development.* New York: United Nations.

Werch, C.E., and DiClemente, C.C. (1994). A multi-stage model for matching prevention strategies and messages to youth stage of use. *Health Education Research, 9*(1), 37–46.

Wodarski, J. (1987). Evaluating a social learning approach to teaching adolescents about alcohol and driving: A multiple variable evaluation. *Journal of Social Science Research, 10,* 121–144.

Zemke, R., and Clark, F. (1996). *Occupational science: The evolving discipline.* Philadelphia: F. A. Davis.

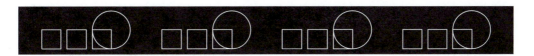

5 CHAPTER

Legislation and Policy Issues

Nancy Van Slyke, EdD, OTR

■ OUTLINE

LEARNING OBJECTIVES

This chapter is designed to enable the reader to:

■ Discuss the need for a basic understanding of legislation pertinent to community-based practice.

■ Compare and contrast legislation supporting reimbursement for services with those providing support and funding for programs.

■ Identify specific legislation that focuses on issues related to each of the following categories: education and development, medical rehabilitation, consumer rights, and environmental issues.

■ Discuss the factors requiring consideration by an occupational therapy practitioner in determining his or her role in a community-based setting.

 ## INTRODUCTION

"Legislation that affects the lives of people with disabilities should be of more than just a passing interest to those who are involved with the disability community. Not only does legislation articulate who is to receive the services, but it also articulates what and how services are to be delivered" (Fifield and Fifield, 1995, p. 38).

Occupational therapists practicing in the more traditional medical model have expected payment from, and therefore been influenced by, the medical insurance providers, including programs offered by federal, state, and private sources. Although this **reimbursement** for services will continue to influence the practice of occupational therapy within the medical model, the current shift from the fee-for-service delivery model to community-based practice will require practitioners to broaden their perspectives to include knowledge of legislation that impacts community service programs. According to Baum and Law (1998), occupational therapists must understand the mechanisms of service delivery for social programs, including the legislative policies and **funding** (provision of money for a specified purpose) resources that support them.

Historically, special-interest groups have impacted legislation and policies, resulting in the development of the majority of community services and programs currently available for special populations. The influence of federal legislation and regulation on the increased availability of community programs for persons with disabilities has been part of the impetus for the interest and shift in occupational therapy practice from the medical model to a variety of other environments within the community (Jacobs, 1996).

This chapter briefly describes the legislation and policies that might influence community-based practice. The legislation described is not intended to be all-inclusive. It should be emphasized that policy is constantly changing and practitioners must be alert to both existing and pending legislation that impacts the practice setting as well as the client population served. The basic themes described are an amalgamation of those described in publications by Fifield and Fifield (1995) and Reed (1992). An extensive outline of the relevant legislation is provided in Box 5–1.

LEGISLATION AND DISABILITIES

To effectively facilitate the shift in practice to the community model and promote the role of occupational therapy, the practitioner must have a basic understanding of the historical background of legislation that affects the lives of people with disabilities. Although most practitioners are generally aware of legislation affecting reimbursement for services, the clinicians' knowledge has been traditionally based on the location of service provision (e.g., inpatient and outpatient). According to Brownson (1998), current legislation and funding mechanisms have moved beyond the medical management of the client to addressing other societal and environmental factors that affect health.

Reed (1992) has thoroughly discussed the history of federal legislation relating to persons with disabilities that has affected the field of occupational therapy both favorably and adversely. Although she categorizes 13 areas impacted by public policy, the following areas seem most pertinent to occupational therapy practice within the community:

- Basic and special education
- Vocational and medical rehabilitation
- Economic support
- Social rehabilitation
- Facility construction and architectural requirements
- Deinstitutionalization and independent living
- Transportation and public accommodation
- Technology-related assistance and civil rights and advocacy

According to Reed (1992, p. 397), "several of these areas have a long history of at least partially successful federal legislation, whereas other areas have just begun to be supported by legislation and governmental efforts."

In a more recent publication, Fifield and Fifield (1995, p. 38) state that "legislation not only articulates who is to receive services, but it also articulates what and how services are to be delivered and reflects the values, philosophies, and concerns of society." According to these authors, much of the early legislation provided compensation programs for military and work injuries, which later led to the emergence of rehabilitation and education legislation that provided funding for services rather than compensation for injury. Fifield and Fifield (1995) state that a majority of the current federal programs for persons with disabilities have evolved from legislation that was initiated under the administration of President John F. Kennedy. Although the work of the President's Panel on Mental Retardation of 1962 focused on mental retardation, it outlined legislative needs and programs that applied to almost all disabilities. These included prevention, education, public resources, research, coordi-

◻◻◻ **BOX 5-1**

Outline of Major Legislation Influencing Community Practice

 I. Protection and care referenced legislation/policy
   A. Social Security Act
     1. Aid to the permanently and totally disabled
     2. Supplemental security income program
   B. Maternal and Child Health and Mental Retardation Planning Amendments (P.L. 88-156)
   C. Mental Retardation and Community Mental Health Center Construction Act (P.L. 88-164)
   D. National Institute of Mental Health Community Support Program
   E. Omnibus Reconciliation Act of 1981 (P.L. 97-35)
   F. Reauthorization of P.L. 102-321 ADAMHA Re-Organization Act Substance Abuse Prevention and Treatment Services Block Grant
 II. Educational and developmental legislation for persons with disabilities
   A. Education
     1. National Defense Education Act (P.L. 85-864)
     2. Maternal and Child Health and Mental Retardation Planning Amendments (P.L. 88-156)
     3. Mental Retardation and Community Mental Health Center Construction Act (P.L. 88-164)
     4. Education for All Handicapped Children Act (P.L. 94-142)
       a. Part H Amendment to P.L. 94-142
   B. Developmental referenced legislation/policy
     1. Developmental Disabilities Act of 1970 (P.L. 91-517)
     2. 1973 Amendments to the Rehabilitation Act (P.L. 93-112)
     3. Education for All Handicapped Children Act of 1975 (P.L. 94-142)
     4. Part H of P.L. 94-142, Early Intervention Provisions
 III. Legislation establishing reimbursement and funding for rehabilitation programs
   A. Rehabilitation Act of 1973 (P.L. 93-112)
   B. Subsequent Amendments to the Rehabilitation Act
     1. 1986 P.L. 99-506 clarified supportive employment
   C. Subsequent Amendments to Social Security Act
     1. 1965 P.L. 89-97 created Medicare and Medicaid
     2. 1972 P.L. 92-223 established intermediate-care facilities for persons with mental retardation
     3. 1972 P.L. 92-603 established supplemental security income to persons on standardized assistance programs
   D. Mental Retardation Facilities and Community Mental Health Center Construction Act of 1963 (P.L. 88-164)
 IV. Civil rights referenced legislation
   A. Civil Rights Act of 1964 (P.L. 88-352) and 1988 Civil Rights Restoration Act
   B. Architectural Barriers Act of 1968 (P.L. 90-480)

C. Amendments to Developmental Disabilities Act
D. Section 504 of the Rehabilitation Act of 1973 (P.L. 93-112)
E. Education for All Handicapped Children Act (P.L. 94-142)
F. Americans with Disabilities Act of 1990 (P.L. 101-336)
V. Environment referenced legislation
   A. Architectural Barriers Act of 1986 (P.L. 90-480)
   B. Independent Living Provisions of the 1973 Vocational Rehabilitation Act (P.L. 93-112)
   C. Education for All Handicapped Children Act (P.L. 94-142)
   D. Technology Related Assistance Act of 1988 (P.L. 100-407)
VI. Consumer referenced legislation
   A. Developmental Disabilities Act of 1970
   B. 1977 Rehabilitation Act Amendments
   C. Education for All Handicapped Children Act (P.L. 94-142)
   D. Technology Related Assistance Act of 1988 (P.L. 100-407)
   E. Americans with Disabilities Act of 1990 (P.L. 101-336)

Sources: Fifield, B., and Fifield, M. (1995). The influence of legislation on services to people with disabilities. In O.C. Karan and S. Greenspan (Eds.), *Community rehabilitation services for people with disabilities* (pp. 38–70). Boston: Butterworth-Heinemann. Reed, K.L. (1992). History of federal legislation for persons with disabilities. *American Journal of Occupational Therapy, 46,* 397–408.

nation of services, and consumer participation. Subsequently, legislation has been developed in almost all of these areas. Fifield and Fifield (1995) categorized the legislation that emerged into five social concerns or themes: (1) protection and care, (2) development and opportunities, (3) civil rights, (4) environmental issues, and (5) consumer responsiveness.

PROTECTION AND CARE REFERENCED LEGISLATION

Protection and care referenced legislation is intended to provide for the safety of those constituencies covered by the legislation. The focus of this type of legislation is on guardianship or protection of the citizenry. Legislation related to protection and care was initially introduced with the **Social Security Act of 1935.** This act was designed as a federally financed program that would be managed by the state to provide relief and assistance to indigent dependent children, elderly adults, and the blind. The Social Security Act originally provided old-age assistance (Title I) and aid to families with dependent children (Title IV). In addition, the act provided programs for the blind (Title VI), established state and public health authorities (Title X), and authorized grants to states for maternal and child health and crippled children services (Title V). The Social Security Act has been amended numerous times (1956, 1972, and 1980) to allow workers with disabilities to receive pensions before reaching retirement, to provide income maintenance for those who are permanently and totally disabled, and to provide income maintenance and health benefits (Medicaid and Medicare) to families and individuals with disabilities living in noninstitutional and community-based settings (Fifield and Fifield, 1995; Reed, 1992).

EDUCATIONAL AND DEVELOPMENTAL REFERENCED LEGISLATION

Educational and developmental referenced legislation is intended to provide for the instructional and training needs of those constituencies covered by the legislation. The focus of this type of legislation is on increasing the productivity and enriching the lives of people with disabilities. Because public education was primarily considered the responsibility of the state, the early education laws for children with disabilities came from the individual state legislatures. The first significant federal support for public education for people with disabilities was provided through the National Defense Education Act in 1957. Amended versions of the National Defense Education Act (Public Law 85-864 and Public Law 85-926) provided funds for mental retardation research and authorized the first federally supported programs to train teachers of children who were mentally retarded (Fifield and Fifield, 1995). Additional public policies, such as the Mental Retardation Facilities and Community Mental Health Center Construction Act of 1963 (Public Law 88-164) and the Developmental Disabilities Act of 1970 (Public Law 91-517), have attempted to better meet the needs of at-risk populations and individuals with developmental disabilities by addressing gaps in services.

The Education of the Handicapped Act Amendments of 1986 (Public Law 99-457) was the most influential piece of legislation for children with disabilities and their families. Part H and Part B of this legislation established services for children from birth through 2 years of age and 3 to 21 years of age, respectively. Subsequent amendments to that law, the **Individuals with Disabilities Education Act of 1990 (IDEA)** (Public Law 101-476) further defined implementation of these services and reinforced the importance of prevention rather than remediation (Stephens and Tauber, 1996).

MEDICAL REHABILITATION REFERENCED LEGISLATION

Medical rehabilitation referenced legislation is intended to provide for the health of those constituencies covered by the legislation. The focus of this type of legislation is on medical care and the development of programs to meet the special health needs of persons with disabilities.

Public funds for rehabilitation services are typically available through either insurance or grant programs. "Between 1965 and 1975, legislation separated itself from protection and care legislation by redefining and broadening these concepts to include intervention, treatment, and therapy which focused on maintaining and restoring physical, social, vocational, and cognitive skills" (Fifield and Fifield, 1995, p. 58). Most significant were the **Title XVIII** (Medicare) and **Title XIX** (Medicaid) **Amendments to the Social Security Act** because they provided health insurance coverage to beneficiaries for services delivered in a wide range of settings, including hospitals, outpatient facilities, skilled nursing facilities, comprehensive rehabilitation facilities, home health agencies, hospices, and clinics (Reed, 1992).

The Mental Retardation Facilities and Community Mental Health Center Construction Act of 1963 (Public Law 88-164) authorized construction of specially designed state facilities for the diagnosis, treatment, education, and training of people with disabilities, specifically individuals with mental retardation or mental illness. In addition, this act provided funding to establish community mental health centers and to increase the accessibility and availability of mental health services to the public (Ellek, 1991; Reed, 1992).

CIVIL RIGHTS REFERENCED LEGISLATION

Civil rights referenced legislation is intended to protect the lawful privileges of those constituencies covered by the legislation. The focus of this type of legislation is on equal protection under the law for all citizens. Social conflict during the 1960s resulted in an initial piece of legislation (Civil Rights Act of 1964) that asserted fundamental human rights and guaranteed numerous protections for all citizens. Subsequent legislative activities, such as the Architectural Barriers Act of 1968, Rehabilitation Act of 1973, and the Americans with Disabilities Act of 1990, included provisions to ensure the rights of people with disabilities. The Architectural Barriers Act of 1968 required all federal buildings to be accessible to persons with disabilities and included standards for accessibility that were later revised and incorporated into Section 504 of the Rehabilitation Act of 1973. Section 504, which provided the foundation for the Americans with Disabilities Act of 1990, prohibits discrimination on the basis of a disability by any program receiving or benefiting from federal financial aid. It also provided the first federal statutory definition of a disability, which has been used extensively in subsequent legislation.

Other legislation that incorporated civil rights provisions were the 1974 amendments to the Developmental Disabilities Act and the Education for All Handicapped Children Act (Public Law 94-142). The 1974 amendments to the Developmental Disabilities Act established protection and advocacy agencies in every state to ensure that state, public, or private service agencies did not violate the rights of persons with disabilities. The **Education for All Handicapped Children Act of 1975** (Public Law 94-142) established the right of children with handicaps to a free and appropriate public education.

Perhaps the most significant disabilities legislation was the **Americans with Disabilities Act (ADA) of 1990** (Public Law 101-336). It expanded the nondiscrimination provisions primarily associated with the Rehabilitation Act of 1973 to include the private sector and public services. Previous legislation affected only government agencies and agencies receiving federal support (Fifield and Fifield, 1995; Reed, 1992; Stephens and Tauber, 1996).

ENVIRONMENT REFERENCED LEGISLATION

Environment referenced legislation is intended to provide physical access to a variety of settings for those constituencies covered by the legislation. The focus of this type of legislation is on the accessibility and usability of programs for all persons but particularly for those with disabilities. Since the implementation of the Architectural Barriers Act of 1968 (Public Law 90-480), legislative provisions have extended the original focus of eliminating environmental barriers to buildings to include better access to information, services, and opportunities. Often, important community services were provided in locations and at times inconvenient to consumers but convenient to providers. The ideology for change has progressed from normalization and mainstreaming to full inclusion of persons with disabilities. The shift in the focus of control from the providers to the consumers was a direct result of the Independent Living Provisions of the 1973 Vocational Rehabilitation Act.

In the 1980s the Education for All Handicapped Children Act (Public Law 94-142) focused on improving the fit between the person with a disability and the regular education environment. As a result, increased attention was placed on mainstreaming children with special needs and providing placement in the least restrictive environment.

The **Technology Related Assistance Act of 1988** (Public Law 100-407) expanded the definitions of assistive technology introduced and defined in the Older Americans Act (1986) and in the Developmental Disabilities Act (1985) to include devices and services used to achieve independence, productivity, and integration (Fifield and Fifield, 1995, p. 63):

Since 1988, assistive technology has been an expanding provision included in the Individuals with Disabilities Education Act of 1990 and the 1992 amendments to the Rehabilitation Act. Advancements in assistive technology have made it feasible to implement many of the provisions of the Americans with Disabilities Act.

CONSUMER REFERENCED LEGISLATION

Consumer referenced legislation is intended to provide for representation in decision making of those constituencies covered by the legislation. The focus of this type of legislation is on autonomy and the individual's right to self-determination.

Historically, society has viewed people with disabilities as different, often using negative descriptors. Throughout the 1970s and 1980s the terms handicapped and client were used interchangeably when referring to people with disabilities. Both terms implied a dependent relationship in which the provider was the decision maker. The Developmental Disabilities Act of 1970 and the 1977 Rehabilitation Act amendments outlined provisions for increased consumer representation on policy and advisory councils, thus introducing the term "consumer" (Fifield and Fifield, 1995; Reed, 1992). The Education for All Handicapped Children Act strengthened the role of parents through the individual education plan process. According to Fifield and Fifield (1995), each successive reauthorization of these pieces of legislation has aggressively strengthened the level and depth of consumer participation in planning, monitoring, setting priorities, and making decisions in the development of service delivery. Both the Technology Related Assistance Act of 1988 and the Americans with Disabilities Act of 1990 also strengthened consumer responsiveness by "using 'people first' language that addressed dignity, choice, and participation" (Fifield and Fifield, 1995, p. 64).

 ## CONCLUSION

Historically, federal legislation concerning persons with disabilities has developed from a focus on adults to a focus on children. Federal legislation has progressed from concerns for primarily physical disabilities to concern for all types of disabilities and expanded from assistance for primarily medical management to assistance that also includes nonmedically based programs for citizens with disabilities (Reed, 1992). Because community-based programs are unique to the community served and are often based financially and programmatically on a variety of local, state, and federal policies, practitioners shifting from the more traditional practice arena must research the environment of their intended practice to ensure optimum service provision to their clients. A readily accessible source for researching both current state and federal legislation that might impact occupational therapy practice is the American Occupational Therapy Association's Website (*www.aota.org*). In some community-based programs the role of occupational therapy may not be clearly defined. It is then incumbent upon the practitioner to determine the role of occupational therapy. Both the roles and responsibilities should be based on personal expertise, program and consumer needs, and applicable legislation/policy. Following are questions that practitioners should consider in determining the appropriate role for occupational therapy:

● What is the mission of the community-based program?
● What client populations are served?
● What local, state, and federal regulations impact the program and/or service?
● Are there limitations in the number and types of services or visits provided?

- Are there restrictions in the number or type of sites at which services may be received?
- How is the program funded?
- Are there limitations or caps on annual costs for specific services?
- Is there a network of providers from whom clients must obtain service?
- What unique services can the occupational therapist provide that fit within the parameters identified?

This information is essential for practitioners to provide the optimal care. In changing times and with changing societal needs, occupational therapists must be responsive to the needs of consumers and the community programs that serve them. According to Powell (1992, p. 562), "Occupational therapists must forge stronger bonds with consumers, increase consumer independence, and hasten consumer community integration to refocus and develop new programs."

 STUDY QUESTIONS

1. Discuss the differences in the terms "reimbursement" and "funding." For each, identify an example of federal legislation that provides this type of financial resource.
2. Describe the basic features of the following pieces of legislation: the Social Security Act, the Americans with Disabilities Act (ADA), Individuals with Disabilities Education Act (IDEA), and the Technology Related Assistance Act.
3. Identify a community-based setting and discuss the policies that may affect practice in this setting.
4. Identify a community-based program and discuss the factors that an occupational therapy practitioner might consider in determining his or her role in that setting.
5. What resources are available to research legislative changes that may impact occupational therapy practice?

REFERENCES

Baum, C., and Law, M. (1998). Community health: A responsibility, an opportunity, and a fit for occupational therapy. *American Journal of Occupational Therapy, 52,* 7–10.

Brownson, C. (1998). Funding community practice: Stage 1. *American Journal of Occupational Therapy, 52,* 60–64.

Ellek, D. (1991). The evolution of fairness in mental health policy. *American Journal of Occupational Therapy, 45,* 947–951.

Fifield, B., and Fifield, M. (1995). The influence of legislation on services to people with disabilities. In O.C. Karan and S. Greenspan (Eds.), *Community rehabilitation services for people with disabilities* (pp. 38–70). Boston: Butterworth-Heinemann.

Jacobs, K. (1996). The evolution of the occupational therapy delivery system. In *The occupational therapy manager* (pp. 3–48). Bethesda, MD: American Occupational Therapy Association.

Powell, N.J. (1992). Supporting consumer-mandated programming for persons with developmental disabilities. *American Journal of Occupational Therapy, 46,* 559–562.

Reed, K.L. (1992). History of federal legislation for persons with disabilities. *American Journal of Occupational Therapy, 46,* 397–408.

Stephens, L.C., and Tauber, S.K. (1996). Early intervention. In J. Case-Smith, A. Allen, and P. Pratt (Eds.), *Occupational therapy for children* (pp. 648–653). St. Louis: Mosby.

ADDITIONAL READINGS

Albrecht, G.L. (1997). The health politics of disability. In T.J. Litman and L.S. Robins (Eds.), *Health politics and policy* (pp. 367–383). Albany, NY: Delmar.

Bachelder, J. M., and Hilton, C. L. (1994). Implications of the Americans with Disabilities Act of 1990 for elderly persons. *American Journal of Occupational Therapy, 48,* 73–81.

Burke, J.P., and Cassidy, J.C. (1991). Disparity between reimbursement-driven practice and humanistic values of occupational therapy. *American Journal of Occupational Therapy, 45,* 173–175.

Hanft, B.E. (1991). Impact of federal policy on pediatric health and education programs. In W. Dunn (Ed.), *Pediatric occupational therapy: Facilitating effective service provisions* (pp. 273–294). Thorofare, NJ: Slack.

Kalscheur, J.A. (1992). Benefits of the Americans with Disabilities Act of 1990 for children and adolescents with disabilities. *American Journal of Occupational Therapy, 46,* 419–425.

Rochefort, D.A. (1997). Health politics and mental health care. In T.J. Litman and L.S. Robins (Eds.), *Health politics and policy* (pp. 352–366). Albany, NY: Delmar.

Sankar, A., Newcomer, R., and Wood, J. (1986). Prospective payment: Systematic effects on the provision of community care for the elderly. *Home Health Care Services Quarterly, 7*(2), 93–117.

Thomas, V.J. (1996). Evolving health care systems: Payment for occupational therapy services. In *The occupational therapy manager* (pp. 577–602). Bethesda, MD: American Occupational Therapy Association.

Thomasma, D.C. (1996). The ethics of managed care: Challenges to the principles of relationship-centered care. *Journal of Allied Health, 25*(3), 233–246.

Verville, R.E. (1990). The Americans with Disabilities Act: An analysis. *Archives of Physical Medicine and Rehabilitation, 71,* 1010–1014.

6 CHAPTER

Program Development for Community Health: Planning, Implementation, and Evaluation Strategies

Carol A. Brownson, MSPH

■ OUTLINE

Ecological perspective
Formative evaluation
Goal
Group processes
Impact
Implementation
Interventions
Institutionalization
Needs assessment
Objectives
Outcome

Preplanning
Process evaluation
Program development
Program evaluation
Program planning
Secondary data
Societal levels
Stakeholders
Summative evaluation
Theory

LEARNING OBJECTIVES

This chapter is designed to enable the reader to:
- Define the key steps in community health/health promotion program development.
- Describe three sources of data for needs assessments.
- Identify four factors that impact the selection of needs assessment strategies.
- Demonstrate understanding of the role of health behavior theories in community health/health promotion program planning using examples of theories.
- Define "goal" and "objective."
- List examples of different types of objectives.
- Describe the five levels of the ecological approach to community health/health promotion programs.
- Give examples of implementation strategies at the different levels of intervention.
- Identify the purposes for each of the three levels of program evaluation.
- Describe three program evaluation designs.
- Discuss the importance of disseminating the results of program development and evaluation.

 ## INTRODUCTION

Program development, including planning, development of implementation strategies, and evaluation, emerged in the 1980s as a key component of health education and health promotion (Timmreck, 1995, p. xv). With growing concerns about health-care costs and access to care, health promotion and disease/injury prevention activities will likely play a major role in the future of health services. Planning, implementation, and evaluation skills are essential to the delivery of successful health promotion, health education, and prevention services.

Programs are distinguished from clinical services in that programs are primarily educational. Sometimes referred to as **interventions,** programs are systematic efforts to achieve preplanned objectives such as changes in knowledge, attitudes, skills, and behaviors to maintain or improve function and/or health. These interventions can occur in a number of settings such as schools, worksites, community agencies, and health-care environments.

Among the barriers to occupational therapists developing and/or providing health education and health promotion programs listed by Johnson and Jaffe (1989, pp. 63–65) were lack of training in health promotion and lack of training in designing and implementing effective educational interventions.

This chapter describes and explains the steps involved in developing community health and health promotion programs. It also introduces some of the theoretical foundations and models on which these programs are based.

 # *PROGRAM PLANNING PRINCIPLES*

Program planning has been described as a process of establishing priorities, diagnosing causes of problems, and allocating resources to achieve objectives (Green, 1980). People have always planned, with or without a systematic method. As knowledge accumulates, planning continues to become more sophisticated. Although no one perfect model exists, Breckon, Harvey, and Lancaster (1994) point to seven principles common to all planning models.

PLAN THE PROCESS

Preplanning is an important step that, if overlooked, can undermine the success of an otherwise effective intervention strategy. During the preplanning phase, consideration is given to who should be involved, when the planning should occur, what resources are needed, and what process will be followed. Internal and external resources are assessed, including attitudes, policies, available expertise, time, space, money, priorities, and fit with the organization's mission.

PLAN WITH PEOPLE

Experience has demonstrated the importance of involving clients in the planning process. Two community health promotion principles are encompassed here: (1) the principle of relevance and (2) the principle of participation. Similar to the concept of client-centeredness in occupational therapy, the principle of relevance, or "starting where the people are," tells us that successful programs begin by considering the perceived needs of clients rather than those of the planners or their organizations.

Participation and influence are considered essential for developing effective programs and are considered health enhancing in and of themselves. People meet and sustain their goals more effectively when they are actively involved in the process (Baker and Brownson, 1998; Minkler and Wallerstein, 1997). Client participation can range from responding to requests for feedback on program plans to taking an active role in the design, implementation, and evaluation of program activities.

Planning with people also encompasses the concept of collaboration. Program planning generally begins with a group of people who have a vested interest in the issues (**stakeholders**). Working with people and agencies who have shared interests and goals offers many advantages: resources and workload can be shared, duplication of effort can be minimized, and more creative problem solving can occur. The end result is a program that provides better service to clients.

PLAN WITH DATA

Sound planning decisions are based on a thorough knowledge of the health issue and associated factors, the service area or site, the target population, social and environmental support systems, and existing or former programs addressing the same issue. Much of the quantitative information can be gathered from existing sources such as health departments, libraries, the National Center for Health Statistics, Chambers of Commerce, and health systems. Planners may also identify the need for additional data, perhaps more qualitative data that would help to identify attitudes, beliefs, or barriers. A review of available and gathered data provides a context in which planning and prioritizing can occur logically.

PLAN FOR PERFORMANCE

This principle speaks to long-range planning. Given that most serious health challenges will not completely disappear with one program, approaching the planning process with the idea of permanence, or institutionalization, makes sense. That means considering how the program might be staffed and financed after the initial intervention or how it might ultimately become an integral part of an agency's services.

PLAN FOR PRIORITIES

The most effective programs are those that address the greatest need and are designed or known to have the greatest effect within given resources. Prioritization should flow naturally from planning with people and planning with data. It assumes a comprehensive needs assessment and input from all stakeholders.

PLAN FOR EVALUATION

Evaluation is a continuous process of asking questions such as "Are we doing the right thing?" and "Are we doing things right?" and "What do we need to measure to know what and how we're doing?" These questions are usually answered through the systematic collection and analysis of program and client information (data). Evaluation methods, depending on the goals and objectives of the program, should be built into the program design and spelled out in the program plan. Once the needed information is determined, record-keeping systems and evaluation instruments need to be selected and put in place to ensure that data are properly collected. The planning process should address who will be responsible for both data collection and analysis. It should also establish time frames for all steps.

PLAN FOR MEASURABLE OUTCOMES

This principle speaks to the importance of having clearly articulated and measurable program objectives with some baseline data against which to judge program accomplishments. The format for the objective and the evaluation should match. For example, if the objective of a program is to reduce the risk of developing a secondary condition, then the outcome would be stated in terms of risk reduction, not reduced mortality or reduced hospitalization.

THE PLANNING PROCESS

A typical program planning process follows steps that are very similar to the occupational therapy process (Table 6–1). Program planning is a process involving continuous cycles of needs assessment, planning the intervention, implementation, and evaluation (Dignan and Carr, 1992). Although these planning subtasks have discrete roles, in good programs they are interdependent and interwoven, using feedback at each step to revise or improve previous steps, as depicted in Figure 6–1 (Simons-Morton, Greene, and Gottlieb, 1995).

 TABLE 6–1

COMPARISON OF THE PROGRAM PLANNING PROCESS AND OCCUPATIONAL THERAPY PROCESS

Program Planning Process	Occupational Therapy Process
Preplanning (Exploration)	*Chart Review*
● Identify/state the problem and the target population (also called "issue identification").	
● Identify existing information regarding issue of concern.	
● Assess the internal and external resources and barriers.	
● Determine the goals of, and an approach for, the needs assessment.	
Needs Assessment (Data Gathering and Analysis)	*Client Evaluation*
● Collect relevant data.	
● Analyze and synthesize data.	
● Determine priorities.	
● Identify and evaluate alternative solutions.	
● Formulate an action plan.	
Plan Development	*Treatment Planning*
● Establish goals and objectives.	
● Develop the details of the intervention strategies, procedures, and timelines.	
● Develop a plan for evaluation.	
● Pretest materials and procedures.	
Implementation	*Treatment Implementation*
● Implement/offer the program or service.	
Evaluation	*Re-evaluation*
● Monitor and evaluate the program process, its impact, and ultimately the outcome.	
Institutionalization	*Carry Over to Home and Community*
● *Share the results with stakeholders, peers, and clients.*	
● Revise program as indicated and plan next steps (e.g., continue, terminate, and expand).	

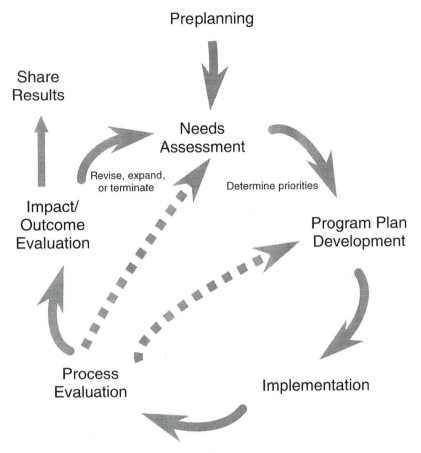

FIG. 6–1. The Cycle of Program Development.

PREPLANNING

The preassessment or preplanning phase is an exploratory step during which existing data on the issue are identified and reviewed, resources are assessed, and the goals of the needs assessment are established. Identifying an issue to address can come from data, professional judgment, observation, existing literature, concerned individuals, or agencies.

Key questions of who, what, and why are answered. For example, *who* are the key players (e.g., service receivers, service providers, experts in the field, policy makers, agency representatives) with a vested interest in the issue; *what* do they hope will come from the needs assessment; and *why*—what prompted their concern, and how important is it (Soriano, 1995)? Answers to these questions will help define the key questions for the needs assessment. Planning often occurs through a group of stakeholders forming a planning committee. However broad or narrow the group, the perspectives of all stakeholders—particularly those of potential clients—must be considered and integrated into the planning process.

Every program planning initiative is influenced by factors that can support or inhibit the process. Considering these internal and external factors early in the process is important to avoid unnecessary pitfalls. First, a need must be analyzed for consistency or "fit" with the organization's mission. Assuming it fits, how important is the need relative to other issues? Is there a commitment of time and resources to see the project through? What is the potential for effecting a positive change? What do the other stakeholders want or expect? Are there other programs addressing this issue of concern?

Assessment of resources goes beyond the question of whether or not there is funding. Depending on the nature of the program being planned, other considerations may include location, space, materials, appropriately trained personnel, transportation for clients, and access to experts for certain phases of the process. Finally, preplanning should include an assessment of existing regulations and policies that might have an impact on the issue or the approach(es) being pursued.

NEEDS ASSESSMENT

The occupational therapy practitioner evaluates needs of clients daily in the delivery of direct care. In the context of program planning, however, a needs assessment is not intended to provide diagnostic information about individuals. Instead, the purpose is to make decisions about priorities for programs and services that affect groups of people.

A *need* is generally defined as the gap between the present state of affairs (what is) and some desired future state for a particular group with an identified issue (McKillip, 1987; Witkin and Altschuld, 1995). **Needs assessment** may be defined as a systematic set of procedures that serves to identify and describe specific areas of need and available resources in a given population, discover factors that contribute to the identified problem, establish priorities, and devise criteria for interventions that will address the need (Witkin and Altschuld, 1995). If done properly, the needs assessment will lead to a clear set of program goals and objectives.

Data Collection

Key to the needs assessment process is the gathering of accurate and comprehensive information for making decisions about the best use of resources to resolve high-priority needs. Methods for gathering data vary. Only a few of the methods will be briefly described here. Before collecting new data, a review of the scientific and intervention literature for background on the issue of concern and identification of strategies that have been used in similar situations are necessary.

Some common data sources and methods, such as secondary data, surveys, and group processes, are outlined in Table 6–2. The use of secondary data is one of the simplest and most cost-effective methods. **Secondary data,** also called archival data, are existing data collected by agencies for other purposes. Examples include birth and death records; census data; prevalence data on diseases, disability, illness, injury, and risk; demographic data; social indicators; and special surveys and reports. Secondary data are generally easy to obtain and particularly useful in the exploratory phase of the needs assessment process to determine what is already known about an issue. These data give a sense of the current status and give the planner an idea of what further information to gather. By themselves, secondary data do not constitute a needs assessment. To provide context and client perspective, they are best used in conjunction with qualitative data.

Surveys, the most frequently used tool for gathering information for the needs assessment, are a cost-effective method for gathering information from large numbers of people who represent the target population. They may take the form of written questionnaires or interviews (in person or by telephone). Surveys should be administered to obtain information that doesn't exist elsewhere and should be designed so that inferences can be drawn about priorities and seriousness of needs. The most effective type of survey for a needs assessment asks people for their opinions based on their own experiences, background, expertise, or knowledge or for facts about themselves and others about whom they have direct knowledge (Witkin and Altschuld, 1995).

TABLE 6–2

AN OVERVIEW AND COMPARISON OF COMMONLY USED DATA COLLECTION METHODS FOR NEEDS ASSESSMENT

Data Source/Method	Description	Resulting Information	Advantages	Disadvantages
Secondary (archival) data, i.e., records and logs, prior studies, demographic data, social indicators, risk-factor data, epidemiologic studies, census data, and rates under treatment	Existing data usually found in city, county, state, and national organizations and government bureaus	Quantitative data that help determine the status of a target population with regard to a need; may furnish information on causal or contributing factors	Relatively low in cost; generally available; minimal investment of time or staff; unbiased; complements other sources of data	No client input; possibly not representative for given target audience; technical assistance for statistical interpretation possibly needed
Survey methods, i.e., written questionnaire, face-to-face interview, telephone interview, and key informant interview	Techniques for gathering information directly from individuals using structured forms or protocols	Mainly qualitative—values, perceptions, opinions, judgments of importance, and observations	Client input achieved; quantitative data complemented	Generally more time and labor intensive than using secondary data sources
1. Written questionnaire			Easy to administer; relatively low in cost; time efficient; quantifiable; broad reach into community/target population	Possible low return rates; may not be representative; not useful for people who are illiterate or not fluent in English; prone to design problems; technical assistance for questionnaire construction and data processing/analysis possibly necessary

Method	Advantages	Disadvantages
2. Face-to-face interview	High response rate; greater flexibility for answers and interviewer probing; opportunity to observe non-verbal responses; ability to include people who are illiterate or who have vision problems; rapport building	Smaller sample size; costly in terms of time and travel; trained interviewers required; possible difficulty with scheduling; time consuming; opportunity for bias; possibility to raise client expectations; data more difficult to interpret and summarize; technical assistance for questionnaire construction, data processing/analysis possibly necessary
3. Telephone interview	Easy to administer; no travel time and cost; perceived anonymity; fairly good response rate	Sampling challenges; may not be representative; not as suitable for long questionnaires; inability to observe non-verbal reactions; possible rise in client expectations; trained interviewers necessary to avoid bias; computer capability and technical assistance for questionnaire construction, data processing/analysis possibly needed

(Continued)

T A B L E   6 – 2

AN OVERVIEW AND COMPARISON OF COMMONLY USED DATA COLLECTION METHODS FOR NEEDS ASSESSMENT (*Continued*)

Data Source/Method	Description	Resulting Information	Advantages	Disadvantages
4. Key informant	Surveys (written and/or interview) of a select group of key community leaders, informal lay leaders, and professional persons who are aware of, and in touch with, the target population and the given issue		Limited number of participants necessary	Possible difficulty in identifying informal leaders; biased results possible; participants may have vested interests
Group processes, i.e., community forums, focus groups, and nominal group processes	Techniques that involve small or large groups of stakeholders (e.g., service receivers, service providers, experts in the field, policy makers, and agency representatives) in varying degrees of interaction	Mainly qualitative—opinions and expert judgments; group perceptions and perspectives regarding values, importance of need; information on causes/barriers; decisions on priorities; feedback or consensus on goals or courses of action	Opportunity for fluid, natural discussion around an issue; complementary to other data	

Method	Description		Advantages	Disadvantages
1. Community forum	An open public meeting with all interested parties invited; a large group discussion	Ideas and input from a broad segment of the population	Broad range of views and concerns provided; natural discussion format; facilitation of dialogue among people with different viewpoints	Possibly not reflective of opinions of general population; participation possibly low; domination by a few possible; difficult to analyze; logistics
2. Focus groups	Groups of 8 to 12 clients/potential clients responding to a structured set of questions	Individual and group perspectives on a focused area or theme	Possible in-depth probing of themes	Skilled facilitators needed; technical assistance in data analysis possibly required; logistical challenges getting group together; groups variable, thus, more than one needed for reliable results
3. Nominal group process	The most structured of the group methods; a combination of written responses, voting, and discussion used in small groups of 10 or less	Ranking by the group of what they perceive to be the most important issues and/or solutions	Highly effective for getting at a large number of issues in a short amount of time; equitable participation	Expensive in terms of time and results; skilled leadership required; limited ability to generalize

Sources: Simons-Morton, B.G., Greene, W.H., and Gottlieb, N.H. (1995). Introduction to health education and health promotion. Prospect Heights, IL: Waveland. Soriano, F.I. (1995). Conducting needs assessments: A multidisciplinary approach. Thousand Oaks, CA: Sage. Witkin, B.R., and Altschuld, J.W. (1995). Planning and conducting needs assessments: A practical guide. Thousand Oaks, CA: Sage.

The specifics of survey methodology are beyond the scope of this chapter. While surveys look deceptively simple to construct, obtaining meaningful and reliable information requires considerable expertise in questionnaire development and administration. Questions need to be simple, straightforward, and carefully worded to elicit the desired information. The survey also must include people who are representative of the target audience and the stakeholders. Additionally, effort must be made to ensure that the method itself doesn't exclude segments of the population. Decisions need to be made about how the results will be analyzed. The survey also should be pretested on a sample of respondents. These tasks may require additional study (recommended are Witkin and Altschuld, 1995, chap. 6) or the input of professionals with expertise in survey methodology.

Aside from surveys, **group processes** are the most frequently used method of collecting qualitative data for needs assessments (Witkin and Altschuld, 1995). Group processes provide face-to-face interactions with groups of stakeholders in a variety of discussion formats, most commonly open forums, focus groups, and nominal group processes. Group processes also provide direct interaction between the agency representatives and the target population, which can serve to build rapport. Like the other methods, group processes are most valuable when used in conjunction with other methods and sources. For further explanation of these techniques, the reader is referred to Witkin and Altschuld (1995), Krueger (1994), and Dignan and Carr (1992).

There is no inherently perfect or best method of data collection for needs assessment. The selection of methods depends on several factors (Witkin and Altschuld, 1995; Soriano, 1995), including:

- The characteristics of the target group and the survey respondents. For example, socioeconomic factors, literacy, language, availability, and level of ability are among the factors that may influence the manner in which information is gathered.
- The type of information desired. It makes sense to choose a combination of methods that yield different types of information, both qualitative and quantitative.
- Resources available, e.g., time, financial and human resources, and expertise. Trade-offs between the desired comprehensiveness of the needs assessment and the resources available may be necessary.
- The amount of interaction desired with the audience. Some methods offer greater opportunity for dialogue with members of the target audience. Those same methods may be more costly or harder to analyze. Advantages and disadvantages of each approach should be considered.

Data Analysis and Interpretation

The data-gathering methods yield raw data. The next step is to analyze the data and use it in a practical way for planning. Even though the needs assessment is a form of survey research, the analysis is more of a planning tool than a statistical exercise. As such, the needs assessment relies less on inferential statistics and more on identification of need, risk, seriousness of a problem, and access to services (Timmreck, 1995). Once analyzed, the data should be presented to stakeholders in an easily understandable manner. Charts, graphs, and tables are useful techniques.

Interpretation of the data for planning purposes is the last step in the needs assessment process. The goal of this intermediate step is not to make final decisions about the intervention strategy but to interpret findings, set priorities regarding needs, suggest ways of addressing needs, weigh the alternatives based on a set of predetermined criteria, and propose a plan to implement the best solution (Witkin and Altschuld, 1995). This final step in the needs assessment process provides the direction and rationale for program planners to develop an effective intervention.

PROGRAM PLAN DEVELOPMENT

While needs assessments focus on the *ends* to be attained, the development of a program plan focuses on the *means* or solutions (Witkin and Altschuld, 1995). Ideally, the development of program components is based on a merging of the findings of the needs assessment, theories, and available resources (Simons-Morton et al., 1995).

The Role of Theories

Any time a program or service is planned, planners make assumptions about the causes of the problem and the best ways to effect change. If those assumptions are not made in terms of an explicit theory or theories, and there is no conceptual framework behind the choice of intervention, then there is no way to link the intervention to the intended outcome (Posavac and Carey, 1997). As a result, program design would be much less effective and evaluation would be less informative.

Simply stated, a **theory** is an explanation of why a phenomenon occurs the way it does (Freudenberg et al., 1995). Good theories complement practical skills and technologies by taking the program beyond simply conducting activities to actually solving problems. Theories can provide answers to a program developer's questions about *why* people engage or do not engage in specific health behaviors and *how* to engage people in changing and maintaining behaviors. Programs devised to address expected behaviors according to a theory help to determine *what* factors to focus on in the evaluation (van Ryn and Heaney, 1992; Posavac and Carey, 1997).

No single theory exists on which to base health education and health promotion programs. Populations, environments, cultures, and health issues vary broadly, so different theories or different combinations of theories may be useful in addressing a particular issue. Some theories focus on individual behavior; others focus on groups, organizations, or communities as the unit of change. The dominant theories currently used in health education have roots in social psychology and deal with health behavior at the individual level. These include the health belief model; self-efficacy, a construct of social learning theory; and the transtheoretical model. Bridging the individual, group, and community levels is social learning theory, also called social cognitive theory (see Chapter 4 for a discussion of these theories).

Theories that address organizations and communities include organizational change theory (Goodman, Steckler, and Kegler, 1997), community organization (Minkler and Wallerstein, 1997), community empowerment (Minkler and Wallerstein, 1997), diffusion of innovations (Oldenburg, Hardcastle, and Kok, 1997), and media advocacy (Wallack, Dorfman, Jernigan, and Themba, 1993). These are not described here due to space constraints but are well described in the references noted.

Learning how to analyze the fit of a theory to the issue or problem identified is challenging. According to Glanz and Rimer (1995, p. 12), "a working knowledge of a handful of theories and how they have been applied will go a long way to improve one's skill in this area." She further suggests that if a theory is a good fit, the theory will make assumptions about a behavior, health problem, or condition of people or the environment that are: (1) logical, (2) consistent with everyday observations, (3) similar to those used in previous successful programs, and (4) supported by past research in the same or related area (Glanz and Rimer, 1995). For more detail on the theories just described and others, and for a better understanding of their applications, the reader is referred to Glanz, Lewis, and Rimer (1997) and Glanz and Rimer (1995).

Putting the Plan Together

The general form of the written program plan includes:

● Goals
● Objectives

● Strategies
● Evaluation plan

GOALS. Despite commonality of plan components, terminology is often confusing and used differently from one discipline to another. In health and social services planning, a **goal** is a quantified statement of a desired change in the status of a priority health need. Goals are long term and broad in scope. As such, they are not directly measurable, but should be considered attainable. Programs may have more than one goal.

OBJECTIVES. **Objectives** are used to reach goals. Unlike goals, objectives are specific, measurable, and performance based. "They specify who, to what extent, under what conditions, by what standards, and within what time period certain activities are to be performed and completed" (Timmreck, 1995, p. 32). They outline the tasks and activities essential to accomplish the established goals. One goal may have several objectives, with each objective representing one aspect of accomplishing the goal. Well-written objectives typically answer the following questions:

● Who (clients/participants)?
● What (action/performance)?
● When (time frame)?
● How much (to what degree/standard of performance/level)?

For example, an objective might read: Within six months of completing the fall prevention course, 75 percent of participants will be continuing their balance exercises. Using the questions listed,

● *Who* refers to the participants of the fall prevention course.
● *What* refers to the action of continuing their balance exercises.
● *When* is identified as within six months of completing the course.
● *How* much is denoted as 75 percent of participants.

Programs that employ multiple approaches to reaching their goals may have different types of objectives. Some are directed at changes in the participants—their knowledge, behavior, or health status. Others may be directed at changes in resources or services. Examples of different types of objectives that pertain to the same goal are listed in Table 6-3.

Program plans may identify objectives by type and group them as such. Others may consider one type of objective as a "subobjective" of another. The important element is that the program plan clearly identify its health objective(s), what the program will do to accomplish the objective(s), and what change in knowledge, skill, or behavior is expected in participants.

Strategies

The next task is to develop specific strategies for accomplishing the objectives that will be effective with the intended audience. Participation by members of the intended audience in the selection of methods is crucial to ensure that the methods are acceptable and effective. Other factors to consider include literacy of the potential participants; degree of auditory or visual stimulation in their everyday lives; ways they customarily obtain information; cost; convenience; cultural relevance; feasibility; and anticipated effectiveness (Dignan and Carr, 1992).

The most comprehensive programs go beyond the individual level, addressing systems that affect the ability of an individual to achieve work, leisure, and social goals. Socioecologic approaches to improving health recognize the interrelationships be-

TABLE 6–3

DIFFERENT TYPES OF OBJECTIVES FOR ONE GOAL

Goal: By 2005, reduce injury from falls by half among older adults in Johnson County.

Objectives	Type
Within two years of the program's inception, admissions due to injury from falls in adults over age 60 will be reduced by 15 percent at Johnson County Hospital.	This is an example of a *health objective*. This objective specifies a change in health status (i.e., fewer injuries from falls). Health objectives define the specific health outcomes the program aims to accomplish and are sometimes referred to as "outcome objectives." There may be several for each goal.
By January 2000, the occupational therapist will reach 300 adults over age 60 through a fall prevention course taught in 15 senior housing complexes and nutrition centers in Johnson County.	This is an example of a *program objective*. It deals with the new service that is planned. These often address the "process" of the intervention.
By the end of the course, participants in the fall prevention program will be able to identify at least four risk factors for falls and develop an action plan for addressing their personal risks.	This is an example of a *learning objective*. It addresses knowledge, attitudes, or skills the program will attempt to effect to encourage specific behaviors in the intended population.
Within six months of completing the course, 75 percent of participants will be continuing their balance exercises at their goal level.	This is an example of a *behavioral objective*. Behavioral objectives, closely related to learning objectives, describe what the program will encourage people to do to reduce risk or improve health. Learning and behavioral objectives are sometimes called "impact objectives"; they do not directly address the health outcome but deal with factors that affect outcomes. They reflect the specific program strategies.
Home assessments will be provided to all interested clients who attend the fall prevention course.	This is an example of a *resource objective*. It addresses material support or essential services the program plans to provide.

tween people and their physical, social, cultural, economic, and political environments. Key to the **ecological perspective** in health promotion is that health behavior both influences and is influenced by the environment (reciprocal causation). This concept is well recognized in occupational therapy and evident in the theories and models of person-environment-occupation that guide occupational therapy practice (Law et al., 1997). In an ecological health promotion planning model, Simons-Morton et al. (1995) described five **societal levels** in which planners could intervene:

1. **Intrapersonal:** individual characteristics that influence behavior, such as knowledge, attitudes, beliefs, values, and personality

2. Interpersonal: family, friends, peers, and groups that provide social identity, support, and role definition
3. Organizational: agencies and their rules, regulations, policies, procedures, programs, and resources
4. Community: social networks, norms, trends, and standards that constrain or promote desired action
5. Public policy: local, state, and federal policies, laws, and programs that regulate or support desired action

An example of addressing the same health concern, physical activity for people with disabilities, from the different levels is provided in Table 6–4.

Popular health promotion planning models that offer ecological frameworks for planning programs include PRECEDE-PROCEED (Green and Kreuter, 1991), social marketing (Lefebvre and Rochlin, 1997), and MATCH (Simons-Morton et al., 1995). They address all societal levels and can be used to integrate diverse theories.

Some common methods used in the different societal levels are described in Table 6–5.

Most occupational therapy practitioners are involved in smaller subpopulation interventions (levels 1 and 2), as opposed to working at changing systems, community norms, or policies (levels 3 to 5). Even at the interpersonal or group level, understanding and maintaining an ecological perspective of the issue is useful. It becomes a "mindset" for viewing an issue of concern. At the very least, seeing clients as part of larger systems can provide guidance for improving transitions between and among programs and services and for identifying gaps. Having an ecological perspective should also encourage collaboration with agencies and systems that focus more clearly on other levels of intervention.

Trying to address all levels in one program initiative may not be feasible or even desirable. However, using their experience, knowledge, and expertise to influence others along the continuum can be every effective for occupational therapy practi-

 TABLE 6–4

ECOLOGICAL HEALTH PROMOTION MODEL AND OCCUPATIONAL THERAPY

Level of Intervention	Potential Occupational Therapy Role
Intrapersonal/individual	Adapt physical activities/exercises for people with functional limitations to encourage fitness and promote health.
Interpersonal	Offer adapted exercise classes for specific populations; provide education to family members and friends.
Organizational	Work with existing gyms, YMCA/YWCAs, and exercise facilities to make their facilities accessible to people of all abilities; train staff.
Community	Work with appropriate health agencies and health professions to develop messages about the importance of physical activity for everyone; use appropriate channels to raise awareness; join others in advocating for accessible community facilities and transportation; offer professional consultation on adaptations and accommodations.
Government/policy level	Advocate for funding to support making public parks, trails, and facilities accessible to people with disabilities.

TABLE 6-5

SOCIETAL LEVELS AND METHODS USED

Societal Level	Method	Description
Individual/group level (educating, training, and counseling)	Lecture-discussion	Combination of prepared remarks by leader/facilitator and guided discussion or question-answer session
	Audiovisual aids	Cassettes, compact discs, booklets, posters, flipcharts, models, display boards, overhead transparencies, slides, videotapes, computers, and interactive multimedia programs
	Peer group discussion	Use of small groups for discussion of topic common to group
	Simulation and games	Games, role-playing, dramatizations, case studies, storytelling, and songs
	Skill development	Explanation, demonstration, and practice of a psychomotor competency
	Mass media	Information provided through television, radio, newspapers, magazines, billboards, direct mail (Dignan and Carr, 1992; AMC Cancer Research Center, 1994; Simons-Morton, Greene, and Gottlieb, 1995; Office of Cancer Communications, 1992)
Interpersonal level (educating, training, and facilitating)	Enhancing/developing social ties	Interpersonal relationships that provide emotional, instrumental, or informational assistance (Heaney and Israel, 1997)
	Use of natural helpers	Members of social networks that other members go to for advice, support, and other assistance (Eng, 1992)

(Continued)

TABLE 6-5

SOCIETAL LEVELS AND METHODS USED (*Continued*)

Societal Level	Method	Description
Organizational level (consulting, networking, training, and advocating)	Organizational development	Implementation of planned change within organizations (Goodman, Steckler, and Kegler, 1997)
Community level (marketing, organizing, developing, and advocating)	Media advocacy	The strategic use of mass media to increase public support for a social or policy initiative (Wallack, Dorfman, Jernigan, and Themba, 1993)
	Community coalitions	An alliance of organizations or individuals working together to achieve a common purpose (Butterfoss, Goodman, and Wandersman, 1993)
	Community organization	A set of processes and procedures by which community groups are helped to identify problems, mobilize resources, and in other ways develop and implement strategies to solve a common problem or pursue a common goal (Minkler and Wallerstein, 1997)
	Community empowerment	A social action process through which individuals, communities, and organizations gain mastery over their lives in the context of changing their social and political environment to improve equity and quality of life (Minkler and Wallerstein, 1997; Rappaport, 1984)
Governmental and policy level (advocacy, lobbying, and political action)	Policy development/advocacy	Changes in, or development of, local, state, or federal policies, programs, practices, regulations, and laws on behalf of a particular interest group or population

tioners. Encouraging advocacy, providing information to clients, employers, and policy makers, and joining community organizations and coalitions are examples of how one might extend his or her "reach" and leverage action at other levels. Doing so can also generate new partners and possibly new funding for programs that meet mutual goals (Brownson, 1998). Although not addressed in this chapter, another approach is to expand occupational therapy's role in community, environmental, policy, and social arenas.

Evaluation Plan

An evaluation strategy, developed as part of the overall program plan, should be done with input from the key stakeholders, including potential participants or clients. Several steps for developing an evaluation plan are as follows:

1. Determine who will coordinate data collection and who will analyze it.
2. List the strategies, methods, or materials of interest for evaluation (i.e., the evaluation questions) and the anticipated results based on program standards and objectives.
3. Construct "dummy" tables or charts to help visualize how the information collected might be organized and summarized to show results.
4. Make a list of all the information needed.
5. Develop a timeline or work schedule for the remaining steps (6 to 11).
6. Identify the data collection techniques that are appropriate and feasible for the information needed (e.g., assessments, surveys, medical records, reports, questionnaires, observations, tests, interviews, etc.).
7. Identify sources of existing data that may be used, existing tools or instruments for data collection, and instruments that need to be developed.
8. Develop and test needed instruments.
9. Establish a data collection plan, including what will be collected, when, and by whom (this should be incorporated into the overall program timeline).
10. Establish a data analysis plan, including timelines and responsible parties.
11. Develop a plan for disseminating the results (presentations, program reports, and papers) (Green and Kreuter, 1991; Dignan and Carr, 1992).

LEVELS OF EVALUATION. Programs can be evaluated at one or more of three levels: (1) process, (2) impact, and (3) outcome. Each level asks different questions, addresses different aspects of the program, and considers different indicators, as shown in Table 6–6. Note that, in this taxonomy, **impact** refers to the intermediate effects and **outcome** to the long-term effects of a program or process (Green and Kreuter, 1995). Others have delineated two levels of program evaluation: **formative** or **process evaluation,** which focuses on program development, and **summative evaluation,** which focuses on program results.

EVALUATION DESIGNS. Evaluation designs range from simple to complex. The decision about the level and depth of evaluation to undertake is based on a number of factors, including the program's objectives, time, money, and expertise available, and management or funding agency priorities. **Process evaluation,** which should be done on every program, tends to be the least complex. A record-keeping approach or "historical design" provides an ongoing account of what is occurring in the program. "The critical product from process evaluation is a clear, descriptive picture of the quality of the program elements being put into place and what is going on as the program proceeds" (Green and Kreuter, 1995, p. 230). Information of interest can be plotted on charts and graphs to show changes as they occur.

As one moves along the continuum to measure the impact and outcome of a program, evaluation tends to become more complex and costly in terms of time, money,

TABLE 6–6

CHARACTERISTICS OF AND DISTINCTIONS AMONG THE LEVELS OF PROGRAM EVALUATION

Level of Evaluation	What Is Being Evaluated	Timeframe for Evaluation	Outcome of Evaluation
Process	Program processes and procedures	Short term—during and immediately following intervention	Feedback on program implementation (planned versus actual), audience participation and response, quality and appropriateness of materials, resources expended, staff response, etc.
Impact	Program objectives	Intermediate—end of program and periodically thereafter	Feedback on changes in knowledge, attitude, behavior, and/or performance of participants; changes in environment; policies enacted, etc.
Outcome	Program goals	Long term—varies, depending on issue; may be years	Feedback on changes in health status—morbidity, mortality, disability, and quality of life

Sources: Dignan, M.B., and Carr, P.A. (1992). *Program planning for health education and health promotion* (2nd ed.). Philadelphia: Lea and Febiger. Green, L.W., and Kreuter, M.W. (1991). *Health promotion and planning: An educational and environmental approach* (2nd ed.). Mountain View, CA: Mayfield. Simons-Morton, B.G., Greene, W.H., and Gottlieb, N.H. (1995). *Introduction to health education and health promotion.* Prospect Heights, IL: Waveland.

and expertise required. Program evaluation designs are classified in a number of ways, but generally fall into the three broad categories listed here, beginning with the least complex:

1. Nonexperimental designs (also called *pretest-posttest designs, before-and-after designs,* or *time-series designs*) involve participants serving as their own controls. Evaluation measures are gathered on participants before and after the intervention program.
2. Quasi-experimental designs (also called *nonrandomized controlled trials* or *controlled comparisons*) compare two groups. The group receiving the intervention is matched to a population that is similar demographically but is not receiving the program. Data are collected from both groups at the same time points and compared.
3. Experimental designs (also called *randomized controlled experiments, true experiments,* or *controlled experiments*) randomly assign people to two groups. One group receives the intervention and the other does not. Data are collected from both groups at the same time points and compared (Fink, 1993; Simons-Morton et al., 1995; Green and Kreuter, 1991).

These methods all yield quantitative data that help to assess the impact/outcome of the program. They do not necessarily tell *how* and *why* the program had its effect on participants. To get at that level of discovery and understanding, one can employ qualitative evaluation measures to complement and support the quantitative data. Qualitative methods include in-person interviews, surveys, direct observations, and written documents (such as client journals) (Fink, 1993; Dignan and Carr, 1992).

PROGRAM IMPLEMENTATION

Once the evaluation plan is complete and built into the overall program plan, the implementation phase of the program can begin. **Implementation,** the process of putting a program into effect, is the most critical phase of the program development process. As such, it requires an implementation plan. This plan is a document that spells out the details of each procedure and activity necessary for successful execution of the program and specifies who is responsible for each. Staffing, materials, equipment, space, marketing, contracts, and approvals are some of the areas around which planning may need to occur. The use of planning matrices, worksheets, and timelines can provide organization to tasks in easy-to-read formats and facilitate monitoring of the program processes. To assemble such charts, following these steps is helpful (Timmreck, 1995):

1. List all of the activities and tasks to be done.
2. Determine the order in which they need to occur.
3. Determine how long each activity will take.
4. Set an expected beginning and ending time for each activity or task.
5. Assign responsibility for each activity to ensure accountability.

PROGRAM EVALUATION

Fink (1993, p. 2) defines **program evaluation** as

> a diligent investigation of a program's characteristics and merits. Its purpose is to provide information on the effectiveness of projects to optimize the outcomes, efficiency, and quality of health care. Evaluations can analyze a program's structure, activities, and organization and examine its political and social environment. They can also appraise the achievement of a project's goals and objectives and the extent of its impact and costs.

While program evaluation employs research methods and uses statistical tools, it should not be confused with basic research. The purposes are very different. Basic research concerns questions of theoretical interest, while program evaluation is a management tool for making decisions about which programs and services to offer or how to improve them (Posavac and Carey, 1997; Simons-Morton et al., 1995).

Program evaluation also should not be confused with individual assessment. Assessments may, indeed, be conducted to gather information on individuals' levels of function, knowledge, or health status. But the purpose is not to diagnose or "track" individuals; instead, it is to learn *how well the program helped people to improve* on those variables (Posavac and Carey, 1997). According to Fink (1993, p. 132):

> Program evaluators use statistical methods to analyze and summarize data and to come to conclusions that can be applied to program planning and policy. The statistical methods are derived from the fields of statistics and epidemiology. Biostatistics refers to the application of statistics to biological and health sciences. Epidemiology includes the study of health and illness in human populations (not individuals).

> Choosing a method to analyze program evaluation data is an intellectual process in which statistical technology and the outcomes of health interventions converge.

Fink (1993) goes on to say that the choice of analysis is as much a function of the characteristics of the evaluation questions and the quality of data available as it is on the planner's ability to identify appropriate statistical techniques. This speaks to the need to involve experts in biostatistics and evaluation design early in the program planning process if the planners are not well versed in these areas. These experts can assist in choosing or developing measures that are reliable and valid, selecting appropriate statistical tools for the analyses and interpreting the findings once data are collected.

 ## INSTITUTIONALIZATION

Program developers often think of evaluation as the last step in the process. However, to ensure the **institutionalization,** or integration of the program into service delivery systems, two additional steps can be taken. The first is to use the evaluation findings to make appropriate decisions about the program. Simply stated, there are three options: (1) replication, (2) modification, or (3) termination.

The second step is to disseminate the results, no matter what the outcome. Sharing the results of the evaluation with those who funded the program and other key stakeholders is important and often required. Beyond meeting a requirement to ensure accountability, there are several reasons to prepare reports, abstracts, and manuscripts about the program and its results. Most important, contributing knowledge to the field or adding to the literature can improve practice. Others can model programs based on your experience or learn from your mistakes. Also, publishing together can improve partnerships with those who shared in the process. It is a way to acknowledge everyone involved and let them see the fruits of their labors. Publishing can also have the effect of enhancing the credibility of the planners and their program, particularly if the work is peer reviewed.

 ## CONCLUSION

King (1993, p. 50) writes, "The therapist's role is to facilitate the entire educational process from needs assessment to evaluation." The level of responsibility for the different phases in the process will be determined by the occupational therapy practitioner's role, for example, program coordinator, educator, or project consultant. Moreover, the steps themselves will occur at varying degrees of rigor and depth, depending on the setting, the issue, the level of intervention, and the desired outcome. To further establish the role of occupational therapy practitioners in community health, health promotion, and disability/disease prevention, more studies are needed to identify the occupational factors that affect health and well-being and to document the effectiveness of occupation-based community health and health promotion interventions. By being skilled in the steps of program development, from preplanning to publication, occupational therapy practitioners can strengthen their position in the provision of health education and health promotion programs and increase their marketability in the evolving health-care arena.

 ## STUDY QUESTIONS

1. Discuss the reasons why occupational therapy practitioners need to acquire community health/health promotion program development skills.

2. Assume you are treating children in day care. You observe that many of the parents are single, teen-aged mothers and many have sought your advice on parenting issues. The day care has hired you to develop programs. Some funding is available. What steps would you take to assess need? Who would you involve? What questions would you want answered?

3. How would you use occupational therapy concepts to shape an intervention strategy for the teen mothers?

4. Write a goal, two learning objectives, and two behavioral objectives for this program.

5. For the same program, describe possible interventions at each of the five societal levels.

6. List several specific pieces of information you would record to conduct process evaluation of your program.

REFERENCES

AMC Cancer Research Center. (1994). *Beyond the brochure: Alternative approaches to effective health education.* CDC Cooperative Agreement U50/CCU806186–04.

Baker, E.A., and Brownson, C.A. (1998). Defining characteristics of community-based health promotion programs. *Journal of Public Health Management and Practice, 4*(2), 1–9.

Breckon, D.J., Harvey, J.R., and Lancaster, R.B. (1994). *Community health education: Settings, roles, and skills for the 21st century.* Gaithersburg, MD: Aspen.

Brownson, C.A. (1998). Funding community practice: Stage 1. *American Journal of Occupational Therapy, 52*(1), 60–64.

Butterfoss, F. D., Goodman, R.M., and Wandersman, A. (1993). Community coalitions for prevention and health promotion. *Health Education and Research Theory and Practice, 8*(3), 315–330.

Dignan, M.B., and Carr, P.A. (1992). *Program planning for health education and health promotion* (2nd ed.). Philadelphia: Lea and Febiger.

Eng, E., and Young, R. (1992). Lay health advisors as community change agents. *Family and Community Health, 151,* 24–40.

Fink, A. (1993). *Evaluation fundamentals: Guiding health programs, research, and policy.* Newbury Park, CA: Sage.

Freudenberg, N., Eng, E., Flay, B., Parcel, G., Rogers, T., and Wallerstein, N. (1995). Strengthening individual and community capacity to prevent disease and promote health: In search of relevant theories and principles. *Health Education Quarterly, 22*(3), 290–306.

Glanz, K., Lewis, F.M., and Rimer, B. (Eds.). (1997). *Health behavior and health education: Theory, research, and practice* (2nd ed.). San Francisco: Jossey-Bass.

Glanz, K., and Rimer, B.K. (1995). *Theory at a glance: A guide for health promotion practice.* National Cancer Institute, U.S. Department of Health and Human Services, National Institutes of Health.

Goodman, R.M., Steckler, A., and Kegler, M. (1997). In K. Glanz, F.M. Lewis, and B. Rimer (Eds.), *Health behavior and health education: Theory, research, and practice* (2nd ed., pp. 287–312). San Francisco: Jossey-Bass.

Green, L.W. (1980). *Health education planning: A diagnostic approach.* Mountain View, CA: Mayfield.

Green, L.W., and Kreuter, M.W. (1991). *Health promotion and planning: An educational and environmental approach* (2nd ed.). Mountain View, CA: Mayfield.

Heany, C.A., and Israel, B.A. (1997). Social networks and social support. In K. Glanz, F.M. Lewis, and B. Rimer (Eds.). *Health behavior and health education: Theory, research, and practice* (2nd ed.). San Francisco: Jossey-Bass.

Johnson, J.A., and Jaffe, E.J. (Eds.). (1989). *Occupational therapy: Program development for health promotion and prevention services.* New York: Haworth.

King, P.M. (1993). A program planning model for injury prevention education. *Occupational Therapy Practice, 4*(4), 47–53.

Krueger, R.A. (1994). *Focus groups: A practical guide for applied research* (2nd ed.). Thousand Oaks, CA: Sage.

Law, M., Cooper, B.A., Strong, S., Stewart, D., Rigby, P., and Letts, L. (1997). Theoretical contexts for the practice of occupational therapy. In C.H. Christiansen and C.M. Baum (Eds.), *Occupational therapy: Enabling function and well-being* (2nd ed., pp. 73–102). Thorofare, NJ: Slack.

Lefebvre, R.C., and Rochlin, L. (1997). Social marketing. In K. Glanz, F.M. Lewis, and B. Rimer (Eds.), *Health behavior and health education: Theory, research, and practice* (2nd ed., pp. 384–402). San Francisco: Jossey-Bass.

McKillip, J. (1987). *Need analysis: Tools for the human services and education.* Newbury Park, CA: Sage.

McLeroy, K.R., Bibeau, D., Steckler, A., and Glanz, K. (1988). An ecological perspective on health promotion programs. *Health Education Quarterly, 25,* 351–377.

Minkler, M., and Wallerstein, N. (1997). Improving health through community organization and community building. In K. Glanz, F.M. Lewis, and B. Rimer (Eds.), *Health behavior and health education: Theory, research, and practice* (2nd ed., pp. 241–269). San Francisco: Jossey-Bass.

Office of Cancer Communications. (1992). *Making health communications work: A planner's guide.* U.S. Department of Health and Human Services, National Cancer Institute, NIH Publication No. 92–1493.

Oldenburg, B., Hardcastle, D.M., and Kok, G. (1997). In K. Glanz, F.M. Lewis, and B. Rimer (Eds.), *Health behavior and health education: Theory, research, and practice* (2nd ed., pp. 270–286). San Francisco: Jossey-Bass.

Posavac, E., and Carey, R. (1997). *Program evaluation: Methods and case studies* (5th ed.). Upper Saddle River, NJ: Prentice Hall.

Rappaport, J. (1984). Studies in empowerment: Introduction to the issue. *Prevention in Human Services, 3*(2–3), 1–7.

Simons-Morton, B.G., Greene, W.H., and Gottlieb, N.H. (1995). *Introduction to health education and health promotion.* Prospect Heights, IL: Waveland.

Soriano, F.I. (1995). *Conducting needs assessments: A multidisciplinary approach.* Thousand Oaks, CA: Sage.

Timmreck, T.C. (1995). *Planning, program development, and evaluation.* Boston: Jones and Bartlett.

van Ryn, M., and Heaney, C.A. (1992). What's the use of theory? *Health Education Quarterly, 19*(3), 315–330.

Wallack, L., Dorfman, L., Jernigan, D., and Themba, M. (1993). *Media advocacy and public health: Power for prevention.* Newbury Park, CA: Sage.

Witkin, B.R., and Altschuld, J.W. (1995). *Planning and conducting needs assessments: A practical guide.* Thousand Oaks, CA: Sage.

7 CHAPTER

Accessibility Issues

Felecia Moore Banks, MEd, OTR

◼ OUTLINE

Accessibility
American National Standards
 Institute (ANSI)
Americans with Disabilities Act
 (ADA)
Americans with Disabilities Act
 Accessibility Guidelines
 (ADAAG)

Architectural barriers
Assistive technology
Augmentative communication
Environmental control units
Negotiability
Uniform Federal Accessibility
 Standards (UFAS)

LEARNING OBJECTIVES

This chapter is designed to enable the reader to:
- Discuss the political, attitudinal, and architectural barriers that interfere with equal access to the community.
- Identify the major legislation enacted to provide access to people with disabilities.
- Describe the relationship between assistive technology and accessibility.
- Discuss the role of occupational therapy in promoting accessibility in community-based settings.
- Compare and contrast the concepts of accessibility and negotiability.
- Identify strategies needed for global change.

 ## INTRODUCTION

Over the years, a wide range of initiatives have significantly influenced how accessibility issues are addressed in the community today. **Accessibility** refers to the degree to which an environment (i.e., site, facility, workplace, service, or program) can be approached, entered, operated, and/or used safely and with dignity by a person with limitations (American Occupational Therapy Association, 1996; Dattilo, 1994; Trombly, 1995). Advocacy movements mandating public laws and state regulations have contributed considerably to the enforcement of legislation, promoting equal access and reasonable accommodations for persons with disabilities. Legislation, such as the Architectural Barriers Act of 1968, the Rehabilitation Act of 1973, the Fair Housing Act as amended in 1988 (P.L. 100-420), and the Americans with Disabilities Act (ADA) of 1990, has played a key role in facilitating subsequent growth in the availability of services to persons with disabilities.

Moreover, educational initiatives and current technology have provided a more level playing field, promising better access to the community and greater consumer control for many persons with disabilities. However, despite the many initiatives, the drive for equal access to the community still presents barriers.

This chapter presents an overview of the major legal and technological issues associated with accessibility. The major legislation impacting accessibility is highlighted. The chapter also describes important educational initiatives and the role of occupational therapy in creating a barrier-free environment. Doing so empowers the client to achieve functional independence in the community and improves quality of life.

A CYCLE OF INACCESSIBILITY

Passage of the Americans with Disabilities Act of 1990 has helped foster efforts to provide a barrier-free environment, allowing for greater freedom for persons with disabilities in the community. However, efforts to provide access to persons with disabilities began long before the 1990s. The fight for a barrier-free environment that meets the needs of persons with disabilities has been a slow, steady, and ever-changing process. For decades, lack of established standards and noncompliance of facilities with existing accessibility standards have contributed to this slow process, making access to the community difficult to achieve.

Persons with disabilities are faced with various barriers, including architectural, attitudinal, communication, time, economic, and technologic barriers. Of these, **architectural barriers** (physical structures that present obstacles for individuals who have mobility, visual, or sensory limitations) have been most apparent (Box 7–1). For example, inaccessible doorways, ramps, high shelves, narrow aisles, and poorly adapted rest rooms delay smooth transition from hospital to community, particularly for persons who are experiencing life from a wheelchair.

Barriers of communication, time, and attitudes have challenged persons with disabilities. More recently, companies have begun to make provisions that allow persons who are hearing and/or speech impaired or those who have difficulty assimilating information, to communicate effectively. The development of augmented communication devices has played a significant role in addressing these needs. Nonetheless, attitudinal barriers continue to remain prevalent in society. The attitudes of coworkers, supervisors, trainers, and even health-care practitioners can present the most difficult

---

BOX 7–1

Common Architectural Barriers in the Community

- Inaccessible doorways
- Heavy doors
- Stair barriers
- Poorly adapted/absent ramps
- High shelves
- Narrow aisles
- Poorly adapted rest rooms
- Inaccessible buses, vans, and rapid-rail systems
- Altered sidewalks
- Crowded sidewalk cafes
- Grocery store fences
- Unreachable store merchandise
- Inaccessible post office buildings
- Buildings without adequate signs to access points
- Poor lighting
- Lack of handicap parking

and limiting problems for persons with disabilities. Some individuals may have had little exposure to, and therefore little experience in, working with a person with a disability, and may be operating under misconceptions and false assumptions about the person's abilities and capabilities. Sometimes well-intentioned actions can actually restrict the opportunities available for disabled persons and may result in inequality in their treatment (Gadbow and DuBois, 1998).

Only after World War II did services for people with disabilities increase significantly. The Architectural Barriers Act of 1968 (P.L. 91-480) and Section 504 of the Rehabilitation Act of 1973 (P.L. 93-112) required programs and buildings receiving federal funds to be accessible to people with disabilities. The Rehabilitation Act of 1973 and the Social Services Act of 1974 particularly emphasized the pertinence and urgency of developing comprehensive programs for individuals who were homebound to promote independent living (Jackson and Banks, 1996). Life as a homemaker became a viable occupation and was considered for governmental funding. In 1978, amendments to the Rehabilitation Act of 1973 established Title VII, called "Comprehensive Services for Independent Living." The Comprehensive Services for Independent Living under the jurisdiction of the state provided grants for independent living centers, independent living programs for the older blind person, and protection and advocacy programs to guard the rights of persons with severe disabilities (Walker, 1979).

The Fair Housing Act as amended in 1988 (P.L. 100-420) played a significant role in establishing accessibility requirements for all buildings with four or more housing units. Under this law, landlords were prevented from screening out people with disabilities. As a result of the many legislative acts regarding the rights of people with disabilities, the independent living movement emphasized making the community more accessible for persons with disabilities (Jackson and Banks, 1996).

 ## LEGAL ISSUES

Legal issues, such as personal disputes, lawsuits and claims, lobbying for or against new bills, amendments to current laws, and the establishment of local and state regulations, often determine the removal of barriers to accessibility. While federal laws require accessibility of structures, buildings, and facilities for persons with disabilities, the enforcement of these regulations is far from simplistic. For example, in 1998, the U.S. Department of Transportation reported that violations of accessible parking laws represented the largest single category of complaints. The Disability Rights Bureau disputes regulations since 1968 that require any facility offering marked parking for employees or visitors to provide accessible parking for persons with disabilities.

Occupational therapists have long served as advocates for a barrier-free environment. Today more than ever before, occupational therapists have taken the lead as policy makers, advocates, presidents of nonprofit organizations, and business owners of companies with a vested interest in the removal of barriers to accessibility.

THE POLITICAL PLATFORM

According to President Clinton (May 13, 1994),

> Information, which will be education, which will be employment, which will be income, which will be possibility, must flow to all Americans on terms of equal accessibility without regard to physical condition. And we are committed to doing that.

Fifty-four million Americans have physical or mental disabilities (U.S. Department of Health and Human Services, 2000), too often being excluded from the mainstream of American life by attitudes and inaccessible environments. Sixty-seven percent of all people with disabilities are unemployed, even among college graduates (National Council for Disability Rights, 1999). The Civil Rights Division of the U.S. Department of Justice and the National Association of Attorneys General Disability Rights Task Force are designed to promote and protect the rights of individuals with disabilities. This task force, along with federal and state regulatory boards and committees charged with the enforcement of laws designed to meet the needs of persons with disabilities, are examples of the committed efforts of federal and state governments to achieve a barrier-free environment.

Probably the strongest commitment from Congress was the passage of the **Americans with Disabilities Act (ADA)** of 1990. This law, one of the most democratic and flexible civil rights laws in the history of this nation, has served as a strong catalyst for change, benefiting every individual. According to statistics reported by the National Council for Disability Rights (1999), each person has a 20 percent chance of becoming a person with a disability and a 50 percent chance of having a family member with a disability.

Other examples of committed political efforts include the *National Information Infrastructure (NII): Agenda for Action*. On September 15, 1993, the Clinton Administration issued this agenda, which formalized several federal policy development mechanisms and enumerated the guiding principles and goals for future policy development. Agenda for Action addresses responsiveness to the usage requirements of people with disabilities as a founding principle.

Since the early 1970s, the Federal Election Commission (FEC) Act of 1971 recognized that corporations and professional and trade associations have a vital and legitimate interest in the operation of government. This initiative became especially important to advocacy corporations dedicated to providing equal access to persons with disabilities. Occupational therapists are very much an integral part of this vested interest. The American Occupational Therapy Political Action Committee (AOTPAC), a voluntary, nonprofit, unincorporated committee of members of the American Occupational Therapy Association (AOTA) authorized by the Representative Assembly in 1976, has as its goal to further legislative initiatives that impact the occupational therapy profession.

LAWS AND AMENDMENTS

Architectural Barriers Act (ABA) of 1968

This law was the first federal legislation on accessibility protecting the rights of persons with disabilities. The ABA requires that buildings and facilities designed, constructed, or altered with direct or indirect federal funds must conform to accessibility standards issued by the U.S. Access Board and four other federal agencies. The standards currently in effect are the **Uniform Federal Accessibility Standards (UFAS).** The UFAS are guidelines for accessible design that assure compliance with federal accessibility legislation in all federally funded facilities. The ABA also covers residential design, construction, and alterations supported by federal funds.

Rehabilitation Act of 1973

This legislation ensures the rights of individuals to have equal access to employment, education, housing, and transportation programs and facilities receiving federal funds. The Rehabilitation Act of 1973 specifically covers federally assisted or conducted housing programs and services. Like the ABA, this act requires conformance to the UFAS accessibility provisions in new construction and alterations. This act was later reauthorized by the Workforce Investment Act.

Fair Housing Amendment Act of 1988

This legislation prohibits discrimination against persons with disabilities in housing and requires accessibility in federally funded facilities. Accessibility in multifamily residential facilities is covered by the Fair Housing Amendments Act of 1988 (FHAA) and its related regulations and standards. More information about FHAA can be obtained from the Department of Housing and Urban Development. All housing, even single-family residences, constructed or altered by, or on behalf of, state and local governments must meet ADA Title II requirements.

Americans with Disabilities Act (ADA) of 1990

The ADA extended the federal mandate for accessibility to include not only publicly funded facilities and programs but also facilities and programs in the private sector. The ADA's broad scope includes equal access to employment, public accommodations, state and local government, public transportation, and telecommunications.

The **Americans with Disabilities Act Accessibility Guidelines (ADAAG)** for buildings and facilities provides specific recommendations for accessibility in restaurants, businesses, medical-care facilities, hotels, libraries, and transportation facilities (Dattilo, 1994). These guidelines were published in the *Federal Register* (July 26, 1991).

The Architectural and Transportation Barriers Compliance Board and the Department of Transportation amended the accessibility guidelines and standards under the Americans with Disabilities Act for over-the-road buses (OTRBs) to include scoping and technical provisions for lifts, ramps, wheelchair securement devices, and moveable aisle armrests. Revisions to the specifications for doors and lighting were also adopted. The specifications describe the design features that an OTRB must have to be readily accessible to, and usable by, persons who use wheelchairs or other mobility aids.

ADA enforcement is divided among several federal agencies, including the Department of Justice (DOJ), the Department of Transportation (DOT), the Equal Employment Opportunities Commission (EEOC), and the Federal Communications Commission (FCC).

Telecommunications Act of 1996 (Section 255)

The Architectural and Transportation Barriers Compliance Board issued guidelines for accessibility, usability, and compatibility of telecommunications equipment and customer premises equipment covered by Section 255 of the Telecommunications Act of 1996. This act requires manufacturers of telecommunications equipment and customer premises equipment to ensure that the equipment is designed, developed, and fabricated to be accessible to, and usable by, individuals with disabilities, if readily achievable. When not readily achievable to make the equipment accessible, the act requires manufacturers to ensure that the equipment is compatible with existing peripheral devices or specialized customer premises equipment commonly used by individuals with disabilities to achieve access. The effective date was March 5, 1998.

The Workforce Investment Act of 1998

The Workforce Investment Act (WIA) included amendments that reauthorize the Rehabilitation Act for five years (FY 1999 to 2003). The bill was signed by President Clinton and became law on August 7, 1998. The changes made to both the Rehabilitation Act and the major job training programs will have profound impact on the delivery of all these services over the next five years. The most noticeable change likely will be the divergence among states in the ways that they implement the redesigned programs. Some states have already made significant changes in their employment training systems while others have changed little.

REGULATORY AGENCIES

Governmental agencies are charged with the responsibility for ensuring adherence to the major legislation. Some examples of committed efforts by federal and state governments to address issues of inaccessibility are described here (National Council for Disability Rights, 1999).

Department of Transportation (DOT)

Design, construction, and alteration of public transportation facilities and specifications for public and private transportation vehicles are covered by Department of Transportation regulations. These include the provision of complementary paratransit and general service requirements for public transit agencies under the ADA.

The Department of Transportation also has published a separate rule that addresses when OTRB operators are required to comply with the specifications (the effective date was October 28, 1998). Answers to some commonly asked questions regarding transportation accessibility provided by the Department of Transportation (1999) are highlighted in Box 7–2.

Department of Justice (DOJ)

The Disability Rights Section of the Civil Rights Division of the Department of Justice provides practical information and technical assistance on how to comply with the ADA. ADA technical assistance publications update and highlight specific topics of interest to business owners and managers, state and local government officials, architects, engineers, contractors, product designers and manufacturers, and all others seeking a better understanding of accessible design and the intent of the ADA. The goal of the publication series is to clarify potential misunderstandings about the requirements of the ADA and to highlight its flexible, commonsense approach to accessibility.

The Department of Justice generally enforces the ADA, including Title II, which applies to state and local governments, and Title III, which applies to accessibility of public accommodations and commercial facilities. Almost half of U.S. states reference and utilize the **American National Standards Institute** (ANSI 117.1) accessibility standard. ANSI provides detailed specifications for barrier-free design in its publication *American National Standards for Buildings and Facilities—Providing Accessibility and Usability for Physically Handicapped People* (American National Standards Institute, 1986). Several have developed unique codes and a few reference the UFAS. The remaining states have adopted ADAAG as their accessibility code, implementing its requirements through state and local building code officials in the same way as other applicable building regulations are applied, reviewed, and enforced. ADA compliance does not relieve the designer from complying with the provisions of a state or local access code or other accessibility regulation. Where such a code or document contains more stringent requirements, they must be incorporated. Conversely, adoption of ADAAG or certification of the equivalency of a state/local code will not relieve covered entities of their responsibilities to meet the accessibility standards of the ADA (or other accessibility requirements).

Although publicly operated airports are not subject to DOT's ADA regulation, they are covered by the DOJ Title II rule. Additionally, the ABA covers airports that receive federal financial assistance (for facilities designed, constructed, or altered with federal funds). As with housing, UFAS is the generally referenced standard. Privately op-

□□◁◯ *B O X   7 – 2*

The DOT's Answers to Frequently Asked Questions about Transportation Accessibility

Question: The vehicle guidelines for buses and vans specify that one or two wheelchair securement areas be provided, depending on the size of the vehicle. If more than the required number is provided, must the additional ones meet all of the requirements?
Answer: No, with one exception. Additional securement areas and devices must all be oriented to face forward or rearward even though they need not meet the other requirements.

Question: The vehicle guidelines require sufficient maneuvering room in a vehicle to reach the securement area from the lift. Does this mean a wheelchair must be able to turn around?
Answer: No. Because a vehicle is constrained in size by factors like roadway or track right-of-way width, vehicles cannot meet design considerations normally imposed on buildings. Depending on the location and orientation of the wheelchair area, the maneuvering space available in a vehicle may force a wheelchair user to back into a securement location.

Question: Is a three-wheel scooter required to be accommodated on a new bus?
Answer: The vehicle specifications define a wheelchair as any three- or four-wheel mobility device designed for, and used by, a person with a disability. A common wheelchair is any such device that is not more than 30 inches wide and 48 inches long, measured 2 inches above the floor, and does not weigh more than 600 pounds when occupied. Notice that the width and length are not measured at the floor. A complying lift must have a clear width of 28½ inches at the surface but 30 inches clear at 2 inches above the platform. This allows handrail-mounting hardware and some mechanisms needed to operate safety barriers to intrude partly into the area at the platform surface. Any wheelchair or mobility aid that fits these parameters, including a scooter, must be accommodated on a lift meeting the ADA standards. However, many lifts are still in service that were purchased before the standards took effect and are smaller than the current standard. There is no requirement to retrofit these older vehicles.

Question: Why must a new bus pad be 96 inches deep, measured from the curb face?
Answer: This dimension is based on Board-sponsored research that examined how much space is needed for a wheelchair or mobility aid to exit a lift and make a 90° turn. It is the same dimension as the width of the access aisle for a van-accessible parking space.

Question: Must new subway cars have specific spaces and securement devices for wheelchairs?
Answer: No, the spaces for two wheelchairs or mobility aids can be provided in the normal space allotted for standing passengers as long as there is an accessible path to them from an accessible door. No securement devices are required on rail vehicles.

Question: Must all the characters on a new bus stop sign be 3 inches high?
Answer: The character height requirement applies only to the route designation, usually a number or number/letter combination. Other information, such as "Express," "via Downtown," or "Sat. and Sun. Only" may be any size. Some stops serve many lines, such as a transfer stop, so that having all the route numbers 3 inches high would make the sign bigger than allowed by local sign ordinances. The exception permits the route designations to be as close to 3 inches as possible within the allowable sign size.

Question: Must an accessible bus display the international symbol of accessibility?
Answer: No, buses are not required to display the symbol.

Question: Must people using crutches be allowed to use a bus lift?
Answer: Yes. The guidelines require lifts meeting the ADA to be designed to accommodate standees and the DOT regulation requires bus drivers to allow standees to use all but one particular type of old lift.

Question: Are there specifications for vehicle step riser height and tread depth?
Answer: No, because individuals who would have difficulty using steps must be allowed to use the lift. The undercarriage of a vehicle together with required ground clearance does not permit vehicles to meet requirements appropriate for building stairs. The only requirements for steps are that they be slip resistant and have contrasting color step edges.

erated airports are covered by subpart A of DOT's transportation regulation and by the DOJ's Title III rule as commercial facilities. Most airports also contain places of public accommodation in shops, restaurants, and rest rooms that must meet ADA standards. Airline operations are subject to the Air Carrier Access Act of 1986 and its implementing regulations, which include some facility provisions. Most new construction and alterations projects, and work undertaken as barrier removal or to provide program accessibility where a local building department requires a permit, will be subject to state accessibility requirements as well as those of the ADA.

The National Information Infrastructure (NII): Agenda for Action

The (NII): Agenda for Action provides choices in the modes of information representation and manipulation. It is designed to break down existing barriers and accelerate progress toward the full participation of people with disabilities in society as envisioned by the Americans with Disabilities Act (ADA).

Federal Communications Commission (FCC)

The ADA Title IV requirement for relay services and the requirements of Section 255 of the Telecommunications Act of 1996 are regulated by the Federal Communications Commission. All telephone companies were required to provide telecommunication relay services by 1993. Relay services enable a person with a hearing impairment, using a telecommunication display device (TDD), to communicate, through a voice operator, with someone using a telephone. In addition, the FCC enforces the Hearing Aid Compatibility Act (P.L. 100-394) which requires that all new telephones have an inductive coil that is compatible for use by persons with hearing aids (National Center for Access Unlimited, 1991). The ADA provides for a "private right of action" so individuals can file lawsuits to enforce the act. However, the Telecommunications Act does not provide a private right of action, and complaints must be filed with the FCC.

U.S. Access Board

The U.S. Access Board enforces the Architectural Barriers Act (ABA) of 1968 but not the Americans with Disabilities Act (ADA). The board investigates complaints and has an excellent record of achieving voluntary compliance.

Recently, the Access Board issued accessibility guidelines for telecommunications and customer premises equipment under the Telecommunications Act of 1996. The Telecommunications Access Advisory Committee submitted its final report to the board with recommendations, and the board published a final rule on February 3, 1998.

The Access Board is a member of the ANSI A117.1 Committee and shares its interest in more uniform national accessibility specifications. As ADAAG, ANSI A117.1, UFAS, and state and model codes are periodically reviewed and revised, it will be possible to achieve greater consistency among the several documents in provisions that design professionals must apply to new construction and alterations.

Design professionals can track these and other regulatory actions of the Access Board through professional membership organizations, trade publications, and updates posted on the Access Board Website.

 ## TECHNOLOGICAL ISSUES

Technology has resulted in a dramatic change in providing better access to the community for persons with disabilities. Approximately 7.4 million Americans use assistive technology devices to accommodate mobility impairments (National Center on Accessibility Technical Assistance Program, 1994). Today, the most sophisticated scientific developments in design and manufactured technology are available for persons with disabilities. Not only are scientists and technicians responsible for these developments, but consumers, advocates, and planners in the public and private sectors have also made significant contributions to the advancements in technology.

At present, technology is redefining the way people view disability. Computers are capable, to a considerable extent, of adapting to input, throughput, and output so that the disability of today may not be a disability tomorrow.

Even with today's sophisticated technology, it is not the magic solution to all problems in the community of persons with disabilities. Matching technology to the individual's needs through careful assessment, design, and proper assistance is critical to its success as a tool to improve functional independence and access to the community. Box 7–3 lists some myths shared by concerned consumers, educators, and advocates on technology and the disabled.

Historically, occupational therapy and technology have had a close relationship, evolving from a low technological base in the 1950s to today's high technology that includes computers, robotics, adapted vehicles, and electrical circuitry (Smith, 1991). Occupational therapists use technology to help persons improve functional independence in the community by enhancing performance and minimizing barriers that make independence in everyday living difficult to achieve. This type of technology is often referred to as *assistive technology*.

Today, occupational therapy service delivery models for the use of technology rely heavily on close collaboration with private rehabilitation technology firms and/or expert centers in the community. Service delivery models are moving more toward a system built on regional expert centers (Smith, 1991). Occupational therapists working in community-based settings might be employees or owners of regional expert

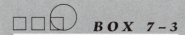

BOX 7-3

Myths Associated with Technology

Myth 1: Because of the availability of technology, all facilities must be equally accessible.
As noble as this may sound, facilities are not required to be equally accessible. Even with the use of technology, new construction must be designed with accessibility concerns in mind. However, all existing buildings need not be made equally accessible.

Myth 2: People with disabilities need high-tech assistive devices or services to live independent lives.
Simple inexpensive devices are often the most critical in helping people with disabilities live independently. For example, assistive devices can be as affordable as modified eating utensils or a button hook.

Myth 3: Easy access to the technology is made available to persons with disabilities.
Access to computers and other technology for people with disabilities can often lag behind. This is characteristic of other services that lag behind, such as education, employment, or income.

Myth 4: If a person has a disability, a funding market is easily available for the person's technology needs.
Mechanics of funding assistive technology, providing for appropriate professional assessments, and training in its availability and use present a barrier that is not easily addressed. Assistive technology can be very expensive and is not easily paid for through traditional reimbursement mechanisms. Finding the right funding source is very important.

Myth 5: Corporations make easy access to new technology available for persons with disabilities.
Rapid changes in technology may present barriers, particularly in the workplace. New technology may not integrate well with older technology, and economics often preclude regular and frequent replacement with newer technologies and innovations.

Myth 6: Persons with disabilities look forward to technological changes and new innovations.
It may be harder for some persons with a disability to change as rapidly as other individuals. The claims of a technological world are demanding for some people with disabilities.

centers or refer clients to local centers where special technological services are available. Regional expert centers should consist of multidisciplinary, interdisciplinary, or transdisciplinary team approaches with members of the team including positioning specialists, augmentative communication specialists, special educators, rehabilitation engineers, architects, funding specialists, and rehabilitation suppliers.

Assistive Technology

Assistive technology, as defined by the Technical Assistance to the States Act (P.L. 100-407), is (Cook and Hussey, 1995):

> Any item, piece of equipment or product system whether acquired commercially off the shelf, modified, or customized that is used to increase or improve functional capabilities of individuals with disabilities.

Assistive technology has significantly increased the ability of persons with disabilities to lead independent lives. For example, computer-based **environmental control units** permit persons with disabilities to operate lights and appliances and open doors from wheelchairs. For persons who cannot speak to voice thoughts, **augmentative communication** devices that use touch- or light-activated keyboards coupled to synthetic speech systems have provided access to a new world of communication. Screen magnification systems for those with low vision, screen reading programs for the blind, and special ability switches that allow a person with a mobility impairment to use computer-based systems are among examples of how assistive technology has offered greater access to the community (Angelo, 1997).

Ineffective and Inappropriate Technology

The high volume of products on the market today for persons with disabilities can be overwhelming. Consumers typically recognize that products come with flaws. The good products stay on the market and are used over and over again, while the bad products break down. A wide range of vending options is available to consumers. Thousands of selected items are available to choose from, requiring careful selection. Guidelines for the selection of appropriate equipment are important to the occupational therapist and the consumer. Box 7–4 offers some suggested guidelines modified from Dicky and Shealey (1987).

Overdependency on Technology

Technology can significantly enhance a person's ability to perform in everyday living. However, the belief that technology is the only choice available can sometimes encourage overuse of or dependency on a product. When a person with a disability is unable to accomplish daily life tasks in the usual way, adapted techniques or equipment may enable him or her to accomplish them. Adapted techniques are preferred to equipment because they make the person's life more flexible and independent and are associated with a less handicapping status. This common rehabilitation principle is consistent with concepts of compensation, adaptation, and teaching.

For some clients, permanent use of adaptive equipment will be necessary. For others, temporary use of a product is needed. The occupational therapy practitioner is responsible for working collaboratively with the client to establish goals that involve grading the use of a product so that overdependency does not occur and maximum independence is achieved.

 # *EDUCATIONAL INITIATIVES*

People with disabilities are entitled to comprehensive education that provides a continuity of services, including early detection and early intervention. However, some institutions continue to be inaccessible for persons with disabilities. The use of technology can make education much more accessible and inclusive through environmental control systems, computerized instruction, supported communication with classmates, "schools without walls," and other creative innovations.

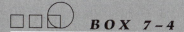 **BOX 7-4**

Suggested Guidelines for Selection of Appropriate Assistive Technology

- Match the product with the personal needs of the individual.
- Examine cost benefits. If the item is not that costly and could really improve a person's level of independence, then it might result in savings.
- Avoid being fooled by the pretty advertisement. Check out the product and make sure that it does what it is supposed to do.
- Find out the reputation of the product. Is it reliable?
- Inquire from others who have used the device. Listen to people whom you trust.
- Avoid vendor bias. Purchase products based on recommendations or decisions made jointly by the occupational therapist and consumer.
- Make sure there is a will and a desire to use the product.
- Find out how difficult the product will be to install.
- Find out how difficult the product will be to operate.
- Find out what is involved in the care of the product.
- Find out if the product is portable or stationary.
- Look at return policies and warranties.
- Review consumer reports for complaints of ineffective products.
- Find out if the product may soon be obsolete.
- Know that buying a product may not be the best answer. Rental or adaptation of a common item might do the job.

Source: Dickey, R., and Shealey, S.H. (1987). Using technology to control the environment. *American Journal of Occupational Therapy, 41,* 717–721.

The passage of the Goals 2000: Educate America Act in 1990, and subsequent federal legislation such as the Improving America's Schools Act, has focused the nation's attention on accountability and the need for standards-based education reform. The passage of the 1997 Amendments to the Individuals with Disabilities Education Act (IDEA) has placed even greater emphasis on education for persons with disabilities. States are required to have established goals for the performance of students with disabilities and to assess progress toward achieving those goals. The performance of students with disabilities will be accounted for by indicators such as test scores, dropout rates, and graduation records.

The United Nations Educational, Scientific, and Cultural Organization (UNESCO) has taken the lead in promoting lifelong learning as a master concept for persons with disabilities. "Lifelong learning for all" was chosen in 1994 as the major term of reference for the UNESCO midterm strategy covering the period 1996 to 2001. This hallmark event occurred during the Fifth International Conference on Adult Education by UNESCO in Hamburg, Germany, in 1997. Adults with disabilities were put on the world education agenda for the first time. As a result, an aim for a worldwide commitment to adults and continuing education through lifelong learning was established as a major objective (United Nations Educational, Scientific, and Cultural Organization, 1997).

THE ROLE OF OCCUPATIONAL THERAPY

Successful integration into the community requires access to community facilities. In the home and community, the role of the occupational therapist includes self-care training, use of adaptive equipment, and psychosocial and emotional support. Occupational therapists are concerned with clarification of values, development of obtainable life goals, and instillation of positive attitudes toward independent living. Occupational therapy programs that prepare for discharge allow persons to practice overcoming barriers in the community. Realistic activities encourage skill practice in various environments, encourage the client to develop solutions to problems and barriers, and diffuse the fear of returning to the community. Restoration of functional skills may be accomplished through treatment aimed at diminishing the disability, compensatory strategies taught by the therapist, or the therapeutic application of assistive devices (Mann and Lane, 1991). Occupational therapists evaluate barriers in the community and develop solutions for the removal of barriers to accessibility.

The National Center on Accessibility Technical Assistance Program (NCA) is a resource service that provides the latest information regarding the inclusion of people with disabilities in parks, recreation, and tourism. The technical assistance staff have provided services to occupational therapists, architects, interpretive specialists, exhibit designers, recreation specialists, program and facility managers, as well as individuals with disabilities. The following questions illustrate the broad scope of technical assistance available:

- I work at a national battlefield. How do I obtain a three-dimensional tactile map of my site?
- What types of materials can be used to make accessible trail surfaces at our nature center?
- How do I make a zoo experience accessible to a person who is blind?
- Our wildlife refuge has an orientation video. When are assistive listening devices required and what types are available?

Many ways are available to change an inaccessible home environment. However, these changes will depend on financial resources, building codes, availability of experts, approval of landlord (if renting), and personal choice. For access to public facilities, the U.S. Department of Justice has established four priorities (National Center for Access Unlimited, 1991):

1. Accessible approach and entrance
2. Access to goods and services
3. Access to and usability of rest rooms
4. Additional devices and communication equipment as needed

Box 7–5 is a checklist with recommendations for access solutions based on the ADA Title II regulations.

NEGOTIABILITY VS. ACCESSIBILITY

Noris-Baker and William (1978) proposed the concept of "negotiability." **Negotiability** refers to the person's ability to access a feature of the environment and use it for its intended purpose with only one's usual adaptive equipment. Bates (1994) proposed that this definition be amended to read: "the ability to access a feature of the environment in a manner acceptable to the individual." Bates (1994) further discusses the importance of considering the functional interaction of the individual as he or she becomes an integral part of the community. She states that "negotiability involves

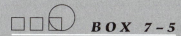 **BOX 7-5**

Survey for a Museum, Theater, or Sports Arena

Arrival at facility (drop off, independent arrival or parking)
- Number and placement of accessible handicapped spaces, drop off, and curb cuts by parking lot
- Path of travel to entrance (walkway or ramp)
- Accessible entrance—signage indicating accessible bathrooms
- Teletype (TTY) devices, phones, etc.

Directional signage (to accessible entrance, goods, and services)

Entry area (ease of entrance)
- Entry door weight and width
- Coatroom counter height
- Information booth height and informational materials
- Ticket counter height and enhanced sound system

Accessible bathrooms (male/female; unisex)
- Complete surveys
- Path of travel

Elevators/stairways (interior ramps to access programs and exhibits)

Auditorium and theater (accessible seating)
- Number and placement of seats
- Accessible stage and dressing room
- Enhanced listening system (FM, LOOP, INFRARED)

Exhibition signage (check one gallery)
- Height of signs: 45 inches in the front and 54 inches on the side
- Raised characters
- Braille text of same information

Programs (alternative formats)
- Large print
- Braille
- Audio description tapes

Public phones (clear floor space of at least 30 by 48 inches in front of at least one)
- TTY's with TTY symbol signage
- Volume control
- Hearing-aid compatible

Drinking fountains (availability and height)

Education (visual and auditory alarm systems)

Gift shop (if appropriate)
- Path of travel
- Shelving at accessible heights
- Signage checkout counter

Food concessions or restaurant (if appropriate)
- Heights of counters and tables
- Clear path of travel
- Menus in alternate format
- Table legs to accommodate wheelchairs

a functional interaction among the person, environment, and equipment. Failure to consider all three aspects and their impact on one another results in a less-than-optimal outcome." Relevant to occupational therapy is an example of this concept, according to Bates' definition, presented as follows:

> A woman in a sports wheelchair enters the cafeteria. She is able to access the short-order counter. She gets as close to it as a walking person, but she can not use it independently for its intended purpose. She can not place her order with the cook unless a standing person gets the cook's attention first. The counter is accessible but not *negotiable*. Conversely, the woman is perfectly capable of opening the beverage case and obtaining a soda can independently but the case is too high to be *accessible*.

To assess if an environment is negotiable, a therapist should examine all of the features within the environment. If the structures are accessible according to ADA guidelines, but the feature cannot be used for its intended purpose, then further accommodations will be needed. The therapist can begin by asking the client to perform the task needed in the environment. According to Bates (1994), the examiner, based on the following calculation example, can record a percentage of negotiated features:

1. Number of environmental features = 76
2. Number negotiable = 42
3. Calculation = $(42/76) \times 100$
4. Negotiable environment = 55.26 percent

The occupational therapist could use these types of calculations to demonstrate changes from intervention by indicating the number of environments assessed ($N = 76$), what was negotiable upon assessment ($N = 42$), followed by an increase in negotiability based on occupational therapy intervention ($N = 6$). The negotiable environment score would then be 63.15 percent.

EDUCATION AND RESEARCH NEEDS

With the rapid changes in technology, merging systems of integrated care, new education initiatives, and an increasingly diverse workforce, professions should embrace the concept of lifelong learning. Occupational therapists need to continually update their skills through training programs that emphasize creative problem solving and technological advancement in the context in which clients live. Increasing awareness of community resources, developing more effective ways to network, building partnerships, and developing greater collaborative relationships with consumers are critical. The process occupational therapists use to create accessible environments is not gained simply by prescribing a piece of equipment but rather by giving individuals the necessary tools for the "job of living."

Additional dialogue and research are needed on emerging accessibility issues. Research designed to explore better assessment tools, accessibility standards, and efficacy studies in practice warrants further investigation. In addition, empirical studies that examine curriculum inclusion of current trends regarding accessibility issues, problem-solving strategies, and innovative solutions to inaccessibility locally and around the world are needed.

 ## CONCLUSION

Approximately 750 million people in the world have disabilities (Adams and Benson, 1990). Disabled people are usually among the poorest of all populations, and this is particularly true in Third World countries. Medical and educational facilities are not available to everyone, and literacy rates for people with disabilities are significantly below average (National Institute on Disability and Rehabilitation Research, 1990). Poverty and lack of suitable and affordable educational opportunities force many children with disabilities to abandon their education. Despite the United Nations' Declaration of Human Rights, the Bill of Rights, and other significant charters throughout the world, societies have not enjoyed an exemplary reputation in the treatment of this underserved population.

Today, concern about the kinds of social and health-care services, and the way in which they are delivered, is evident. People with disabilities seek better access to regular schools and housing, instead of spending a lifetime in segregated settings such as group homes, sheltered workshops, and specialized schools. Moreover, U.S. technology companies that provide goods and services for people with disabilities have positioned themselves as early competitors in the global marketplace. The movement to promote human performance by creating accessible communities for all people in all parts of the world will require the committed responsibility of all citizens.

Inaccessibility is a problem that affects the global community. Occupational therapists are skillful in dealing with problems of inaccessibility. In their roles as adaptation specialists, advocates, policy makers, educators, business owners, and concerned citizens, occupational therapists can play a key role in the fight for a barrier-free environment.

 ## STUDY QUESTIONS

1. What are the most frequent types of architectural barriers encountered in the community by persons with disabilities? List potential solutions to these barriers.
2. Which federal laws address accessibility for persons with disabilities and what accessibility concerns do they cover?
3. What are the roles and responsibilities of the occupational therapist regarding community accessibility for persons with disabilities?
4. How does assistive technology improve access to the community?
5. Define negotiability and its relationship to accessibility. Which is a better measure of a community's response to the needs of persons with disabilities? Why?

REFERENCES

Adams, P.F., and Benson, V. (1990). *Current estimates from the National Health Interview Survey, 1989.* Washington, DC: National Center for Health Statistics.

American National Standards Institute (1986). *American national standards for buildings and facilities—providing accessibility and usability for physically handicapped people.* New York: American National Standards Institute.

American Occupational Therapy Association. (1996). ADA and occupational therapy education informational packet. Bethesda, MD: Author.

Americans with Disabilities Act (ADA) of 1990. *Federal Register, 56*(156).

Angelo, J. (1997). *Assistive technology for the rehabilitation therapist.* Philadelphia: F. A. Davis.

Bates, P. (1994). The self-care environment: Issues of space and furnishing. In C. Christiansen, *Ways of living: Self-care strategies for special needs.* Bethesda, MD: American Occupational Therapy Association.

Cook, A.M., and Hussey, S.M. (1995). *Assistive technologies: Principles and practice.* St. Louis: Mosby.

Dattilo, J. (1994). *Inclusive leisure services: Responding to the rights of people with disabilities.* State College, PA: Venture.

Dickey, R., and Shealey, S.H. (1987). Using technology to control the environment. *American Journal of Occupational Therapy, 41,* 717–721.

Gadbow, N., and DuBois, D. (1998). *Adult learners with special needs: Strategies and resources for postsecondary education and workplace training.* Malabar, FL: Krieger.

Jackson, S., and Banks, F. (1997). Home management. In J. Van Deusen and D. Brunt (Eds.), *Assessment in occupational therapy and physical therapy.* Philadelphia: Saunders.

Mann, W., and Lane, J. (1991). *Assistive technology for persons with disabilities: The role of occupational therapy.* Bethesda, MD: American Occupational Therapy Association.

National Center for Access Unlimited. (1991). Achieving physical and communication accessibility. Washington, DC: Author.

National Center on Accessibility Technical Assistance Program. (1994). *Update.* Washington, DC: Author.

National Council for Disability Rights. (1999). *Disability Report.* Chicago, IL: Author.

National Institute on Disability and Rehabilitation Research. Levine, D.B., Zitter, M., and Ingram, L. (Eds.). (1990). *Disability statistics: An assessment.* Committee on National Statistics, National Academy Press.

Noris-Baker, C., and Williams, E.P. (1978). Environmental negotiability as a direct measurement of behavior-environment relationships: Some implications for theory and practice. In A.D. Seidel and S. Danford (Eds.), *Proceedings of the Tenth Annual Conference of the Environmental Design Research Association* (pp. 209–214). Houston: Environmental Design Research Association.

Rehabilitation Act of 1973, 29 U.S.C. 01 et seq. (1973).

Smith, R. (1991). Technology approaches to performance enhancement. In C. Christiansen and C. Baum, *Occupational therapy: Overcoming human performance deficits.* Thorofare, NJ: Slack.

Trombly, C.A. (1995). Occupational therapy for physical dysfunction. Baltimore: Williams and Wilkins.

United Nations Educational, Scientific, and Cultural Organization. (1997). *Proceedings, Fifth International Conference on Adult Education,* Hamburg, Germany.

U.S. Department of Health and Human Services. (2000). *Healthy People 2010* (Conference ed.). Washington, DC: Author.

U.S. Department of Transportation (1999). *Update Report.* Washington, DC: Author.

Walker, J.M. (1979). *A guide to organizations, agencies, and federal programs for handicapped Americans.* Washington, DC: Handicapped American Reports.

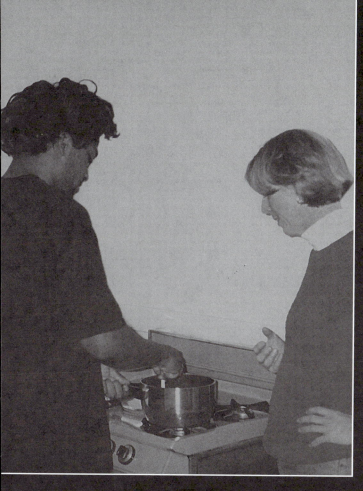

II

SECTION

*A Variety of
Community-Based
Practice Settings*

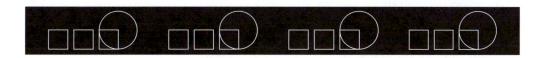

8

CHAPTER

Community-Based Work Programs

Brent H. Braveman, MEd, OTR
Supriya Sen, MS, OTR
Gary Kielhofner, DrPH, OTR, FAOTA

■ OUTLINE

KEY TERMS

Assessment of Communication
  and Interaction Skills (ACIS)
Client centered
Community
Community centered
Identificational communities
Occupational behavior settings
Occupational competence
Occupational identity
Occupational Performance
  History Interview (OPHI-II)

Occupational Self-Assessment
  (OSA)
Team approach
Work capacity evaluation
Work Environment Impact Scale
  (WEIS)
Work hardening
Worker role
Worker Role Interview (WRI)

LEARNING OBJECTIVES

This chapter is designed to enable the reader to:
- Identify the main factors that influence work success.
- Describe the trends within and outside of occupational therapy influencing vocational rehabilitation practice.
- Identify the advantages of community-based work programs as compared to clinic-based programs.
- Describe the characteristics of high-quality community-based work programs.
- Explain the psychosocial and environmental factors impacting an injured worker's ability to return to work.
- Discuss the role of the occupational therapist in community-based work programs.

 INTRODUCTION

To understand current vocationally oriented practice, some of the trends that have shaped it must be considered. This chapter provides an overview of developments both within and outside of occupational therapy that have influenced the nature of vocationally oriented programs provided in the community. In addition, the chapter identifies the contributing factors and general characteristics of high-quality community-based work programs. Two examples of such programs are presented.

 INFLUENCES ON WORK-RELATED PRACTICE

Tremendous changes occurred in the U.S. health-care system in the second half of the 20th century. In the decades following World War II, dramatic improvements in technology led to an increased understanding of the underlying causes of disease and impairments and an increased emphasis on strategies to reduce impairments that restricted function. Occupational therapy's approach to treatment paralleled this emphasis on minimizing underlying impairments (Kielhofner, 1997). Therapists participated with other health-care professionals in developing and implementing "work- hardening" programs. These programs sought to assist workers who were injured or disabled to return to employment by reducing biomechanical incapacity for work activity (Matheson, Ogden, Violette, and Schultz, 1985; Niemeyer and Jacobs, 1989; Hanson and Walker, 1992).

During this time in occupational therapy, vocational rehabilitation approaches were biomechanical in nature and focused on improving strength, range of motion, coordination, and dexterity as a means to improve work performance (Lohman and Peyton, 1997). Efforts to improve the evaluation of the person's physical ability to complete tasks led to the development of formal **work capacity evaluation.** Work capacity evaluations simulate the physical demands of a job and assess a wide range of physical capabilities. This evaluation tends to emphasize physical capacity while ignoring aptitudes, interests, and vocational skills (Matheson, 1982). At the same time, work-hardening programs were being developed to remediate the deficits identified in work capacity evaluations. According to Niemeyer and Jacobs (1989), **work hardening** was defined as:

> An individualized, work oriented treatment process that involves the client in simulated or actual work tasks that are structured and graded to progressively increase physical tolerances, stamina, endurance and productivity with the eventual goal of improved employability.

Although the American Occupational Therapy Association (AOTA) adopted a definition that was broader and included references to improving "psychological and emotional tolerance" as goals of work hardening (American Occupational Therapy Association, 1986), the emphasis of work hardening continued to be biomechanical.

Work-hardening programs led to a refinement of principles and methods for increasing biomechanical fitness for work. However, increasing concern was raised over the limitations of an exclusively biomechanical approach to improving function after the onset of injury or disability. Specifically, it was argued that such an approach failed to address the full range of problems faced by persons with disabilities (Kielhofner, 1997).

Contemporary thinking in occupational therapy recognizes that occupational dysfunction is multidimensional, resulting from the interplay of biological, psychological, and ecological factors. Consistent with this approach, in addition to previously considered biomechanical factors, such as joint range of motion, muscle strength, and endurance, research has begun to identify psychosocial factors, such as job satisfaction or relationships with others in the workplace, as possibly playing a critical role in influencing the success of an attempt to return to work after injury or the onset of a disability (Braveman, 1999; Bigos et al., 1991; Appelberg, Romanov, Heikkila, and Honkasalo, 1996).

Moreover, the occupational therapy profession has also begun to return to its original focus on occupation as both the "means" and "ends" of therapeutic intervention (Trombly, 1995). This emphasis has led occupational therapists to be more cognizant of work as a component of the individual's total occupational life and to consider dimensions of work beyond the issues of underlying capacity.

THE TRANSITION TO COMMUNITY-BASED WORK PROGRAMMING

Changes have arisen in not only "how" to intervene but also "where" to intervene. Traditional work-related programs took place within traditional rehabilitation programs or in settings designed for work-focused intervention. However, increasingly, work programs are located in the community in which the client resides or specifically within the work setting itself.

Traditionally, work-related interventions occurred primarily in medical model clinics rather than at the site where the worker actually performed his or her role. Ordinarily, the worker only returned to the work site after a period of work hardening in a clinic-based program (Matheson, Ogden, Violette, and Schultz, 1985). Concerns over the costs of such traditional vocational rehabilitation, combined with emerging views of work disability, have led to interventions at the actual work environment at a much earlier stage.

In contrast to earlier descriptions of interventions, current descriptions of "on-site" vocational rehabilitation programming for the injured worker find the therapist and client in the workplace often within days of the onset of the injury (Kenny, Powell, and Reynolds-Lynch, 1995). Such early intervention at the job site can prevent significant disruption in habits that support work, prevent fears of reinjury from becoming major barriers, and limit the antagonism that may develop between the injured worker and the worker's supervisor or peers over prolonged absences.

The trend toward increased practice in the community is most likely the result of changes within the field of occupational therapy and external forces influencing practice. The advent of vocational rehabilitation programs based in community agencies or at the work site represents incorporation of an understanding of the multidimensional nature of occupational dysfunction into current practice. Also, changes in reimbursement and health-care policy, such as the increased use of managed care strategies by payers, have also played a role (Braveman and Fisher, 1997). For example, decreasing reimbursement in traditional medical model settings and skilled nursing facilities has resulted in an increased number of therapists exploring opportunities to practice in the community.

A broad definition of the term **community** is useful in understanding community-based programs. The concept of community has varied widely in social science literature. Towns and cities have been called communities but so have prisons and religious groups. Even corporations, factories, and trade unions have been referred to as communities (Minar and Greer, 1969). Fellin (1993) described the useful concept that the persons we encounter may also have membership in nonplace **identificational communities.** These communities include groups such as ethnic or cultural groups, patient groups, friendship groups, and workplace groups. Members of such communities need not reside in the same neighborhood, catchment area, or municipality. Although membership in these communities often overlaps with geographic communities, it is not determined by place but rather by interest or identification with the group (Longres, 1990; Germain, 1991).

One of the two program examples in this chapter is an "on-site therapy" program that focuses on providing vocational rehabilitation at the employment site of the injured worker or worker with a disability. Thinking of the workplace as a community is particularly useful when considering the psychosocial factors relating to an injured worker's attempt to return to work, such as the injured worker's relationship to his or her supervisor and shared concerns about issues such as safety within the worker's peer group. The second example is a program provided to a community of individuals living with HIV/AIDS. While the program is provided at two locations and draws clients from multiple geographic communities, each program participant is also a member of a community of individuals with a shared need and a shared social dilemma.

 HIGH-QUALITY COMMUNITY-BASED WORK PROGRAMS

Many factors may contribute to a high-quality community-based program. These factors may be general or specific to the discipline of occupational therapy. Regardless, they influence the value and effectiveness of any community-based service. In addition, high-quality community-based work programs share three characteristics: (1) they utilize a team approach, (2) they are client-centered, and (3) they have a community-centered focus. These factors and characteristics are important to consider in the development of community-based work programs.

CONTRIBUTING FACTORS

Three factors influencing the development of a high-quality, contemporary work program include:

1. Considering the worker role in relationship to other roles in the client's role repertoire
2. Addressing work dysfunction as a multidimensional problem in assessment
3. Employing an occupational therapy theory that addresses the multifactorial nature of work dysfunction

Worker Role in Relation to Other Roles

Community-based practice, by its nature, tends to make therapists increasingly aware of the client's total life. This has led to greater awareness that work, disability, and success at work are interconnected with other dimensions of a person's life.

Through an increased understanding of the factors influencing the success of an attempt to return to work, occupational therapists have recognized the limitation inherent in the assumption that if physical capacity is restored, then the worker with a disability will be successful in returning to work. Unfortunately, sufficient research about the influence of other life roles on attempts to return to work is lacking. Hammel (1999) presented the results of an initial qualitative study that investigated how members of a group of individuals with spinal-cord injuries went about reinstating their **worker roles** (patterns of behaviors and tasks required for job performance). Hammel (p. 49) noted that a key insight from this study was that "participants were struggling with maintaining and balancing multiple roles and interweaving these roles together." She utilized the metaphor of a rope to symbolize the interrelationship of roles in individual lives. "Each role is like a strand within a rope. Strands take up and leave off at different points in time and under different situations or environmental expectations" (Hammel, p. 49). Based on this study, Hammel (p. 59) concluded that "the key to a strong yet flexible life rope was not necessarily related to the number or type of roles so much as the ability to flexibly bring roles in and out of the role repertoire, create new ones, and continue to develop competence in existing roles to fit individual short and long term needs and environmental expectations. Thus, the worker role must be considered in the context of the person's entire life rope and social world."

While further formal investigation is needed, it seems clear that to truly understand the injured worker or worker with a disability, one must understand the full complement of roles within that worker's life.

Work Dysfunction as a Multidimensional Problem

When an occupational therapist completes a work-related evaluation, the result is to frame or name the problems currently interfering with a person's engagement in work. If the conclusions of assessment are to reflect the interplay of biological, psychological, and ecological factors, therapists must use assessments that capture information on such factors.

Velozo (1993) pointed out that the case for a broad evaluation approach was supported by research. He noted that of the studies that have included biomechanical factors in their predictive models of return to work, none has shown physical performance factors (e.g., trunk range of motion, trunk flexor-extensor strength, lifting ability) to be statistically related to return to work. Based on these results, he suggested that it is unwise to base evaluations of return to work entirely on physical capacity and work capacity assessments. Similar to Velozo's finding concerning biomechanical factors, Anthony, Cohen, and Danley (1988), through a review of related research, asserted that neither measures of psychiatric symptoms nor psychiatric diagnosis predict vocational rehabilitation outcome.

These arguments support the concept that, in addition to standard work evaluations that provide only information on the physical or mental capacities of a worker, therapists should also use psychosocial and environmental assessments. Fortunately, a number of assessments now exist to provide information on the psychosocial and environmental dimensions of a worker's experience. These assessments are based specifically on an occupational therapy conceptual practice model, the model of human occupation. Examples include the Occupational Performance History Interview (OPHI-II), the Occupational Self-Assessment (OSA), the Assessment of Communication and Interaction Skills (ACIS), the Worker Role Interview (WRI), and the Work Environment Impact Scale (WEIS). These assessments are highlighted in Table 8–1.

The **Occupational Performance History Interview (OPHI-II)** is a semistructured interview designed to provide information about the occupational performance and history of clients. The instrument consists of three scales: (1) **occupational identity** (how persons see themselves), (2) **occupational competence** (how well persons feel they perform), and (3) **occupational behavior settings** (the environments in which persons act). After completing the scales, a mechanism within the assessment allows therapists to identify the type of life history pattern that the respondent exhibited and write a qualitative description of the person's life-history narrative. The OPHI-II was not designed specifically for assessment of the worker role or for clients who have experienced work disability. However, the OPHI-II allows exploration of the client's roles, social contacts, and the environments in which the client operates. Because of the wide range of information gathered through the OPHI-II, the therapist is able to investigate the full range of factors that have been shown to influence return to work after a disability experience (Kielhofner et al., 1998).

The **Occupational Self-Assessment (OSA)** is a self-administered assessment designed to capture clients' perceptions of their own occupational competence and the impact of the environment on their occupational adaptation. It elicits a process for establishing goals based on the clients' priorities. The assessment includes a two part self-rating form. The first part includes a series of statements about the client's occupational functioning. The client responds by labeling each as an area of strength, adequate functioning, or weakness. The client also identifies the importance that he or she places on each item. The second part includes a series of statements about one's environments to which similar responses are given. Clients are then led through a process to establish priorities for change. These are then translated into therapy goals (Baron, Kielhofner, Goldhammer, and Wolenski, 1998).

The **Assessment of Communication and Interaction Skills (ACIS)** is an observational assessment that provides information on the client's skill when communicating and interacting with others in an occupation. The ACIS is used to gather data on skills as exhibited by the client during the performance of an occupational form and/or within a social group. The assessment is composed of behaviors or action "verbs" representing performance skills. The skill items represent three communication and interaction domains: (1) physicality, (2) information exchange, and (3) relations. Observation of the client's skills in each domain by the therapist allows the client and therapist to identify the impact of skill level on social interaction and to establish goals to improve effectiveness (Forsyth, Salamy, Simon, and Kielhofner, 1998).

The **Worker Role Interview (WRI)** is a semistructured interview for gathering data from injured workers about the psychosocial and environmental components of the

ASSESSMENTS FOR USE IN COMMUNITY-BASED WORK PROGRAMS*

Assessment	Usefulness/Administration	Yield
Occupational Performance History Interview (OPHI-II) (Kielhofner et al., 1998)	Useful as an initial assessment in combination with assessments of physical, cognitive, or other performance components. Semistructured interview that can be administered over multiple sessions requiring 40 to 90 minutes, depending on the client.	Provides narrative information on the client's occupational performance and history, including the client's roles and physical and social environments. Includes scales on three constructs measured by the instrument: 1. Occupational identity (how persons see themselves) 2. Occupational competence (how well persons believe they perform) 3. Occupational behavior settings (the environments in which persons act)
Occupational Self-Assessment (Baron, Kielhofner, Goldhammer, and Wolenski, 1998)	Useful as part of an initial assessment battery and as part of a goal-setting process. Especially useful when time is limited; client may complete portions of the assessment outside of therapy sessions. Two sections that may be given in different sessions requiring 30 to 60 minutes of therapist time for explanation and discussion/interpretation.	Provides data on occupational competence, environmental impact, and values. Provides a sense of how satisfied the client is with items that describe occupational competence and environment. Permits examination of the difference between how much a client values an item and his or her perception of competence for incorporation into a process of goal establishment for change.
Assessment of Communication and Interaction Skills (Forsyth, Salamy, Simon, and Kielhofner, 1998)	Useful for measuring the consequences of disease/illness on communication and interaction skills. Observation of a social interaction mutually agreed upon by the client and the therapist. Time range for observation and scoring is variable, from 20 to 60 minutes.	Provides scores on 20 skill verbs in three domains: 1. Physicality 2. Information exchange 3. Relations Does not provide information as to the underlying causes of skill deficits but yields identification of problem areas for exploration and intervention through remediation or compensatory strategies.

(Continued)

TABLE 8-1

ASSESSMENTS FOR USE IN COMMUNITY-BASED WORK PROGRAMS* (*Continued*)

Assessment	Usefulness/Administration	Yield
Worker Role Interview (Velozo, Kielhofner, and Fisher, 1998)	Useful for gathering information on the psychosocial/environmental components during an initial assessment process in conjunction with observations made during physical capacity evaluation. Semistructured interview requiring 30 to 60 minutes and 10 to 15 minutes for scoring.	Provides scores on six content areas including: 1. Personal causation 2. Values 3. Interests 4. Roles 5. Habits 6. Environment. Is intended for use during initial assessment and discharge to allow comparisons (although a second administration is not required).
Work Environment Impact Scale (Corner, Kielhofner, and Olson, 1998)	Useful for gathering information on clients' experience and perceptions of their environments, specifically individuals currently employed or those not presently working but anticipating a return to a specific job or type of work. Semistructured interview requiring 40 to 50 minutes for interview and scoring. Useful independently as part of the treatment process or in conjunction with other assessments such as the worker role interview during initial assessment.	Provides scores on 17 individual items such as the physical space, social contact and supports, temporal demands, objects utilized, and daily job functions indicating how the environmental factor impacts the worker's performance, satisfaction, and well being (physical, social, and emotional). Provides information on how qualities and characteristics of the work environment impact a worker.

*Each of these assessments may be purchased through the American Occupational Therapy Association Product Division at *http://www.aota.org*.

Sources: Kielhofner, G., Mallinson, T., Crawford, C., Nowak, M., Rigby, M., Henry, A., and Walens, D. (1998). *A user's manual for the occupational performance history interview (version 2.0)*. Chicago: Department of Occupational Therapy, University of Illinois at Chicago. Baron, K., Kielhofner, G., Goldhammer, V., and Wolenski, J. (1998). *A user's manual for the OSA: The occupational self-assessment*. Chicago: Department of Occupational Therapy, University of Illinois at Chicago. Forsyth, K., Salamy, M., Simon, S., and Kielhofner, G. (1998). *A user's guide to the assessment of communication and interaction skills (ACIS) (version 4.0)*. Chicago: Department of Occupational Therapy, University of Illinois at Chicago. Velozo, C., Kielhofner, G., and Fisher, G. (1998). *A user's guide to the worker role interview (version 9)*. Chicago: Department of Occupational Therapy, University of Illinois at Chicago. Corner, R. A., Kielhofner, G., and Olson, L. (1998). *A user's guide to the work environment impact scale (version 2.0)*. Chicago: Department of Occupational Therapy, University of Illinois at Chicago.

work experience. The WRI combines information from an interview with observations made during the physical and behavioral assessment procedures of a physical and/or work capacity evaluation. The intent of the WRI is to identify the psychosocial and environmental variables that may influence the ability of the injured worker to return to work (Velozo, Kielhofner, and Fisher, 1998).

The **Work Environment Impact Scale (WEIS)** is a semistructured interview for gathering data about how individuals with impairments or disabilities experience their work settings. The focus of the interview is the impact of the work setting on the client's performance, satisfaction, and well-being. A scale allows the therapist to translate the information gathered in the interview into quantitative ratings. Overall, the scale provides a measure of the work environment's impact on a continuum from negative to positive. In addition, when individual items are scored, a profile of how the environment negatively or positively impacts the client emerges (Corner, Kielhofner, and Olson, 1998).

Use of Occupational Therapy Theory

A successful and replicable program of services needs to be guided by an explicit, comprehensive theory that addresses the multiple factors impacting work success. One such theory, the model of human occupation (MOHO) (Kielhofner, 1995), has been applied to the study of injured workers (Azhar, 1996; Corner and Kielhofner, 1996; Corner, Kielhofner, and Lin, 1997; Kielhofner and Brinson, 1989; Velozo, Kielhofner, and Fisher, 1990; Munoz and Kielhofner, 1995; Salz, 1983; Olson, 1995; Mallinson, 1995).

According to this model (Kielhofner, 1995), four main factors influence work success: (1) motivation, (2) life roles and habits, (3) capacities, and (4) environmental contexts. Motivational factors include individuals' cultural values, interests, and beliefs about personal capacity that influence decisions concerning work, commitment to working, ability to cope with work stress, and levels of satisfaction with working. The second factor, lifestyle, includes life roles and habits. Roles refer to the entire complex of social relations on and off the job that may support or interfere with work and to the individual's identification with the worker role and related social roles. Habits refer to overall patterns of typical behavior and work-specific patterns influencing work success or failure. The third factor, capacities, refers to physical, mental and social skills, as well as work-specific skills. The fourth factor, environmental contexts, includes the specific work environment, its human and nonhuman influences on work performance satisfaction, and larger community and societal influences.

Braveman (1999), who reviewed 44 predictive studies of return to work, concluded that the factors most often shown to have predictive power could be organized to support many of the underlying assertions made within the model of human occupation. Because not all of the model's tenets have been investigated as to their relationship to return to work, further specific investigation needs to be conducted to fully justify the use of this model as the primary theory supporting interventions with persons with work-related disability. However, based on Braveman's findings, this model appears to hold great promise. The use of a unifying model provides a strong framework both for evidence-based program development and the evaluation of program outcomes. The relationship of the primary components of the model of human occupation to factors commonly investigated in research on predicting return to work is summarized in Table 8–2.

GENERAL CHARACTERISTICS

Three general characteristics are essential to a sound community-based work program: (1) a team approach, (2) client-centered focus, and (3) community-centered focus.

TABLE 8–2

THE RELATIONSHIP OF MOHO COMPONENTS TO PREDICTIVE FACTORS IN RETURN TO WORK STUDIES

Model Subsystem	Primary Model Components	Related Factors Commonly Investigated as Predictive of Return to Work
Volition	Personal causation	Level of perceived disability Perceived control over environment Educational level Perception of fault for injury
	Values	Age Gender Culture
	Interests	Job satisfaction prior to injury
Habituation	Roles	Work status at time of study (light duty vs. nonworking)
	Habits	Time at job prior to injury Attendance record at work prior to injury
Mind-brain-body performance	Physical capacities	Nature and severity of injury Perceived level of pain Surgery history Diagnosis
Environment	Social groups	Supervisor interaction Peer interaction Work environment/work stress

Team Approach

Most effective vocational rehabilitation programs use a team approach. The term **team approach** has been chosen specifically to differentiate from the term "interdisciplinary." The term "team approach" incorporates the injured worker or worker with a disability, the work supervisor, and significant others as equal members of the team. The membership of the community-based vocational rehabilitation team will vary significantly, depending on the location and focus of the program.

Client-Centered Focus

Six critical components for planning effective community-based services have been identified by Cohen and Anthony (1988). These components, which are **client centered** (focused on the client), include:

1. Program values that maximize choice, increase competency, and provide unconditional support
2. A focus on client goals rather than solely on service system goals
3. A focus on the clients' "perceived" needs for assistance rather than on needs for predetermined services
4. A focus on the clients' preferred level of intervention rather than requiring that consumers take "all or nothing"
5. Identification of the essence of service delivery in terms of what intervention is pro-

vided by whom for what purpose, not simply the configuration or structure of the services

6. A vision of consumer involvement and growth in the community rather than one of community care and maintenance

Community-Centered Approach

In addition to those components offered by Cohen and Anthony (1988), Barker (1994) also suggested two essential ingredients:

1. Services must be an integral part of the community in which they are based by meeting the needs of specific individuals within the community, building on the strengths and unique resources of the community, and developing relationships with multiple businesses rather than adopting any single marketing approach (**community centered**).
2. Services must offer a broad array of choices or a "continuum" of options for individuals at different levels of functioning.

Occupational therapists are well suited to develop community-based vocational rehabilitation programming that meets the criteria of community and client centeredness. Flexibly designed services that tailor intervention, based on client-identified needs and provided at the work site or in the community, can be effective in terms of cost and outcome.

Two such programs have been developed by the Department of Occupational Therapy at the University of Illinois at Chicago. Descriptions of the Worksite Program (an on-site therapy program for injured workers) and the Employment Options Program (a vocational rehabilitation program for persons living with HIV/AIDS) are provided here as examples.

EXAMPLES OF COMMUNITY-BASED WORK PROGRAMS

The Worksite Program

The Worksite Program, established in 1997 as a collaboration between the Occupational Therapy and Physical Therapy Departments at the University of Illinois at Chicago (UIC), was developed with the primary objective of providing cost-effective and comprehensive vocational services to businesses for their workers. Demographic analysis of UIC injured workers highlighted the need for a coordinated rehabilitation service on campus. Although work-related services, including prevention, rehabilitation, pre-employment screenings, and ADA consultation, were available, they were fragmented and not well coordinated. Additionally, injury prevention services were available but not routinely instituted, and return to work for injured workers occurred at the discretion of the department supervisor. A cost analysis of UIC workers' compensation reflected this lack of coordinated services in increased costs, high lost-time injury rate, and continued reinjury. Data from Liberty Mutual Insurance Company show that on-site industrial rehabilitation has demonstrated successful return to work rates exceeding 85 percent—significantly higher than the national average (Foster, 1995). Based on available data, the benefits of establishing the Worksite Program seemed like a logical choice for UIC because its own workers' compensation costs continued to increase.

The benefits of on-site rehabilitation have long been recognized. However, only in recent years has industry been compelled to re-evaluate its return-to-work programs due to increasing workers' compensation costs. From 1992 to 1994, the total costs of workers' compensation in the United States rose 7.9 percent, growing from $111.9 billion to $120.7 billion in costs to employers. In the State of Illinois, total indemnity and medical benefits paid in workers' compensation between 1984 and 1993 increased 102 percent (Foster, 1995). This new concern is an indirect result of the growth of managed care. When medical costs are audited and controlled, previously overlooked injury- and disability-related expenditures become impossible to ignore. Employers are beginning to realize the need to manage employee disability as well as they would their core business. This means redirecting existing therapy budgets into mechanisms such as on-site programs. While therapeutic intervention with work-related injuries has been occurring for decades, therapists have been migrating out of the hospitals and private clinics into on-site clinics housed within industry itself. Therapists are bringing with them new aspects of treatment that are active, functionally based, and related to the physical demands of the job.

On-site rehabilitation programs use a variety of assessment tools to evaluate a person's vocational possibilities and physical functional status, with the aim of returning the injured person back to work. Evaluation strategies range from the use of standardized work assessments associated with vocational rehabilitation to highly technical physical capacity and work capacity equipment. Methods are utilized to identify pain and abnormal pain behavior (Velozo, 1993). The Worksite Program, not unique in its philosophy of recognizing the benefits of on-site intervention, uses these traditional work evaluation tools. The uniqueness of this program is its ability to recognize the need to incorporate evaluation tools that address a person's aptitude, performance, and skills in conjunction with the person's environment and the meaning of work to the person.

THE WORKPLACE AS A COMMUNITY. For years, the terms "work hardening" and "work conditioning" have been viewed as viable alternatives in work rehabilitation. In some instances the success rate for "sustained return to work" has been high, typically if the early intervention model was used. Early intervention promotes a sense of priority, telling the injured worker that his or her injury is of concern to the employer. This, in turn, enhances the employer's credibility and creates a foundation for early recovery. Early intervention also promotes the ideal restoration of function rather than alleviation of symptoms as a primary treatment objective. Work hardening/conditioning requires that the client attend a program in a clinic setting where every effort is made to simulate the task and the physical demands of the job. While it makes sense that workers need to be conditioned by participating in a process to increase strength and flexibility to meet the physical demands of the job, the injured workers tend to feel like patients rather than productive workers.

Rehabilitation on-site provides the opportunity for implementation of all the aforementioned ideals. Plus, it fosters the notion of the workplace as a community. As stated earlier, thinking of the workplace as a community is particularly useful when considering the psychosocial factors relating to an injured worker's attempt to return to work or when designing intervention to prevent the occurrence of injuries. While the physical demands of the job, the physical environment (such as lighting and noise levels), and the machinery used at work can be simulated in a clinic, the psychosocial environment cannot be duplicated in such a setting. Employees share strong bonds with their employers and coworkers that arise from the employment relationship. This relationship is crucial, strongly influencing a person's desire to participate in his or her chosen work community and the individual's concept of self-worth in that particular work environment. Hagberg, Silverstein, and Wells (1995) define psychosocial work factors as perceived characteristics of the work environment having an emotional connotation for workers and managers. These factors may result in stress and strain. Examples of psychosocial work factors include work overload, work pressure, lack of control, social support, and job future ambiguity. Research studies of offices and workers using video display units have shown that psychosocial work factors, such as lack of job control, cognitive overload, and monotonous tasks, are similar to work-related musculoskeletal disorders (WRMDs) as causal factors and as hindrances to return to work (Smith, Carayon, and Sanders, 1992). Work organization and psychosocial work factors have been shown to be related to stress and, therefore, could in turn influence musculoskeletal disorders (Cooper and Marshall, 1976; Smith, 1987). The Worksite Program recognizes the importance of addressing psychosocial factors and the benefits of offering appropriate intervention.

COMMUNITIES BEING SERVED. The primary aim of the Worksite Program is to offer prevention and rehabilitation services to industry and businesses at the workplace. At present, clients of the Worksite Program operate in two environments. The UIC Medical Center's Emergency Department, a primary referral source, has a contract with UIC workers' compensation to treat workers injured on the job. The Worksite Program also serves businesses at the Chicago International Airport, by working in partnership with a UIC Medical Center Clinic located at the airport. This clinic currently has agreements to provide services to employees of companies, including Continental Airlines, Host Marriott, United Express Airlines, and US Air.

Geographic communities are also represented within the Worksite Program. Businesses in the area surrounding O'Hare Airport and metropolitan Chicago businesses in proximity to the UIC Medical Center are also referral sources. Other main sources of client referrals to the Worksite Program include members of professional communities. These referral sources are identifiable groups of people originating from certain professions such as physicians, risk management lawyers, workers' compensation case managers, and health insurance case managers. Each of these professional communities has specific identifiable needs in addition to the shared concern of limiting costs related to injuries on the job. Recognizing and addressing these needs is a critical step in marketing the program, maintaining a stream of referrals, and establishing these professionals as functioning members of the Worksite Program team.

THE WORKSITE PROGRAM TEAM. Generally, the Worksite Program team is comprised of service providers, service receivers, and referral sources. Examples of individuals participating as members of the Worksite team include:

1. Service providers: occupational therapists, physical therapists, UIC case manager, program manager, physicians, occupational health nurse practitioners
2. Service receivers: injured worker, the injured worker's family, the employer
3. Referral sources: physicians, workers' compensation case managers, risk management lawyers

The program recognizes the important role that each team member plays in enabling the rehabilitation process and preventing injury. The composition of the team is dependent on the focus of the service being delivered. For example, an injury prevention team will differ from a rehabilitation team because the goal is dictated by the desired outcome. The team required to create and manage a prevention program usually includes health professionals, workers, supervisors, and representatives from human resources management, risk management, and safety departments. The Worksite Program also recognizes that, without the cooperation and commitment of the team members, together with their ideas and expertise, the goals of the program will not be realized.

PROGRAM DESIGN. The Worksite Program, designed using the model of human occupation and the biomechanical model as the theoretical basis for the program, provides a comprehensive continuum of services, including injury prevention, evaluation, work-site intervention, ADA consultation, and program evaluation. The program is set up to customize or individualize services based on client need. This, in turn, dictates the service protocols. An example of a service protocol for rehabilitation of a UIC injured worker is highlighted in Box 8–1.

EXAMPLE OF A PREVENTION PROGRAM. Since its inception, the Worksite Program has implemented several prevention programs. In 1998 the Post-Offer Screen Program was developed for UIC Facilities Management because workers' compensation data indicated increased numbers of back and upper extremity injuries. The aim of this program was to ensure a match between the physical capacity of the person and the physical demands of the job. The goal was to prevent injuries from occurring, thus preventing the associated rehabilitation costs. Over a period of 12 months, job analyses were conducted to identify the potential risk factors and the critical physical demands imposed in each of the department's jobs. New employees from Facilities Management are now tested against these physical demand criteria, using a standardized functional assessment tool. Analysis of the Post-Offer Screen data indicates that 22 percent of new employees are not able to meet one or more of the physical demands criteria. These data clearly substantiate the need for use of functional assessments to identify workers at risk for injury.

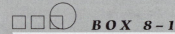

BOX 8–1

Example of a Service Protocol for Work Rehabilitation

1. The injured worker is directed to the UIC Emergency Department promptly after the injury is reported to the supervisor.
2. The Emergency Department physician evaluates the worker's injury and establishes the need for further intervention.
3. Services are requested from the Worksite Program. These are dependent on the nature of the injury and may include: (a) occupational therapy, (b) physical therapy, (c) functional capacity evaluation, (d) job analysis, and/or (e) ergonomics evaluation to identify the mismatch criteria between the person and his or her work environment.
4. Once the service request is initiated, the Worksite case manager collaborates with the therapist, the injured worker, the Emergency Department physician, and, if necessary, the workers' compensation case manager and employer to facilitate a smooth, efficient, and cost-effective transition back to work. The goals for the return to work or any other expected outcomes are the product of a collaborative effort among all parties concerned. Clear goal setting and open communication is imperative.
5. Implementation of injury-prevention strategies are initiated during the transition period between a worker experiencing an injury, receiving rehabilitation, and returning to work. The therapist and the physician actively involve the injured worker in becoming aware of the risks pertaining to his or her work habits, health, and lifestyle, and make the necessary recommendations.
6. After the worker returns to work, follow-up is initiated to ensure success back on the job.

The Employment Options Program

A second example of a community-based vocational rehabilitation program is the Employment Options Program, a vocational rehabilitation program for persons living with HIV/AIDS developed in 1997 through a partnership between the University of Illinois at Chicago Department of Occupational Therapy and the Howard Brown Health Center. The Howard Brown Health Center is a community-based health center located on Chicago's North Side, with a mission of meeting the health-care needs of Chicago's gay and lesbian community.

As a result of promising new pharmacological treatments, huge decreases in HIV-related mortality were seen during the 1990s (Feinberg, 1996; Hogg et al., 1997). In addition to decreases in mortality, many persons receiving combination therapies experienced increases in function and their ability to complete daily activities. In early 1997, the Howard Brown Health Center recognized an evolving need for work-related interventions for persons living with HIV/AIDS. As a result of improved function, some persons living with HIV/AIDS who had been work disabled for periods ranging from months to years began to consider re-entering the workforce. In an effort to respond to the needs of their clients, the Howard Brown Health Center sought and obtained funding from the AIDS Foundation of Chicago and the National AIDS Fund to develop a program to assist persons living with HIV/AIDS to return to work. While the organization had highly developed expertise in meeting the medical and psychosocial needs of persons with HIV/AIDS, they had limited experience in rehabilitation or with work disability.

During this same time period, the Department of Occupational Therapy at the University of Illinois at Chicago was pursuing efforts to develop partnerships with community-based agencies so that the range of occupational therapy services offered by the department would more closely mirror those provided by the profession as a whole. The UIC Occupational Therapy Department has a significant history and considerable expertise in the area of work disability and rehabilitation, including the development of a number of work-related assessments mentioned earlier. Two other vocational rehabilitation programs had previously been developed by the department, including the Work Readiness Program for persons with prolonged disability and no prior significant work history (Olson, 1995), and the Worksite Program described previously. Subsequently, a partnership was forged to develop, implement, and evaluate a pilot program.

Twenty clients were enrolled in the pilot phase of the Employment Options Program. Due to the success of these clients, the UIC Occupational Therapy Department and the Howard Brown Health Center pursued additional funding to continue the program. In the fall of 1998, the program received funding from the U.S. Department of Education's Rehabilitation Services Administration for a three-year period. The funding allowed the program to continue at the Howard Brown Health Center and expand the program to a second site on the UIC campus.

The second site allowed the program to broaden the population of individuals served. While the clients of the Howard Brown Health Center are racially diverse, with a wide range of educational and socioeconomic backgrounds, almost all of the clients referred to the Employment Options Program are male who report contracting HIV through same-sex sexual contact. This population, however, no longer represents the majority of persons living with HIV/AIDS in the United States today. The opening of the second site on the UIC campus allowed the marketing of services to a broad base of clients, including women and clients who self-identified that they most likely became HIV positive through intravenous drug use. In addition, a wider range of racial, educational, and socioeconomic backgrounds were represented among the UIC clients. Some clients at this site were concerned with establishing a vocational role for the first time rather than re-entering the workplace. Clients faced additional dilemmas such as arranging for child care or dealing with a history of arrest in addition to their discontinuous employment history.

COMMUNITIES BEING SERVED. Understanding the communities served by the Employment Options Program requires using a broad definition of community. Clients in the Employment Options Program all belong to the community of persons living with HIV/AIDS and share the common needs and concerns that come with managing a chronic illness. Within this group, however, members also identify with other communities. The Chicago gay and lesbian community is very active, having established communication mechanisms such as gay- and lesbian-oriented newspapers, numerous nonprofit organizations focused on meeting the needs of gay and lesbian consumers, and a wide range of social and political organizations including sports clubs, political action committees, and support groups. Capitalizing on these communication mechanisms helped to identify potential clients, market services, and locate sources of additional support for clients.

Geographic communities are also represented within the Employment Options Program. Chicago is often described as a city of neighborhoods. Many, but not all, of the members of the gay and lesbian community live in a neighborhood area called Lakeview, where the Howard Brown Health Center is also located. Numerous clients who receive services at the UIC site are also members of the same geographic communities or neighborhoods on Chicago's Near West Side or South Side. Specific racial and ethnic groups are also represented within the clients of the Employment Options Program. Some clients identify strongly with these groups as communities. For example, a number of clients reside in Chicago's Pilsen neighborhood, a community with a very strong Latino identity. Membership in multiple communities can provide clients with additional supports that may be helpful in assisting with goal achievement. However, for others, belonging to multiple communities may complicate the vocational rehabilitation process. Having HIV/AIDS or another disability or being homosexual can bring significant stigma and difficulties with acceptance in some communities. Different cultures and ethnic groups may view disability differently and have different strategies for dealing with it (Eisenberg, 1977; Jenkins, 1988; Kleinman, 1988). A significant stigma and prejudice are associated with AIDS that may be pronounced in cultural communities that associate the disease with undesirable behaviors or characteristics such as sexual orientation.

THE EMPLOYMENT OPTIONS TEAM. Two full-time occupational therapists were hired to provide the occupational therapy assessment and intervention. While each therapist is assigned to a primary site, each assists the other to colead groups and provide opportunities for enhanced problem solving. A full-time vocational placement specialist was hired to work with the Chicago business community to develop opportunities for volunteer positions, internships, and paid employment. The vocational placement specialist also collaborates with the occupational therapists to assess client interests, develop employment-related goals, prepare for the job search and interview process, and work with potential employers to maximize chances of success. Other critical members of the team include the client, the client's family, a case manager, the client's physician, and the potential employer. Clients come to the Employment Options Program with varied goals, problems, and expectations. A focus of the program is on maintaining the right of the client to self-determine what constitutes a "successful" outcome. The primary goal of the Employment Options Program is to return clients to paid employment. However, helping a client who decides that returning to paid work is not in his or her best interest to successfully develop other satisfying roles is also considered a success. Clients who have had a prolonged absence from the worker role have often accepted additional responsibilities at home. Thus, returning to work necessitates renegotiation of roles with one's family. Success at an attempt to return to work requires including the family or significant others in the therapy process.

The role of the physician varies, depending on the health status of the client and the complexity of the client's medication regimen. With some clients, this involvement is minimal, while with others, the physician is closely consulted about how to assure compliance with medications while working.

The complexity of the lives of the Employment Options clients and their typical reliance on multiple sources of financial and social assistance often contributes to much confusion about exactly what impact paid employment might have on their benefits. Many clients have a case manager upon referral to the program. Otherwise program staff refers clients to existing social service agencies for case management services. Finally, potential employers who provide internships or paid employment are considered members of the team. Their involvement also varies, depending on how clients initiated contact with the employer and the client's decision regarding disclosure of his or her HIV status. Forgetting to include the employer or supervisor as a member of the team can be the critical missing link in success with some clients.

PROGRAM DESIGN. The Employment Options Program, designed using the model of human occupation as the theoretical basis for the program, is organized in four phases. Phase 1 includes an initial assessment process that begins with a preliminary screening. This screening helps to establish the appropriateness of the program for the client and to determine necessary problem solving and resources to assure program attendance (e.g., child care and transportation). Program staff works with clients who have such difficulties so that program attendance and participation are improved. An example of such intervention would include working with clients to obtain discounted passes for public transportation available to persons with disabilities. Clients are initially assessed using the Occupational Performance History Interview (OPHI-II) (Kielhofner et al., 1998). In addition to the OPHI-II, the Occupational Self-Assessment (OSA), the National Institutes of Health (NIH) Activity Record, and the Assessment of Communication and Interaction Skills (ACIS) are administered to each client (Baron et al., 1998; National Institutes of Health, 1985; Forsyth et al., 1998). The OPHI-II, the OSA, and the ACIS were previously described.

The NIH Activity Record is a self-administered assessment that assists the therapist in gaining an understanding of the clients' routines. Each client completes a log of his or her activity on a half-hour basis for two days, one weekday and one weekend day that represent "normal" days for the client. This assessment provides insights about the client's tolerance for activity and routine social contacts. As clients progress through the program, other assessments are used on an "as needed" basis. These include the Worker Role Interview (WRI) and the Work Environment Impact Scale (WEIS) described earlier, and the Assessment of Motor and Process Skills (AMPS). The AMPS provides information on the impact of motor and process skills on the client's performance during functional activities (Fisher, 1994). Clients' interests and employment-related goals are also assessed by the vocational placement specialist.

Phase 1 also includes client participation in group education and support sessions. The sessions are designed to help the client explore and develop work skills and the daily habits needed to support a vocational role. The sessions include self-assessment and vocational planning, information sharing related to economics, benefits, the Americans with Disabilities Act, other logistics of returning to work, job searching and job skill development exercises, and work task experiences. Program staff have collaborated with numerous existing community-based agencies to develop the educational curriculum for phase 1. Group sessions include presentations and discussions led by representatives of groups such as the SSI Coalition for a Responsible Safety Net, a nonprofit Chicago-based group that advocates for persons relying on public assistance.

Phase 1, which lasts eight weeks, aims to provide:

1. An opportunity for self-assessment and strengthening and refinement of vocational choice
2. A structured routine to develop habits of promptness, consistency, and a commitment to the program
3. A forum for sharing critical information about returning to work
4. A community of emotional support for return to work
5. A context for identifying and addressing factors that may impact on work readiness
6. Opportunities to develop job-relevant skills

Phase 2 focuses on continuing to develop work skills and habits with client placement in volunteer work, an internship, or temporary employment. These opportunities were developed in partnership with Chicago businesses. The placements benefit the client who receives on-the-job training and supervision and the business that receives free labor for the duration of the placement. The business also has access to a fully trained and oriented employee if it wishes to hire the client at the end of phase 2. The duration and intensity of this phase is variable, typically from one to three months, and is adjusted to the clients' needs.

During phase 2 of the program, it is important for clients to develop confidence in their ability to manage the routine of working. It is also a time when challenges associated with working with a chronic disability are identified and addressed in the program. Each of the placements is designed so that the clients receive assessment and feedback concerning job performance. Also, services such as job coaching, assistance in identifying and requesting accommodations, assistance in planning and managing routines, transportation, and finances are provided to the client during phase 2. Program staff works closely with the volunteer or work supervisor in these placements to assure that the client is receiving appropriate supervision and to support the supervisor in responding to any challenges.

Phase 3 consists of direct placement in competitive employment. Clients are placed in jobs developed by the vocational placement specialist or are assisted by program staff to apply for and secure employment. This is the time when clients need to make decisions about the critical issue of disclosing their HIV status. If clients take direct advantage of opportunities developed by the program and request an interview, disclosure of their HIV status is a foregone conclusion. Some clients perceive this as a benefit and appreciate knowing that the employer must be supportive of employing persons with HIV/AIDS by virtue of their participation in the program. Other clients prefer not to disclose their HIV status and seek employment opportunities on their own, with coaching from program staff. Job analysis, adaptation, and on-site job coaching of the client are provided as needed. In addition, the program provides employer education, consultation, and trouble-shooting support for the supervisor and coworkers of the client. When clients secure jobs with employers who are not part of the partnership, the program offers these services to the employers, making them available on request. Clients in this phase may still participate in group support sessions. The intensity and duration of this phase is also variable, averaging approximately four months. Phase 3 is terminated when the client is evaluated as having adjusted to and demonstrated satisfactory performance on the job.

Phase 4 consists of long-term follow-up and support. Because AIDS is a chronic condition and periods of illness or functional limitation may occur, program staff is available to intervene and provide support as needed. Clients can take considerable periods of time to adjust to new and more complicated role repertoires that accompany returning to work. In addition, clients may encounter difficulties after months of successful employment that they might not have anticipated when first returning to work. For example, clients who may not, at first, perceive the need to make requests for reasonable accommodations under the Americans with Disabilities Act may later find this process necessary as they manage side effects, such as fatigue or diarrhea, that might come with changes in medications. Clients also benefit from the emotional support received through ongoing contact with program staff or other clients. Additionally, some clients return to the program to provide peer training and support to other clients.

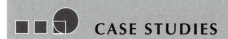 **CASE STUDIES**

THE WORKSITE PROGRAM AND SUE

Sue was a 48-year-old woman, diagnosed with medial epicondylitis in September 1997. She had worked as a hemodialysis technologist for over five years and was assigned an additional task in July 1997. Onset of the symptoms was insidious and not associated with any specific mechanism of injury. Although her symptoms resolved with anti-inflammatory treatment and rest, they recurred with return to her normal work. She was treated at the UIC Emergency Department and then referred to the UIC Worksite Program when symptoms recurred despite medication and rest.

Sue was evaluated by an occupational and a physical therapist to determine her level of functioning and prognosis for a successful return to work. Both therapists recommended a work-site evaluation to identify any confounding risk factors in her physical environment and physical demands of the job that could be interfering with the return to work process.

The ensuing job analysis identified several risk factors related to her physical work environment and work organization. The recommendations stressed the importance of ensuring reduced exposure to risks created by poor configuration of the workstation; work organization issues such as amount of consecutive days worked on the same tasks; and the mismatch between her, the machine, and the physical demands of the job. After some of the recommendations were implemented, particularly the workstation and work organization issues, Sue continued to report symptoms such as elbow pain and inability to "cope" with the physical demands of the job. She also complained about her relationship with her supervisor, which she felt had deteriorated since the onset of her injury. She perceived herself as being singled out by the supervisor to perform the task repetitively and on consecutive days, despite the recommendations of the job analysis.

Though Sue had never been off work, some psychosocial issues at work became apparent, warranting further investigation and attention. Sue was assessed by her occupational therapist, who used the Worker Role Interview (WRI). It was selected as an appropriate tool because it can identify the psychosocial and environmental variables preventing a return to work, or as in Sue's case, preventing her from sustaining a meaningful job (Velozo, 1993). The evaluation identified the following: (1) Sue had fears regarding the risk of reinjury; (2) Sue's decreased performance was noted in maintaining the repetitiveness of one of the tasks; and (3) Sue perceived her supervisor as a barrier to sustaining her job.

The results of the WRI were presented by the occupational therapist and discussed at a team meeting attended by the Emergency Department physician who had been treating her, the physical therapist, and the Worksite case manager. The intervention strategy was as follows:

1. The physical therapist instructed Sue on proper body mechanics and educated her regarding the prognosis of her injury. A work-conditioning program, designed to suit the physical demands of her job, was implemented by the occupational therapist. It

was felt this would also address her decreased performance in maintaining a repetitive motion inherent in her job.
2. The Worksite case manager initiated a conversation with Sue's supervisor regarding the work organization issues identified by the job analysis.

Sue continued with her therapy, which included work conditioning, and reported improvements in her tolerance for the physical demands of the job. The supervisor believed she had done the best she could in accommodating Sue by making necessary changes to the workstation, decreasing exposure to the risk identified, and limiting the number of hours she was exposed to that risk. The supervisor was not able to remove Sue from that particular task due to staff shortage.

After three weeks, Sue was discharged from physical therapy with a home exercise program and the work-conditioning program. Sue returned to her modified job but periodically called the Worksite case manager to express discontent about her relationship with her supervisor. She decided that she was not prepared to leave her job because she was happy with it but believed that she needed to resolve her conflict with the supervisor. Sue sought the services of UIC's Employee Assistance Program. Six months later, Sue informed the Worksite case manager that she was continuing to resolve the conflict with her supervisor with help from employee assistance. Her ultimate goal was to seek transfer to another department.

EMPLOYMENT OPTIONS PROGRAM AND SETH
Seth was a 36-year-old male who had been unemployed for six years due to AIDS before enrolling in the Employment Options Program. While he had had several opportunistic infections prior to leaving work, Seth had begun triple combination drug therapy several years before entering the program and was doing well medically at the time of enrollment. He had lived with a life partner, Sean, for eight years. Sean was supportive of Seth exploring the option of returning to work but also expressed concern that Seth not become ill again as a result of stress. Seth was involved in several community groups and volunteer positions at the time he enrolled in the program but limited his activity to three to four hours at a time due to concern about becoming overfatigued.

Seth was assessed using the OPHI-II to gather information about his life history, his interests and goals, and his perception of how his physical and social environments influenced his day-to-day functioning. He identified the primary roles of spouse, home manager, volunteer, friend, and son. Seth's last employment was as a computer systems analyst. He stated that he enjoyed the job, but that his home life and relationship with his partner were his highest priorities. He saw returning to work as bringing financial benefits to himself and his partner. He also recognized that he valued the independence and feelings of accomplishment that he had received from his worker role. Seth expressed concern that because of changes in technology that had occurred during his period of disability, he might have to pursue considerable training or further education before re-entering the job market. He shared Sean's concern about becoming ill again or overfatigued. Given that he considered his role as spouse as a significant priority, Seth also worried if working full time would have a negative impact on his home life. The assessment identified that Seth had assumed many of the responsibilities for day-to-day management of the home and that he might have to renegotiate homemaker roles with his partner.

Seth began attending the group education and support sessions and was an active participant. In individual sessions, he voiced appreciation for all that he was learning about benefits and his legal rights. He also learned from listening to others who shared his concerns over how to juggle a resumed worker role with their already complicated lives. He worked with his occupational therapist to apply what he was learning about the impact that working would have on his Social Security Disability Income (SSDI) and his private disability health insurance. Because his physical tolerance for work had been identified as a potential barrier to resuming full-time work, his occupational therapist suggested that he negotiate a gradual increase in his hours with one of the organizations with whom he volunteered. He also initiated discussions with his partner, Sean, about the need for Sean to reassume responsibilities for some cooking, cleaning, and errands to accommodate Seth's busier schedule.

Another focus of Seth's individual therapy was helping him to prepare for the job search process. This included updating and improving his resume, honing his job interview skills, brainstorming job search strategies, and exploring opportunities for skill development. The option of an internship was discussed, and his occupational therapist began negotiations with the information technology services of the University Medical Center. During this time, Seth continued to gradually increase the number of hours he was volunteering, reporting an increased confidence in his skills and endurance. A final focus of intervention was helping Seth make difficult decisions about how to explain his absence from the workforce to potential employers and whether or not to disclose his disability and HIV status.

As part of his preparation for job interviews, Seth decided to attend an information technology job fair. His goals for this included becoming more comfortable with interview questions, learning more about whether or not his knowledge base was truly out of date, and experimenting with answering questions about why he had not been employed for the last six years. He carried with him a newly updated resume. Much to his surprise, Seth's inquiries were met with much interest. A large telecommunications company contacted him within days to arrange an interview. Program staff provided intensive coaching and preparation for the interview, while Seth secured a commitment from Sean that he was willing to make the changes necessary to support an attempt at full-time work.

Seth was pleased to find that questions about his six-year absence from the workforce were easily deflected without having to disclose any specifics about the nature of his "illness." In fact, the employer was much more interested in the fact that prior to leaving his last job he had had a stable job history and was able to provide current references from his volunteer position regarding his reliability and professional behavior. Explaining that the resources needed to update Seth's skills were worth finding a stable, motivated employee, the employer offered Seth a full-time position that he accepted.

A year later, Seth is still employed full time and is doing well. He has maintained contact with the program. While his choice not to disclose his status prevented contact or the provision of services to the employer, Seth has occasionally contacted his occupational therapist with questions about managing his new role. In addition, he has acted as a resource for other program participants and has shared his experiences and insights with clients struggling with the same issues he faced.

 ## CONCLUSION

The 20th century was a time fraught with change for the field of occupational therapy. This change was driven by factors from both within and outside of the profession, including: increased focus on the use of occupation in natural environments as the focus of intervention, increased pressure for cost-effective care through the advent of managed care strategies, and ongoing change in worker's compensation policy and administration. If the past is at all predictive of the future, occupational therapists should expect continued pressure to change and adapt the form of work-related practice in the coming years. However, as noted futurist Joel Barker (1992) once remarked, "When a paradigm shifts, everyone goes back to zero." In vocational rehabilitation, paradigm shifts, including a move to providing services at the workplace and in the community, have already been experienced. Future pressures for change may produce constraints on payment for what types of service and how much service may be provided. However, "going back to zero" means that change also brings new opportunities. These opportunities may arise out of the same pressures that are viewed as constraints on traditional practice.

To be prepared to capitalize on opportunities that arise from future change, occupational therapy professionals must keep themselves apprised of outside forces influencing the field, while holding tight to the values and beliefs that are the basis of the profession. Two important areas of effort will help to assure the field's continued success in developing community-based work rehabilitation programming.

The first effort is continued development and testing of sound occupational therapy practice models through empirical research related to assessment of and intervention with workers experiencing impairment or disability. The move toward providing increased service in the community has fostered an increased awareness of the need to fully understand the impact of social and environmental influences on the occupational performance of workers. This awareness has led to changes in practice that have incorporated a multidimensional view of the nature of occupational dysfunction. The second effort is necessary to convince those outside the field, including payers and policy makers, that services such as those described in this chapter should continue to be funded. Occupational therapists must increase efforts to measure and demonstrate the positive outcomes of occupational therapy intervention.

There is no doubt that the future will hold considerable challenges. However, the successes, such as those described in this chapter, are a sound foundation for a promising future for occupational therapy community-based vocational rehabilitation.

 ## STUDY QUESTIONS

1. Describe the components of a comprehensive work evaluation.
2. Identify assessments that could be used in a community-based work program.
3. Discuss the elements of "best practice" in occupational therapy for community-based work programs.
4. Identify worksites in your community that may benefit from occupational therapy services.
5. Develop a proposal/concept paper for a community-based work program in your community.

REFERENCES

American Occupational Therapy Association. (1986). Work hardening guidelines. *American Journal of Occupational Therapy, 40*(12), 841–843.

Anthony, W.A., Cohen, M.R., and Danley, K.S. (1988). The psychiatric rehabilitation model as applied to vocational rehabilitation. In *Vocational rehabilitation of persons with prolonged psychiatric disorders*. Baltimore: Johns Hopkins.

Appleberg, K., Romanov, K., Heikkila, K., and Honkasalo, M.L. (1996). Interpersonal conflict as a predictor of work disability: A follow-up study of 15,348 Finnish employees. *Journal of Psychosomatic Research, 40*(2), 157–167.

Azhar, F.T. (1996). *The relevance of worker identity to return to work in clients treated for work related injuries*. Unpublished master's thesis. Department of Occupational Therapy, University of Illinois at Chicago.

Barker, J.A. (1992). *Paradigms: The business of discovering the future*. New York: Harper-Collins.

Barker, L.T. (1994). Community-based models of employment services for people with psychiatric disabilities. *Psychosocial Rehabilitation Journal, 17*(3), 55–65.

Baron, K., Kielhofner, G., Goldhammer, V., and Wolenski, J. (1998). *A user's manual for the OSA: The occupational self-assessment.* Chicago: Department of Occupational Therapy, University of Illinois at Chicago.

Bigos, S.J., Battie, M.C., Spengler, D.M., Fisher, L.D., Fordyce, W.E., Hansson, T.H., Nachemson, A.L., and Wortley, M.D. (1991). A prospective study of work perceptions and psychosocial factors affecting the report of back injury. *Spine, 16*(1), 1–6.

Braveman, B.H. (1999). The model of human occupation and prediction of return to work: A review of related empirical research. *Work: A Journal of Prevention, Assessment and Rehabilitation, 12*(1), 13–23.

Braveman, B.H., and Fisher, G. (1997). Managed care: Survival skills for the future. *Occupational Therapy in Health Care, 10*(4), 13–31.

Cohen, M., and Anthony, W.A. (1988). A commentary on planning a service system for persons who are severely mentally ill: Avoiding the pitfalls of the past. *Psychosocial Rehabilitation Journal, 12*(1), pp. 69–72.

Cooper, C.L., and Marshall, J. (1976). Occupational sources of stress: A review of the literature relating to coronary heart disease and mental health. *Journal of Occupational Psychology, 49,* 11–28.

Corner, R., and Kielhofner, G. (1996). *The work environment impact scale.* Chicago: Department of Occupational Therapy, University of Illinois at Chicago.

Corner, R., Kielhofner, G., and Lin, F.L. (1997). Construct validity of a work environment impact scale. *Work, 9,* 21–34.

Corner, R.A., Kielhofner, G., and Olson, L. (1998). *A user's guide to the work environment impact scale (version 2.0).* Chicago: Department of Occupational Therapy, University of Illinois at Chicago.

Eisenberg, L. (1977). Disease and illness: Distinctions between professional and popular ideas of sickness. *Culture, Medicine, and Psychiatry, 1,* 9–23.

Feinberg, M.B. (1996). Changing the natural history of HIV disease. *Lancet, 348,* 239–246.

Fellin, P. (1993). Reformulation of the context of community based care. *Journal of Sociology and Social Welfare, 20*(2), 57–67.

Fisher, A. (1994). *Assessment of motor and process skills: Test manual.* Fort Collins: Colorado State University.

Forsyth, K., Salamy, M., Simon, S., and Kielhofner, G. (1998). *A user's guide to the assessment of communication and interaction skills (ACIS) (version 4.0).* Chicago: Department of Occupational Therapy, The University of Illinois at Chicago.

Foster, E. (1995). *Liberty Directions.* Liberty Mutual Insurance Company Newsletter. Hartford, CN: Liberty Mutual Insurance Company.

Germain, C.B. (1991). *Human behavior in the social environment.* New York: Columbia University Press.

Hagberg, M., Silverstein, B., and Wells, R. (1995). *Work-related musculoskeletal disorders (WRMDs): A reference book for prevention.* London: Taylor and Francis.

Hammel, J. (1999). The life rope: A transactional approach to exploring worker and life role development. *Work: A Journal of Prevention, Assessment and Rehabilitation, 12*(1), 47–60.

Hanson, C.S., and Walker, K.F. (1992). The history of work in physical dysfunction. *American Journal of Occupational Therapy, 46*(1), 56–61.

Hogg, R.S., O'Shaugnessy, M.V., Gatarac, N., Yip, B., Craib, K., Schecter, M.T., and Mantaner, J.S. (1997). Decline in deaths from new antiretrovirals (letter). *Lancet, 349,* 1294.

Jenkins, J.H. (1988). Ethnopsychiatric interpretations of schizophrenic illness: The problem of nervous within Mexican-American families. *Culture, Medicine and Psychiatry, 12*(3), 303–331.

Kenny, D., Powell, N., and Reynolds-Lynch. (1995). Trends in industrial rehabilitation: Ergonomics and cumulative trauma disorders. *Work: A Journal of Prevention, Assessment and Rehabilitation, 5*(2), 133–142.

Kielhofner, G. (1995). *A model of human occupation: Theory and application* (2nd ed.). Baltimore, MD: Williams and Wilkins.

Kielhofner, G. (1997). *Conceptual foundations of occupational therapy* (2nd ed.). Philadelphia: F. A. Davis.

Kielhofner, G., and Brinson, M. (1989). Development and evaluation of an aftercare program for young chronic psychiatrically disabled adults. *Occupational Therapy in Mental Health, 9,* 1–25.

Kielhofner, G., Mallinson, T., Crawford, C., Nowak, M., Rigby, M., Henry, A., and Walens, D.

(1998). *A user's manual for the occupational performance history interview (version 2.0)*. Chicago: Department of Occupational Therapy, The University of Illinois at Chicago.

Kleinman, A. (1988). *The illness narratives: Suffering, healing, and the human condition*. New York: Basic Books.

Lohman, H., and Peyton, C. (1997). The influence of conceptual models on work in occupational therapy history. *Work: A Journal of Prevention, Assessment and Rehabilitation, 9*(3), 209–219.

Longres, J. (1990). *Human behavior in the social environment*. New York: Columbia University Press.

Mallinson, T. (1995). *Work programs at Hinsdale Hospital: Addressing work in mental health settings*. Chicago: Department of Occupational Therapy, University of Illinois at Chicago.

Matheson, L.N. (1982). *Work capacity evaluation: A training manual for occupational therapists*. Trabuco Canyon, California: Rehabilitation Institute of Southern California.

Matheson, L.N., Ogden, L.D., Violette, K., and Schultz, K. (1985). Work hardening: Occupational therapy in industrial rehabilitation. *American Journal of Occupational Therapy, 39*(5), 314–321.

Minar, D., and Greer, S. (1969). *The concept of community: Readings with interpretation*. Chicago: Aldine.

Munoz, J.P., and Kielhofner, G. (1995). Program development. In G. Kielhofner (Ed.), *A model of human occupation: Theory and application* (2nd ed.). Baltimore: Williams and Wilkins.

National Institutes of Health. (1985). *Activity record*. Bethesda, Maryland: Department of Rehabilitation Medicine.

Niemeyer, L.O., and Jacobs, K. (1989). *Work hardening: State of the art*. Thorofare, NJ: Slack.

Olson, L. (1995). *Work readiness: Day treatment for the chronically disabled*. Chicago: Department of Occupational Therapy, University of Illinois at Chicago.

Salz, C. (1983). A theoretical approach to the treatment of work difficulties in borderline personalities. *Occupational Therapy in Mental Health, 3*(3), 33–46.

Smith, M.J. (1987). Occupational stress. In G. Salvendy (Ed.), *Handbook of ergonomics/human factors* (pp. 844–860). New York: John Wiley.

Smith, M.J., Carayon, P., and Sanders, K.J. (1992). Electronic performance monitoring, job design and worker stress. *Applied Ergonomics, 23*(1), 17–27.

Trombly, C.A. (1995). Occupation: Purposefulness and meaningfulness as therapeutic mechanisms. *American Journal of Occupational Therapy, 49*(10), 960–972.

Velozo, C.A. (1993). Work evaluations: Critique of the state of the art of functional assessment of work. *American Journal of Occupational Therapy, 47*(3), 203–209.

Velozo, C., Kielhofner, G., and Fisher, G. (1990). *A user's guide to the worker role interview (research version)*. Chicago: Department of Occupational Therapy, University of Illinois at Chicago.

Velozo, C., Kielhofner, G., and Fisher, G. (1998). *A user's guide to the worker role interview (version 9)*. Chicago: Department of Occupational Therapy, University of Illinois at Chicago.

ADDITIONAL READINGS

Gates, L. (1993). The role of the supervisor in successful adjustment to work with a disabling condition: Issues for disability policy and practice. *Journal of Occupational Rehabilitation, 3*(4), 179–190.

Harvey-Krefting, L. (1985). The concept of work in occupational therapy: A historical review. *American Journal of Occupational Therapy, 39*(5), 301–307.

Lougheed, V. (1998). Employer-based rehabilitation. *Canadian Journal of Rehabilitation, 12*(1), 33–37.

Strong, J., and Gibson, L. (1997). A review of functional capacity evaluation practice. *Work, 9,* 3–11.

Shrey, D. (1998). Effective worksite-based disability management programs. In P. King (Ed.), *Sourcebook of occupational rehabilitation* (pp. 389–409). New York: Plenum Press.

Tramposh, A. (1998). On-site therapy programs. In P. King (Ed.), *Sourcebook of occupational rehabilitation* (pp. 275–286). New York: Plenum Press.

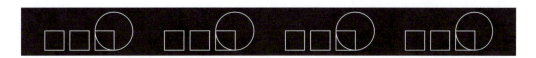

9

C H A P T E R

Adult Day-Care Programs

Nancy Van Slyke, EdD, OTR

■ OUTLINE

Activity program coordinator
Administrator
Adult day care
Case manager
Consultant

Medical/restorative model
    centers
Older Americans Act of 1965
Social model centers

LEARNING OBJECTIVES

This chapter is designed to enable the reader to:
- Substantiate the need for adult day-care programs.
- Discuss the factors that have influenced the development of adult day-care programs in the United States.
- Name and describe the types of adult day-care program models.
- Discuss how adult day-care services might meet the needs of the program participants.
- Describe the various roles of occupational therapy practitioners working in adult day-care programs.

 INTRODUCTION

During the 20th century, the number and proportion of Americans aged 65 years and older rose dramatically. David (1996) indicates that the U.S. Census Bureau reported that the proportion of older Americans increased from 4 percent of the U.S. population in 1900 to almost 13 percent of the population in 1994. By the year 2050, the number of Americans over age 65 is projected to more than double, with individuals who are 85 years and older representing approximately 15 percent of the population (David, 1996). U.S. Census Bureau reports indicate that women now live about seven years longer than men and the ratio of older women to older men increases with age. As a result, women are three times more likely than men to be widowed but are less likely to have a family caregiver assist them during illness (David, 1996). Extended life expectancy increases the likelihood of individuals becoming dependent on others due to poor health or disability and, therefore, requiring additional medical and social support.

This growth in numbers of the older population and longer life spans has significantly impacted individuals, their families, and medical and social systems. Since the early 1980s, the provision of care for the elderly has been gradually shifting from hospitals, nursing homes, and other medical facilities to home and community settings. David (1996, p. 16) states that according to the U.S. Census Bureau (1990), "more than 95% of older adults live in community, rather than institutional, settings." According to Osorio (1991, 1993), growing restrictions on the duration of home health care limit its ability to meet the adult client's long-term needs.

Adult day care, a community-based group program, provides an alternative solution by providing much needed health, medical, social, respite, and rehabilitation services while allowing the elderly individual to remain at home (Conyers, 1996). Although most adult day-care centers serve older adults with functional impairments, a growing number of specialized centers, sometimes referred to as day treatment, day health care, or day hospitals, are available for younger adults with disabilities (Osorio, 1991, 1993; Weissert et al., 1990). Although individual programs may differ in emphasis, all share the goal of enabling clients to function as effectively and indepen-

164

dently as possible within the context of their community (American Occupational Therapy Association, 1986a).

The National Institute on Adult Day Care (NIAD) defines **adult day care** as a community-based group program designed to meet the needs of functionally impaired adults through an individual plan of care that provides a variety of health, social, and related support services within a protective setting during any portion of a day. Since the overall goal of adult day care is to assist the participant to continue living in the community at the highest level of independence possible, support for caregivers should also be an important aspect of services (National Institute on Adult Day Care, 1990). Adult day care, with its holistic approach to meeting the needs of the clients/participants, offers a variety of roles for occupational therapy practitioners (American Occupational Therapy Association, 1986a, 1986b; Osorio, 1991, 1993).

This chapter provides a brief overview of the development of adult day care in the United States and highlights the models of adult day-care programs as a continuum. It also describes the indirect and direct roles assumed by occupational therapy practitioners, which may vary depending on the focus of the program.

 ## DEVELOPMENT OF ADULT DAY CARE IN THE UNITED STATES

Although the concept of adult day care was first introduced in England during the 1950s, it was not until the 1960s and the influence of the **Older Americans Act of 1965** that adult day care was first introduced in the United States (Conyers, 1996; Epstein, 1992; Osorio, 1991, 1993). Initially, the purpose of these programs was to facilitate early hospital discharge for chronically ill elderly patients who required continued restorative services (Conyers, 1996). Legislation in the 1960s and early 1970s led to expanded health services and extended the adult day-care concept to include emphasis on stimulation, activity, and the supportive services needed to maintain the older person in a community setting following rehabilitation (Conyers, 1996; Epstein, 1992). According to Weissert et al. (1990), since the 1980s a tremendous growth in the development of specialized or special-purpose centers for younger adults with physical disabilities, mental retardation, developmental disabilities, mental health needs, and persons with human immunodeficiency virus (HIV) has occurred. With changes in the health-care system and a growing elderly population, adult day care provides an alternative approach to the complex health-care needs of the elderly and special populations, providing a means of postponing or eliminating the need for institutional care.

 ## ADULT DAY-CARE PROGRAM MODELS

Day-care programs offer a wide range of health, social, and supportive services. The type of services provided by an adult day-care center depends on the center's program emphasis or philosophy and the needs of the participants and their caregivers (Conyers, 1996; Epstein, 1992; Johnson, 1981; Osorio, 1991, 1993). Johnson reports that the basic services offered by most programs include general nursing, social work, recreational activities, assistance with activities of daily living, supervision of personal hygiene, lunch, and referral to community agencies. According to the National Institute on Adult Day Care, services provided by adult day-care centers are designed to meet one or more of the following goals:

1. Promote the person's maximum level of independence.
2. Maintain the person's present level of functioning as long as possible, preventing or delaying deterioration.
3. Restore and rehabilitate the person to the highest possible level of functioning.
4. Provide support, respite, and education for families and other caregivers.
5. Foster socialization and peer interaction (National Institute on Adult Day Care, 1990).

A therapeutic milieu and an interdisciplinary focus by the program staff are two of the primary principles of client care identified by the National Standards and Guidelines for Adult Day Care Programs (National Institute on Adult Day Care, 1990). NIAD's standards, as well as individual state regulations, provide guidelines for program development and staffing requirements. Regardless of the day-care model, services provided for an individual participant are based on a functional assessment and developed through an interdisciplinary care planning process. Although the staffing constituents vary with the day-care model and the services provided, the care planning process is often well defined. In states where adult day-care centers are licensed or certified, this planning process may also be regulated (National Institute on Adult Day Care, 1990; Osorio, 1991; Von Behren, 1988). Individual care plans are often problem oriented and include specific goals, activities, time frames, and responsible staff (Osorio, 1991).

Osorio (1991) suggests that the variety of programs can best be conceptualized as a continuum, with **social model centers** serving frail, at-risk, or semi-independent participants on one end and **medical/restorative model centers** serving significantly impaired participants at the other end.

SOCIAL MODEL CENTERS

Social model centers provide supportive, social, and recreational services for participants with stable health conditions who may be at risk due to social isolation, lack of family support, physical frailty, or other similar characteristics. Although screening or periodic health monitoring may be available, services often are limited to the basic provision of meals, transportation, recreation, and social meetings. Prevention is a primary goal (Osorio, 1991). These programs are often funded under Title XX of the Social Security Act or Title III of the Older Americans Act (American Occupational Therapy Association, 1986a; Conyers, 1996; Johnson, 1981). The Older Americans Act, specifically Title III, includes federal grants to state agencies (Area Agencies on Aging) for the provision of nutrition and social services to older individuals through local programs such as senior citizen centers.

MEDICAL/RESTORATIVE MODEL CENTERS

These centers, often classified as day hospitals or day treatment centers, serve participants with unstable health conditions and specific functional impairments. Participants may have a wide range of disabilities including Alzheimer's disease, Parkinson's disease, rheumatoid arthritis, cerebrovascular accident (CVA), or multiple sclerosis (Griswold, 1998). Usually located in hospitals, rehabilitation centers, skilled nursing facilities, or as separate programs in medical model centers, their goal is short-term treatment and timely discharge, frequently to a social model center, where the participant can receive longer-term maintenance and episodic restorative services (Osorio, 1991). Services provided often include on-site nursing care, one or more therapies on a consult or contract basis, medical social work, therapeutic recreation, and adapted social or recreational activities. Occasionally, medical services, such as physical assessments, psychiatry, dentistry, or podiatry, may be available. Maintenance of function and, in some cases, restoration of function are the primary goals. Although medical/rehabilitative day care may be funded through Medicaid and some private insurers, day-care clients often must use their personal financial resources to fund program participation (American Occupational Therapy Association, 1986a; Conyers, 1996; Johnson, 1981; Osorio, 1991).

 ## OCCUPATIONAL THERAPY ROLES

Osorio (1993) suggests that, philosophically, occupational therapy and adult day care both emphasize individual potential for growth and development, and a holistic integration of the mental, physical, social, emotional, spiritual, and environmental aspects of well-being. While occupational therapy services focus on a person's ability to engage in self-care and leisure activities while maintaining or enhancing perceptual, motor, cognitive, and psychological skills (American Occupational Therapy Association, 1986a), the roles of the occupational therapy practitioner may vary according to the emphasis of the adult day-care program. The direct service role includes the typical tasks of providing evaluation and treatment specific to the needs of individual clients. The indirect service roles enacted by occupational therapists in adult day-care settings may include consultant, administrator, and case manager. Additionally, the occupational therapist's role may include that of educator, researcher, or advisory board member (Conyers, 1996).

A recent study completed at the University of Southern California indicated that occupational therapy could provide effective preventive programs as well as rehabilitative services for the elderly (Clark et al., 1997). Results of this extensive study demonstrate that "OT programs could be used in conjunction with other services to proactively manage health care and either generate health improvements or at least slow decline" (Clark et al., 1997, p. 1325). Through this program, the elderly participants "learned to balance their activities, enact healthy decisions in their lives, and face fears that created stagnation by challenging themselves" (Mandel, Jackson, Zemke, Nelson, and Clark, 1999, p. 16).

DIRECT-CARE CLINICIAN

Providing direct care is the most common role for the occupational therapist and the occupational therapy assistant. In centers with a medical/restorative emphasis, the practitioners may provide services similar to those in the traditional medical type of setting, i.e., screening, comprehensive evaluation of the participant's functional performance, treatment, and discharge planning. Treatment interventions might include teaching participants adaptive techniques, training staff in the use of therapeutic activities to improve or maintain the participant's capabilities in self-care, and providing restorative programs when indicated (American Occupational Therapy Association, 1986a, 1986b; Conyers, 1996; Osorio, 1993).

The following is an example of the direct-care clinician's role with a day-care participant:

A 72-year-old retired teacher who had a cerebrovascular accident with resulting left hemiplegia had previously received rehabilitation services at a local hospital and skilled nursing facility. On discharge from the skilled nursing facility, she moved to her married daughter's home, as she was no longer able to live independently in her own apartment. The client's daughter and her family were able to provide supervision and assistance at night, but due to the family's work schedules, were unable to provide adequate supervision during the day. On admission to the adult day-care program, the client required minimal assistance in all activities of daily living (ADL). She ambulated with a quad cane but required continual verbal coaching. She was depressed and often isolated herself from other participants.

The occupational therapy plan consisted of an individualized plan of care that included the following:

● Managing the involved upper and lower extremities to maintain function and prevent contractures through group exercise programs, prescribed activity programs to be followed at the center, and development of a home exercise and activity program
● Increasing psychosocial skills and independent living skills through participation in group activities, including lunch planning and preparation sessions, activities of daily living training to include self-care and basic homemaking skills and community outings
● Establishing and increasing independence within the home environment through home visits for assessment, adaptation, and instruction to facilitate independence and safety, and basic home management training in meal preparation, laundry, and money management

The individualized plan was based on family and participant needs. Since the occupational therapist provided services only three times per week, many of the activities prescribed by the therapist were already included in the center's activity program. In addition, family education and support were an important component of the program.

ACTIVITY PROGRAM COORDINATOR

Occupational therapists and occupational therapy assistants can also serve as activity program coordinators. The **activity program coordinator** assesses the interests of each participant to determine the activity needs and preferences, develops an activities plan that records the client's interests, general activity needs, and goals, and identifies the activities to be used to achieve these goals. Activities programs include planned events and tasks that meet the interests and needs of the participants. These ongoing programs contribute to the prevention of deterioration of mental, physical, and social abilities by providing incentives and opportunities to engage in continuing life experiences and interests (Conyers, 1996). Programs are usually varied so that individual, as well as group, activities are offered (Conyers, 1996; Neustadt, 1985).

CASE MANAGER

The role of **case manager** is a newer role for occupational therapists (American Occupational Therapy Association, 1991). In this role, the occupational therapist may serve as an internal case manager who functions as the liaison between the clinical staff and client/family. He or she coordinates the treatment regimen by assessing, facilitating, planning, and advocating for the client's health needs. More specifically, the case manager is a personal advocate for the participant. He or she performs an initial client screening, leads the interdisciplinary team in preparing and regularly updating a comprehensive treatment plan, monitors intervention by other team members, assesses community support services, and functions as the family or caregiver liaison (American Occupational Therapy Association, 1991; Conyers, 1996).

The following example briefly describes the role of the occupational therapist as an internal case manager:

> The occupational therapist is a team member at an adult day-care facility that provides restorative care for clients with a variety of diagnoses. All clients currently live with family members and require supervision and continuing rehabilitation following discharge from a local rehabilitation hospital or skilled nursing facility. Other team members include a physical therapist, a registered nurse, a recreational therapist, and a social worker. Each member of the team must also assume the responsibilities of internal case manager for a designated number of clients, as well as provide individual therapy (direct services) for referred clients.

Team members functioning as the case manager might perform the following tasks:

- Communicate regularly with the client and family regarding program goals and progress.
- Coordinate the treatment regimen.
- Establish the client's treatment/day-care attendance schedule.
- Lead the interdisciplinary team in preparing and regularly updating the comprehensive care plan.
- Monitor the implementation of the treatment program.
- Act as the liaison with payer sources.
- Assess community support services to assist in the management of the client.
- Coordinate appropriate after-care support services such as personal attendants, chore services, home health care, etc.

The occupational therapist continues as the internal case manager throughout the participant's attendance at the adult day-care center.

CONSULTANT

In the role of **consultant,** occupational therapists do not provide direct treatment. Rather, they use their expertise in the development and delivery of day-care services (Epstein, 1985; Osorio, 1993). According to Osorio (1993), in social model programs where the emphasis is on maintenance of skills and adaptation to impairment, occupational therapists can be effective consultants in the areas of activity adaptation, environmental design, group process, and training paraprofessional staff. Occupational therapy consultants can also provide expertise to enhance the quality of the day-care center by defining and developing specific programs or assisting staff in solving existing or potential problems (Conyers, 1996). Epstein (1985) suggests that key elements in consultation include an understanding of organizational theory and dynamics, proficiency in effective communication, and the ability to diagnose problems and offer appropriate solutions or strategies.

The following is an example of the occupational therapist in the role of consultant:

> In a metropolitan area, a teaching hospital committed to serving the health-care needs of the elderly wanted to develop an adult day-care program. Although the administrative members of the organization understood the concept of adult day care and were sure of its validity for their population, they had no experience in delivering this type of service. To develop the program and the appropriate health and social services, the administration decided to employ a health-care consultant with a rehabilitation background, a local occupational therapist with experience in consulting and in the provision of adult day-care programs.

The consultant's activities included:

- Helping the board understand the variations possible in day-care program models and services
- Providing support and guidance in planning for space
- Designing the program plan and developing policies, procedures, budgets, and staff requirements
- Providing support and guidance in developing community referral sources
- Assisting in the development of public relations materials
- Assisting in the development of grant requests for funding
- Assisting in the search, and participating in the interview process, for the permanent director

The consultant's services were retained for approximately six months following the employment of the director.

ADMINISTRATOR

The adult day-care program's **administrator** or executive director is responsible for the total operation of the agency. This individual assumes responsibility for the financial management, regulatory compliance, and marketing of the facility as well as program planning, implementation, and evaluation (Conyers, 1996; Osorio, 1991). Conyers indicates that while few occupational therapists are currently employed as administrators of adult day-care programs, experienced individuals possess the leadership and management skills to direct such a program. According to Osorio (1991), the supervisory, planning, and documentation skills required are similar to those necessary for managing an occupational therapy department or private practice.

 ## CONCLUSION

As the elderly population steadily increases in number and health-care delivery shifts from institutions to the community, adult day-care programs appear to be an appealing and cost-effective alternative to meet the complex health-care needs of the elderly. The skills and expertise of occupational therapists and occupational therapy assistants afford the practitioner a variety of employment opportunities within this community-based setting.

 ## STUDY QUESTIONS

1. Discuss how legislation has affected the development of adult day-care programs in the United States.
2. Identify the two basic models of adult day-care programs, describing the purpose, potential funding, and services usually provided for each.
3. Justify the need for occupational therapy services in adult day-care programs.
4. Compare and contrast the role of occupational therapy in the adult day-care programs with the role of occupational therapy in the more traditional medical settings, i.e., acute hospital and rehabilitation hospital.
5. Discuss some strategies for developing and funding a new adult day-care program in your community.

REFERENCES

American Occupational Therapy Association. (1986a). Occupational therapy in adult day-care (position paper). *American Journal of Occupational Therapy, 40*(12), 814–816.

American Occupational Therapy Association. (1986b). Roles and functions of occupational therapy in adult day-care. *American Journal of Occupational Therapy, 40*(12), 817–821.

American Occupational Therapy Association. (1991). *Statement: The occupational therapist as case manager.* Rockville, MD: American Occupational Therapy Association.

Clark, F., Azen, S., Zemke, R., Jackson, J., Carlson, M., Mandel, D., Hay, J., Josephson, K., Cherry, B., Hessel, C., Palmer, J., and Lipson, L. (1997). Occupational therapy for independent-living older adults. *Journal of the American Medical Association, 278*(16), 1321–1326.

Conyers, K.H. (1996). Adult day care. In K. Larson, R. Stevens-Ratchford, L. Pedretti, and J. Crabtree (Eds.), *ROTE: Role of occupational therapy with the elderly* (pp. 453–484). Bethesda, MD: American Occupational Therapy Association.

David, D. (1996). Gerontology: The study of aging and older adults. In K. Larson, R. Stevens-Ratchford, L. Pedretti, and J. Crabtree (Eds.), *ROTE: Role of occupational therapy with the elderly* (pp. 15–24). Bethesda, MD: American Occupational Therapy Association.

Epstein, C.F. (1985). The occupational therapy consultant in adult day care programs. *Gerontology Special Interest Section Newsletter, 8*, 3–4.

Epstein, C.F. (1992). Adult day care consultation in a rural community. In E.G. Jaffe and C.F. Epstein (Eds.), *Occupational therapy consultation: Theory, principles and practice* (pp. 419–430). St. Louis, MO: Mosby.

Griswold, L. (1998). Community-based practice arenas. In M.E. Neistadt and E.B. Crepeau (Eds.), *Willard and Spackman's occupational therapy* (9th ed., pp. 810–815). Philadelphia: Lippincott.

Johnson, J. (1981). The community life program: A social model of day care for the elderly. In B. Jacobs (Ed.), *Working with the at-risk older person: A resource manual* (pp. 60–68). Washington, DC: The National Council on Aging.

Mandel, D., Jackson, J., Zemke, R., Nelson, L., and Clark, F. (1999). *Lifestyle redesign: Implementing the well elderly program.* Bethesda, MD: American Occupational Therapy Association.

National Institute on Adult Daycare. (1990). *Standards and guidelines for adult day care.* Washington, DC: National Council on Aging.

Neustadt, L.W. (1985). Adult day care: A model for changing times. *Physical and Occupational Therapy in Geriatrics, 4*, 53–66.

Osorio, L.P. (1993). Adult day care. In H.L. Hopkins and H.D. Smith (Eds.), *Willard and Spackman's occupational therapy* (pp. 60–68). Philadelphia: Lippincott.

Osorio, L.P. (1991). Adult daycare programs. In J.M. Kiernat (Ed.), *Occupational therapy and the older adult* (pp. 241–258). Gaithersburg, MD: Aspen.

Von Behren, R. (1988). *Adult daycare: A program of services for the functionally impaired.* Washington, DC: National Council on Aging.

Weissert, W., Elston, J., Bolda, E., Zelman, W., Mutran, E., and Mangum, A. (1990). *Adult day care findings from a national survey.* Baltimore: Johns Hopkins.

ADDITIONAL READINGS

American Occupational Therapy Association. (1993). *Occupational therapy roles.* Rockville, MD: American Occupational Therapy Association.

Baum, C., and Law, M. (1998). Community health: A responsibility, an opportunity, and a fit for occupational therapy. *American Journal of Occupational Therapy, 52*, 7–10.

Coriensky, M., and Buckley, V.C. (1986). Day activities programming: Serving the severely impaired chronic client. *Occupational Therapy in Mental Health, 6*, 21–30.

Crist, P.H. (1986). Community living skills: A psychoeducational community based program. *Occupational Therapy in Mental Health, 6*, 51–64.

Hall, E.R. (1990). Day care and the continuum of care. *Community long term care services for the elderly* (pp. 25–30). New York: Haworth.

Hasselkus, B.R. (1992). The meaning of activity: Day care for persons with Alzheimer's disease. *American Journal of Occupational Therapy, 46*, 199–206.

Joe, B.E. (1996). Adult day care: A new opportunity. *OT WEEK,* December 12, pp. 18–19.

Levy, L.L. (1991). Occupational therapy in adult day care. *American Journal of Occupational Therapy, 40,* 814–816.

McDonald, K.C., and Epstein, E.P. (1986). Roles and functions of occupational therapy in adult day care. *American Journal of Occupational Therapy, 40,* 817–821.

Sanker, A., Newcomer, R., and Wood, J. (1986). Prospective payment: Systemic effects on the provision of community care for the elderly. *Home Health Care Services Quarterly, 7*(2), 93–116.

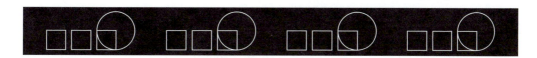

10
C H A P T E R

Independent Living Programs

Robin E. Bowen, EdD, OTR, FAOTA

■ OUTLINE

173

Americans with Disabilities Act of 1990
Community orientation
Consumer control
Freedom of choice
Full participation in society
Handicapping nature of the environment
Independent living
Independent living center
Independent living model
Independent living movement
Independent living residential program

Independent living transitional program
Individualized written independent living plan (IWILP)
Medical model
Normalization
Rehabilitation Act of 1973
1978 Amendments to the Rehabilitation Act
1986 Amendments to the Rehabilitation Act

LEARNING OBJECTIVES

This chapter is designed to enable the reader to:
- Compare and contrast the medical model and the independent living model.
- Describe the history and philosophy of independent living programs.
- Describe legislation that has affected the development of independent living programs.
- Describe different types of independent living programs.
- Discuss the role of the occupational therapist in independent living programs.

 INTRODUCTION

Prior to the 1970s, two service delivery models predominated to address the needs of persons with disabilities: (1) the medical rehabilitation model and (2) the vocational rehabilitation model. Once a person was stabilized following a traumatic injury or after the discovery of a disabling disease, he or she would typically be referred to a medical rehabilitation program. Here, the individual would receive services from physicians, nurses, occupational therapists, physical therapists and/or speech therapists, and a number of other health-care professionals. Under the direction of the physician, the health-care professionals would establish a plan based on their respective areas of expertise to help the individual reach full rehabilitation potential. If adequate supports existed in the home, or if the person became fully independent, the individual was ultimately discharged to his or her home. If not, the individual was transferred to a long-term care facility.

If the person was deemed capable of pursuing employment, referral could be made to a vocational rehabilitation program where additional training or services could be provided to prepare the individual for competitive employment. Yet a gap existed in these two service delivery systems. Because of this, many individuals, who could have lived independently with appropriate community support services, were institutionalized. Others were confined to their home environments if they were lucky enough to find housing that was at least partially accessible. Even those living in their homes were dependent on others to perform tasks necessary for survival, such as getting groceries or prescriptions. In general, communities were not accessible. Few, if any, curb cuts were available to allow a person in a wheelchair to maneuver onto a sidewalk. Accessible bathrooms in restaurants or shopping centers were nonexistent. No advocacy programs to address unmet needs or centralized referral sources for the few available services existed. Persons with disabilities had no united voice other than that given to them by vocational and medical rehabilitation professionals. The independent living movement grew out of a need for persons with disabilities to have more autonomy, better services, and self-determination.

This chapter describes the concepts associated with independent living programs, including how the independent living model differs from the medical model in approach. The chapter briefly highlights major legislation impacting the independent living movement, emphasizing its philosophy and community orientation. Various types of programs are presented in conjunction with a discussion of the occupational therapy roles assumed in independent living programs. The chapter also presents two case studies to illustrate the occupational therapy practitioner's role in independent living programs.

 # INDEPENDENT LIVING

Independent living is "control over one's life based on the choice of acceptable options that minimize reliance on others in making decisions and performing everyday activities, including managing one's affairs, participating in day-to-day life in the community, fulfilling a range of social roles, and making decisions that lead to self-determination and the minimization of physical or psychological dependence upon others" (Frieden and Cole, 1985, p. 735). Advocates of independent living continually work to bridge the gap between medical rehabilitation and vocational programs to allow persons with disabilities to live independently in the community.

COMPARING THE MEDICAL MODEL AND THE INDEPENDENT LIVING MODEL

A comparison of the medical model and the independent living model will help to clarify the differences between the two models. Although both models seek to promote independence among persons with disabilities, the way each model approaches this goal is significantly different.

Occupational therapists have traditionally been educated in, and practice within, the medical model. In the **medical model,** the physician is the primary decision maker and team expert who is ultimately responsible for services provided to the patient by the health-care team. The problems are usually viewed in terms of the persons' inability to perform activities of daily living (ADLs) and/or to participate in gainful employment. In either situation, "the problem is assumed to reside in the individual. Therefore, it is the individual who needs to be changed." The solution lies in the individual's compliance with the prescribed therapeutic program (DeJong, 1981, p. 21).

In the **independent living model,** the consumer (the person receiving services) is the primary decision maker who determines the services in which to participate. The ultimate goal far exceeds ADL performance or gainful employment, with individuals seeking self-direction and full integration into society. In the independent living model, the problem to overcome is not defined as the limited physical, mental, or emotional status of the individual but rather as an inaccessible environment, the negative attitudes of others, and even the rehabilitation process itself. "The problem resides . . . in the solution offered by the rehabilitation paradigm, most notably in the dependency-inducing features of the relationship between professional and client" (DeJong, 1981, p. 22). The solutions to these problems are self-help, consumer control, removal of barriers and disincentives, peer counseling, and advocacy.

THE INDEPENDENT LIVING MOVEMENT

The **independent living movement,** a social movement that advocates equality for disadvantaged individuals, was an outgrowth of several other social movements including the civil rights movement, consumerism, demedicalization, deinstitutionalization, and self-help. "The disability movement therefore originated in the USA (as did many of the social movements in the West in the 1960s and 1970s) because it was in the USA that the social forces described above were most potent" (Craddock, 1996, p. 18). Furthermore, World War II, the Korean War, and the Vietnam War resulted in increased numbers of young people with disabilities, thus facilitating an expansion in medical technology. Persons were now surviving traumas that before would have resulted in death, and even the severely disabled were able to live longer lives (another factor impacting the timing of the movement).

Legislation

As early as the 1950s, rehabilitation professionals recognized that competitive employment was not an option for all people with disabilities. These rehabilitation professionals promoted legislation, albeit unsuccessfully, to provide funding for services to allow a person with a disability to live independently in the community. Similar bills drafted in the 1960s also failed because it was felt that the bills were not consistent with the vocational objectives of the existing vocational rehabilitation program (DeJong, 1983).

In 1973, President Nixon signed the **Rehabilitation Act,** also known as P.L. 93-112. Although the independent living provisions in the bill had been deleted, this legislation was nevertheless vital to the advancement of the independent living movement. The 1973 Rehabilitation Act mandated a service priority for severely handicapped persons, provided civil rights to handicapped persons by mandating affirmative action employment programs within the federal government and by those organizations contracting with the federal government, and banned discrimination on the basis of disability in those programs receiving federal financing (DeJong, 1983). Furthermore, funds were designated for a comprehensive needs assessment study that ultimately identified gaps in services between the medical model, the vocational rehabilitation model, and the ability of a person with a disability to function adequately in society.

The **1978 Amendments to the Rehabilitation Act** (P.L. 95-602), signed by President Carter, "marked the beginning of federal involvement in the independent living movement. For the 1st (sic) time a program was created whose primary goal is to help disabled persons to live independently" (Verville, 1979, p. 447). Title VII—Part A of this law included a provision for comprehensive services in independent living programs such as attendant care, peer counseling, and assistance with housing and transportation. It also allowed for the establishment, operation, and funding of independent living centers in the United States.

The **1986 Amendments to the Rehabilitation Act** (P.L. 99-506) established criteria for individuals receiving independent living services. The criteria include: (1) a physical and/or mental disability which poses a substantial handicap to independence or community integration and (2) a reasonable expectation that the consumer will be able to achieve independence or community integration with services (Wong and Millard, 1992).

The **Americans with Disabilities Act of 1990** (P.L. 101-336) is considered by many to be the most comprehensive legislation affecting the civil rights of persons with disabilities. Signed into law by President Bush, the Americans with Disabilities Act (ADA) extended civil rights protection for persons with disabilities beyond federal programs to both public and private bodies. The ADA addresses five areas: (1) employment, (2) public accommodations, (3) state and local government, (4) public transportation, and (5) telecommunications (American Occupational Therapy Association, 1993a). See Chapter 5, "Legislation and Policy Issues," for details regarding the ADA.

In summary, the study sanctioned by the 1973 Rehabilitation Act identified the need for independent living programs, and the 1978 Amendments to the Rehabilitation Act provided funds for these programs. The 1986 Amendments established criteria for participation in independent living programs, and the civil rights portions of the Rehabilitation Act and the ADA mandated integration of persons with disabilities into society (Table 10–1).

Philosophy

The philosophy of the independent living movement emphasizes freedom of choice and equality for persons with disabilities. "Disabled persons including the most severely disabled have both the capacity and desire to be self directing and independent in all aspects of their lives" (DeJong, 1981, p. 1). The independent living movement espouses **consumer control,** allowing persons with disabilities to decide what course of action, if any, is best. Indeed, no one knows more about the needs of persons with disabilities than persons with disabilities (Shapiro, 1994).

Concepts contributing to the independent living philosophy include normalization, freedom of choice, full participation in society, and access to the physical environment. **Normalization** is simply the right to live as normal a life as one chooses and to have opportunities to live normally. It can be exemplified as the right to live in a home or apartment rather than a group home or nursing home.

Freedom of choice includes both the right of a person with a disability to have the

TABLE 10–1

LEGISLATIVE TIMELINE

Date	Legislation	Key Points
1973	Rehabilitation Act (P.L. 93-112)	Established a service priority for severely handicapped persons Provided affirmative action employment programs within the federal government Banned discrimination on the basis of disability for programs receiving federal funding
1978	Amendments to the Rehabilitation Act (P.L. 95-602)	Provided funding for the establishment and operation of independent living centers Included a provision for comprehensive services
1986	Amendments to the Rehabilitation Act (P.L. 99-506)	Established criteria for individuals receiving independent living services
1990	Americans with Disabilities Act (P.L. 101-336)	Extended civil rights protection for persons with disabilities to public and private bodies

same options as nondisabled persons and the right to make choices for oneself given those options. For example, a person with a disability has the right to get married, have or adopt children, and select a neighborhood in which to live. Each person should have the same opportunity to be financially secure and have equal employment opportunities. A person with a disability should be able to choose to attend or not attend therapy on a given day without externally imposed rewards or consequences.

Allowing **full participation in society** encompasses the right of persons with disabilities to vote and participate in politics or to worship in the setting of their choice. Individuals with disabilities should be able to attend a symphony, a professional football game, or a high school play and be seated with family and friends, not in the "handicapped section."

Finally, the independent living movement attempts to increase awareness of the **handicapping nature of the environment.** A therapist working within the independent living philosophy would focus on changing environmental factors to increase accessibility rather than trying to change the individual. For example, a person who uses a wheelchair for mobility cannot navigate the wheelchair through a doorway because it is too narrow. Using the independent living philosophy, one would advocate widening the doorways rather than increasing the person's balance and upper-extremity strength in an attempt to teach the person to use crutches to get through the small doorway. While this philosophy advocates making the physical environment accessible to persons with disabilities, it expands beyond this narrow interpretation of the "handicapping nature of the environment" to address less visible barriers such as negative attitudes and discriminatory opinions and actions toward persons with disabilities.

Community Orientation

Independent living differs from traditional rehabilitation in its **community orientation**. Traditional medical rehabilitation programs have focused on activities of daily living (e.g., feeding, grooming, dressing, bathing, and toileting) and instrumental activities of daily living (e.g., balancing a checkbook or doing laundry) that primarily enable the person to function in the home environment. Some programs, especially vocational rehabilitation programs, strive to integrate the individual with a disability back into the work environment. Yet both of these rehabilitation programs often stop short of integrating the person back into the greater community. Independent living programs address issues such as housing, personal attendant management, transportation, and physical access to the community and all it offers.

 ## *INDEPENDENT LIVING PROGRAMS*

Independent living programs are community-based service and advocacy organizations designed to meet the needs of persons with disabilities to allow them to achieve and maintain independent lifestyles (ILRU Research and Training Center on Independent Living). Most independent living programs are community based, nonprofit, nonresidential, and consumer controlled (i.e., a majority of persons involved in program development and service provision are persons with disabilities).

In 1992, there were more than 400 independent living programs in the United States (Egan, 1992). Yet many programs provide services to facilitate independent living but do not meet the criteria for being an independent living program. These programs are typically referred to as *independent living service providers.* Medical treatment services, sheltered workshops, and medical equipment suppliers are just a few examples of independent living service providers. Such programs serve as referral sources for independent living programs.

TYPES OF INDEPENDENT LIVING PROGRAMS

Since their origination, three different types of independent living programs have evolved: (1) centers, (2) transitional programs, and (3) residential programs.

The initial concept of an independent living program was that of a nonresidential program, which is also referred to as an **independent living center.** To receive federal funding, an independent living center must provide a minimum of four services. These include: (1) information about and referral to agencies supplying applicable services (such as housing, transportation, and attendant care), (2) peer counseling, (3) advocacy services, and (4) independent living skills training. Furthermore, the program must be nonprofit, nonresidential, and consumer controlled in that "at least 51 percent of any group making decisions, including the center's staff and board of directors" be persons with disabilities (Egan, 1992, p. 15). Some would say that the primary function of an independent living center is to allow persons with disabilities to *continue* to live independently in the community.

In an **independent living transitional program,** the goal is to move the consumer from a more dependent living situation to a more independent situation. Independent living skills training is key to such a program and typically includes training in attendant management, transportation and mobility, money management, medical maintenance, self-advocacy, social skills, living arrangements, sexuality issues, and possibly an exploration of educational or vocational opportunities. Transitional programs are goal oriented (the person learns and practices skills in a supported environment that is similar to the eventual living site) and time linked (support is not designed to be provided on an ongoing or permanent basis). Although consumer participation is encouraged, the transitional program is not necessarily consumer controlled.

Independent living residential programs were designed to allow a person with a severe disability an alternative to being institutionalized or living with family members. Such programs are live-in programs that coordinate or directly provide services such as attendant care and transportation. According to Bachelder (1985, p. 104),

> A variety of arrangements in residential independent living programs exists including individual rooms for several persons in a home or apartment, apartment-type units in a free-standing facility, converted motels or even dormitory-type buildings in which a greater number of persons can be accommodated.

The degree of consumer involvement varies in residential programs although consumers are provided with opportunities for involvement. Only 6 percent of independent living programs are exclusively residential (Bowen, 1994).

VARIATIONS AMONG PROGRAMS

Although independent living programs are usually classified by type of service setting (center, transitional, or residential), they can differ in a number of other ways. One such difference is the service delivery method. In 1994, Bowen found that most programs deliver services themselves or on a contract basis (48 percent). Some offer services primarily on a referral basis (7 percent). Still others use both methods of service delivery (43 percent). Approximately half of the independent living programs require vocational goals as a prerequisite or incidental to participation, while others do not have this requisite (Richards, 1981, p. 36). And, although some programs (28 percent) serve only one population of consumers (e.g., only persons with hearing impairments or only persons with cerebral palsy), most programs (72 percent) serve persons with many different disabilities (Bowen, 1994). Originally, the independent living movement focused on younger adults with physical disabilities. In more recent years, the movement has expanded to include persons of all ages and those with cognitive and emotional disabilities.

Initially, most independent living programs were located near university campuses. As the independent living movement progressed, programs shifted to urban areas and then to rural areas. Currently, most programs serve persons in urban geographic settings (57 percent), some serve rural areas (30 percent), and others (13 percent) provide services to consumers in both settings (Bowen, 1994).

Finally, programs vary according to the primary funding source. Approximately one-third of all programs (31 percent) are funded by a combination of sources, and 29 percent are funded primarily through federal grants. Fourteen percent receive primary funding from a rehabilitation agency, while 11 percent use "other" grant monies. Six percent are primarily funded by charging a fee for services, and less than 1 percent are funded primarily through donations. The remaining 7 percent use other unidentified sources (Bowen, 1994).

INDEPENDENT LIVING PROGRAM PERSONNEL

The staffing patterns in independent living programs vary depending on a number of variables, including the type of program, services to be provided, location, number of persons to be served, and funding. The roles and functions of staff most typically found in independent living programs are described in this section. The 1978 Amendments to the Rehabilitation Act called for substantial involvement of persons with disabilities in the policy direction and management of independent living centers. Although Bowen (1994) found that 90 percent of independent living programs employ some persons who do not have disabilities, every effort is made to find qualified persons with disabilities to fill management, staff, and board positions.

Most independent living programs are headed by a director, who is the chief executive officer of the program. He or she is responsible for the total operation and is the primary spokesperson for the program. The director serves on the board of directors and assists in policy development for the program (Arkansas Rehabilitation Research and Training Center, 1980).

In larger programs, an assistant director, who could assist in program planning and overseeing operations, might be needed. At times, an assistant director is also given the responsibility for developing and directly supervising specific program components such as the peer counseling program, housing, and/or transportation.

The coordinator of personal attendant services is responsible for the recruitment, training, referral, and placement of personal attendants with consumers in the community. The coordinator develops orientation programs for consumers who plan to use personal attendants. The coordinator is also responsible for maintaining current knowledge regarding funding sources for personal attendant services and helping consumers secure these funds.

A coordinator of independent living skills oversees the independent living specialists and creates programming to develop independent living skills as needed by consumers in the community. The coordinator of independent living skills also keeps abreast of services available in the community so that appropriate referrals can be made. The independent living specialist assists consumers in a myriad of services, including skills training, counseling, education, and referral to other agencies. The independent living specialists are usually the staff members who have the most face-to-face contact with consumers.

A financial benefits counselor provides information and counseling on financial benefits and entitlements and is an advocate for persons with disabilities dealing with funding agencies such as Social Security and Welfare (Arkansas Rehabilitation Research and Training Center, 1980). Independent living specialists may also assume this task.

Some independent living programs employ other staff members. If a program has a vocational emphasis, an employment services specialist may be employed. Housing specialists give advice on altering homes to make them accessible, and are also aware of accessible housing available within the community. A transportation specialist is an advocate for accessible transportation and provides information on adapting automobiles and vans. Educational specialists are knowledgeable regarding all areas of education and serve as advocates for persons with disabilities when dealing with educational institutions.

If a large population of consumers with a specific diagnosis resides in the program's geographic catchment area, a special populations coordinator can address the unique needs of a particular population. While many programs have individuals who volunteer to serve as peer counselors (people with disabilities who counsel others with similar disabilities), some employ peer counselors. In either situation, a coordinator for the peer counseling program is needed. Most programs also provide or contract with interpreters for persons with hearing impairments (Bowen, McNally, Kearney-Sadler, and Richards, 1994).

A majority of independent living programs have a board of directors. These governing boards set policies and establish rules for the program. The members are typically individuals who are interested in services for persons with disabilities and who are active members of their respective communities. Most board members of independent living programs are volunteers (Arkansas Rehabilitation Research and Training Center, 1980). Some programs also have advisory committees. Advisory committees often include professionals whom the director of the program can call for information or assistance.

 ## OCCUPATIONAL THERAPY'S ROLE IN INDEPENDENT LIVING PROGRAMS

In its 1993 statement, the American Occupational Therapy Association (AOTA) established that occupational therapy practitioners can serve an important role in independent living programs (American Occupational Therapy Association, 1993b). According to AOTA (1993b, p. 310),

> The philosophy of the independent living movement parallels that of occupational therapy in that both advocate for the right of the individual to live as independently as possible in the community and both work to promote environments and attitudes that will facilitate that process. Occupational therapy practitioners are uniquely qualified to provide services in independent living settings, as they have an understanding of the dynamic interplay between the individual and the environment, and can suggest and implement modifications to enhance the individual's ability to function in a given environment.

An occupational therapy practitioner may assume a number of roles in an independent living program. When working in an independent living program, he or she must be familiar with available community resources in order to make appropriate referrals, must support the philosophy of independent living, and be an advocate of consumer autonomy. The occupational therapy practitioner might work as a consultant, on a referral basis, or as an employee. He or she might function solely as an occupational therapist or as an independent living specialist, a case manager, an administrator, and/or as an advocate for persons with disabilities. Yet the leadership and direction of the program must be allowed to come from within the disabled community as "the able-bodied professional can provide expertise to the program, but cannot provide the essential motivation or role modeling necessary to initiate progress toward independent living" (Berrol, 1979, p. 457).

Services are typically provided in the consumer's home or in the community, not in a clinical setting. This is ideal in that it provides the consumer with the opportunity to learn in the "real environment" and does not require the consumer to generalize information to another setting. However, it may require the occupational therapy practitioner to be more creative in treatment planning and the execution of that plan. Community environments are not as easy to maneuver in or to make adaptations to as clinical environments. Thus, occupational therapy practice in an independent living program is at an advanced level; it is not considered entry-level practice (American Occupational Therapy Association, 1993b).

Independent living legislation does not mandate the use of occupational therapy services. It also does not identify occupational therapy as a primary service (Baum, 1980). Yet almost half of the independent living programs in the United States (46 percent) use occupational therapy personnel in serving their consumers (Bowen, 1994).

OCCUPATIONAL THERAPY EVALUATION AND INTERVENTION PLANNING

The assessment methods used by an occupational therapist in an independent living program typically do not differ significantly from those used in a clinical setting. The occupational therapist would still analyze the activity and the context in which the activity is performed, as well as the consumer's ability to perform the task. The therapist would then identify barriers to performance and make recommendations accordingly. However, in the independent living setting the approach is different. Since referrals for occupational therapy services will not typically come from a physician in an independent living setting, occupational therapists must follow state regulations regarding working with or without a physician's referral (American Occupational Therapy Association, 1993b). If the therapist resides in a state requiring physician referral, the consumer requesting occupational therapy services will need to obtain a physician's referral prior to the onset of services. Working within an independent living model, the occupational therapy practitioner asks the consumer what the consumer's goals are for therapy and assesses only the performance components and contextual issues that might be affecting those aspects of the person's performance in reaching those specific goals. The occupational therapy practitioner then discusses treatment options with the consumer and collaborates with the consumer who ultimately chooses the approach taken to achieve the stated goals. In summary, the consumer identifies strengths and needs and specifies his or her own goals.

If the therapist is unable to ascertain specific goals from the consumer, the therapist may use interviewing techniques outlined in the Canadian occupational performance model (Law et al., 1991) or those published by Payton, Nelson, and Ozer (1990). Using these techniques "will help ensure that activities are indeed purposeful, and that the individual's goals, not the health-care professional's goals for that person, are being addressed" (Bowen, 1996). Collaboration between the consumer and the occupational therapist is critical. In the independent living model, the therapist and consumer collaborate throughout the evaluation and intervention process.

Situations do arise when a consumer is unable to make autonomous decisions. In these situations, a surrogate could make treatment decisions until the person is able to make them. On the other hand, a consumer may request services that the therapist feels are unnecessary or may even do harm. In such cases, the occupational therapy practitioner has an ethical and moral obligation to explain why the services would not be beneficial and stand by that decision unless the consumer is able to provide a rational reason why a certain approach would be best for him or her. At all times, the occupational therapist must abide by the Occupational Therapy Code of Ethics and current Occupational Therapy Standards of Practice.

In an independent living program, "the therapist's principal role [would] be one of support in helping the client to solve problems related to his or her interactions with the environment as opposed to directing therapeutic activities designed to restore certain of the client's abilities" (Frieden and Cole, 1985, p. 738). Consistent with the independent living philosophy, the therapist should strive to make adaptations to the environment rather than trying to change the individual. Yet researchers found that occupational therapists write treatment goals that address changing the person 12 times more often than goals focusing on altering the environment (Brown and Bowen, 1998). Occupational therapists working in independent living settings use assistive devices, adaptive techniques, and environmental modifications in treatment more frequently than restorative treatment techniques.

DOCUMENTATION

The goals and objectives of the consumer's program are documented in an **individualized written independent living plan (IWILP).** While the formats of IWILPs differ somewhat from program to program, they typically include a list of the services to be used by the consumer and identify the consumer's specific goals. Some specify the responsibilities of the consumer and those of the independent living program personnel. IWILPs are then signed and dated by the consumer and a representative of the independent living program.

Beyond the IWILP, no other specific guidelines exist for ongoing documentation in independent living programs. Some programs establish their own internal requirements for documentation, while others have none. Furthermore, occupational therapists contracting with independent living programs may not be advised of internal requirements, seeing ongoing documentation as the choice and responsibility of the contracted therapist.

The recommendation is that occupational therapy practitioners working in independent living programs maintain regular and ongoing documentation of services provided. Occupational therapy practitioners are encouraged to follow the guidelines established by the American Occupational Therapy Association (1995) in the revised "Elements of Clinical Documentation," recognizing that some minor adaptations to these guidelines might be needed based on the uniqueness of the setting.

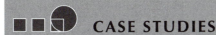 **CASE STUDIES**

TODD

Todd, a 20-year-old male who incurred a C7 spinal cord injury one year ago, had been living at home with his parents since he was discharged from his rehabilitation program. He recently decided that he was ready to return to college and wanted to live in an apartment near the campus as he did prior to his accident. His vocational rehabilitation counselor (to whom he was referred following his hospitalization) provided Todd with the phone number of a local independent living center and that of an independent living center near the college.

When Todd contacted the local independent living center, an independent living specialist discussed Todd's plans with him. He then asked Todd to make a list of what he thought he needed to be able to do to fulfill his primary goals of returning to school and living in an apartment independently.

Todd indicated a desire to use the services of a personal attendant (PA) since his two-hour self-care regime each morning left him with little energy to pursue other activities. The independent living specialist had Todd participate in a seminar on hiring, keeping, or firing (if one has to) a PA that was offered on a regular basis at the center.

Todd was concerned about finding accessible housing near the college and arranging transportation to get him to classes on campus. He had an accessible van but could not functionally use it on campus to go from class to class. The independent living specialist suggested that he contact the Office for Students with Disabilities at the college and see what services already existed and to find out if they could meet his needs. This office identified accessible housing on campus and explained on-campus transportation options. Todd preferred to live off campus and was successful in locating an apartment through the area independent living center. He ultimately decided to commute to campus each day in his van and then use campus buses (which were accessible) to get around campus.

The independent living center also indicated that it maintained a list of potential personal assistants. Todd obtained the list when he moved and he interviewed five candidates. He ultimately chose two personal attendants—one primary provider and another who agreed to serve on an "as needed" basis.

After becoming comfortable with his independent living specialist, Todd voiced some concerns about interacting socially, now that he had a disability. His independent living specialist recommended that Todd talk to a volunteer peer counselor. The man he recommended also had a spinal cord injury and had attended the same college about 10 years earlier. Todd agreed, albeit somewhat reluctantly at first. He found the peer counselor to have a wealth of information, having been in many similar circumstances. He and his peer counselor role-played some awkward situations, providing Todd with some new strategies. Todd also sought information on sexuality, as this was an area that had not been addressed in the hospital or in his rehabilitation program. His peer counselor suggested some written resources and discussed his own experiences openly and honestly.

Todd also stated that he needed some education regarding basic housekeeping and cooking. During rehabilitation, he did not participate in these activities, indicating that his mother would do those tasks. He said that he now wished he had spent his time "in rehab" learning these skills rather than dressing and grooming, as they would serve him better in the long run. He opted to wait until he was in his apartment to receive training in these areas so that he could learn in the actual setting. After moving to his apartment, the independent living center arranged for an occupational therapist to work with Todd to identify assistive devices and adaptive techniques to assist him in completing home-making tasks. Ultimately, he decided to have his personal attendant complete most of the routine cleaning tasks and chose to do his own cooking—an activity he found he thoroughly enjoyed.

While occupational therapy played more of an ancillary role in this situation, an occupational therapist could have performed many of the tasks completed by the independent living specialist. While the independent living specialist or other service providers might suggest a service, the consumer has the right to choose or refuse such an offer. For example, Todd's independent living specialist offered training in money management. Todd declined, citing his ability to manage funds prior to his injury when living independently.

GAYLE

Gayle is a 22-year-old single woman who has had spastic paralysis of both her lower extremities and the left upper extremity since birth. Gayle gave birth to a son who was born six weeks premature. Her son was placed on a breathing monitor. Due to Gayle's physical limitations, she was unable to perform cardiopulmonary resuscitation (CPR) as demonstrated by hospital staff. The physician was hesitant to allow her son to go home with her if she could not perform this task. Reluctantly, Gayle agreed to allow her son to go into a foster home until his lungs had developed adequately and the breathing monitor was no longer necessary. Gayle continued to see her son twice weekly.

At the age of 7 months, her son was medically stable and was no longer using the monitor, yet the state social services agency was averse to allow her son to return to her due to her physical limitations. Gayle contacted the independent living center. The center, in turn, put her in contact with an occupational therapist with whom the center contracted.

The occupational therapist worked with Gayle to identify alternative methods to perform basic care tasks for her child and assisted in identifying funding sources to pay for adaptive equipment. Much of the adaptive equipment Gayle needed was not available commercially and had to be custom made. For example, it was easiest for Gayle to take her son from his baby bed when she was in her wheelchair using a side approach in order to use her stronger right arm. When she lowered the rails vertically, she was afraid her son would fall from the bed before she could retrieve him. Collaboratively, Gayle and the therapist decided that it would be best if the bed rail released horizontally along a "track" from either end. This would allow Gayle options on removing her son from the bed, depending on his position, and give her more control over how much of the bed rail space was open.

The occupational therapist and Gayle also collaborated on choosing the best car seat for her son and methods for getting her son in and out of her van and in and out of his car seat. Gayle initially chose to bathe her son in the kitchen sink, as it was easier to get him in and out, and was at an accessible height for her. Later, a new strategy had to be developed because her son got too big to fit in the sink. Soon he was able to climb in and out of the tub by himself. Gayle would then transfer out of her chair onto the floor to assist him in bathing.

Gayle chose to hold her son in her lap during meals rather than trying to get him in and out of a high chair. She was able to use her left arm to hold her son steady, especially if she had rolled in close to the table for added stability, and use her right arm to feed him. She chose pull-over bibs so she would not need to spend time tying a bib with one hand.

Gayle was already adept at dressing and diapering her son and made clothing choices for him based on their ease in donning and doffing. The therapist assessed ADLs, IADLs, and safety measures in response to requests by the state social services agency. The occupational therapist was asked to testify at the custody hearing in regards to Gayle's ability to care for her son. Gayle received custody of her son just prior to his first birthday.

 ## CONCLUSION

In recent health-care literature, "consumerism" is a much debated topic with health-care professionals debating the pros and cons of individuals with disabilities having the right to choose the services in which they participate. As such, the independent living movement is finally permeating the traditional medical model and the greater health-care system. "These changes are perceived as new and innovative by many health-care professionals, although they originated in the 1960s and 1970s" (Bowen, 1996, p. 24). Although this chapter describes how "consumerism" does work in independent living programs, these same concepts can be used in all treatment settings. Perhaps the greatest contribution of the independent living movement is the philosophy that the person with a disability can be an autonomous individual and a fully participating member of society—a goal mutually supported by occupational therapists.

STUDY QUESTIONS

1. Compare and contrast the role of occupational therapy in the independent living model with the role of occupational therapy in the medical model.
2. Discuss how legislation has impacted the development of independent living programs.
3. Define the concepts of consumer control, full participation, and normalization, and describe how they relate to the independent living movement.
4. Identify three types of independent living programs, and describe the benefits and limitations of each type.

REFERENCES

American Occupational Therapy Association. (1993a). Position paper: Occupational therapy and the Americans with Disabilities Act (ADA). *American Journal of Occupational Therapy, 47,* 1083–1084.

American Occupational Therapy Association. (1993b). Statement: The role of occupational therapy in the independent living movement. *American Journal of Occupational Therapy, 47,* 1079–1080.

American Occupational Therapy Association. (1995). Elements of clinical documentation (revision). *American Journal of Occupational Therapy, 49,* 1032–1035.

Arkansas Rehabilitation Research and Training Center. (1980). *Implementation of independent living programs in rehabilitation.* Hot Springs, AR: Author.

Bachelder, J. (1985). Independent living programs: Bridges from hospital to community. *Occupational Therapy in Health Care, 2*(1), 99–107.

Baum, C. (1980). Independent living: A critical role for occupational therapy. *American Journal of Occupational Therapy, 34*(12), 773–774.

Berrol, S. (1979). Independent living programs: The role of the able-bodied professional. *Archives of Physical Medicine and Rehabilitation, 60,* 456–457.

Bowen, R.E. (1994). The use of occupational therapists in independent living programs. *American Journal of Occupational Therapy, 48,* 105–112.

Bowen, R.E. (1996). Practicing what we preach: Embracing the independent living movement. *OT Practice, 1*(5), 20–24.

Bowen, R.E., McNally, S., Kearney-Sadler, R., and Richards, L.G. (1994). *Model curricula for teaching occupational therapists about independent living and vocational rehabilitation for persons with head injuries.* Kansas City, KS: University of Kansas Medical Center.

Brown, C., and Bowen, R.E. (1998). A comparison of models in occupational therapy treatment planning. *Occupational Therapy Journal of Research, 18*(1), 44–62.

Craddock, J. (1996). Responses of the occupational therapy profession to the perspective of the disability movement, part 1. *British Journal of Occupational Therapy, 59*(1), 17–22.

DeJong, G. (1981). *Environmental accessibility and independent living outcomes.* East Lansing, MI: The University Center for International Rehabilitation, Michigan State University.

DeJong, G. (1983). Defining and implementing the independent living concept. In N.M. Crewe and I.K. Zola (Eds.), *Independent living for physically disabled people.* San Francisco: Jossey-Bass.

Egan, M. (1992). IL movement puts clients in control. *OT Week,* February 13, pp. 14–15.

Frieden, L. (1980). Independent living models. *Rehabilitation Literature, 41*(7–8), 169–173.

Frieden, L., and Cole, J.A. (1985). Independence: The ultimate goal of rehabilitation of spinal cord-injured persons. *American Journal of Occupational Therapy, 39,* 734–739.

ILRU Research and Training Center on Independent Living at TIRR. An orientation to independent living centers (Brochure). Houston: Author.

Law, M., Baptiste, S., Carswell-Opzoomer, A., McColl, M., Polatajko, N., and Pollock, N. (1991). *The Canadian occupational performance measure manual.* Toronto: CAOT Publications.

Payton, O.D., Nelson, C.E., and Ozer, M.N. (1990). *Patient participation in program planning: A manual for therapists.* Philadelphia: F. A. Davis.

Richards, L. (1981). Characteristics and functions of independent living programs: A national perspective. In G.T. Milligan (Ed.), *Implementing independent living centers: Conference proceedings.* Hot Springs, AR: Arkansas Rehabilitation Research and Training Center.

Shapiro, J.P. (1994). *No pity: People with disabilities forging a new civil rights movement.* New York: Times Books.

Verville, R.E. (1979). Federal legislative history of independent living programs. *Archives of Physical Medicine and Rehabilitation, 60,* 447–451.

Wong, H.D., and Millard, R.P. (1992). Ethical dilemmas encountered by independent living service providers. *Journal of Rehabilitation, 58*(4), 10–15.

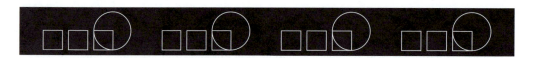

11 CHAPTER

Home Health

Kathy G. Lemcool, MA, OTR
Donna A. Wooster, MS, OTR, BCP
Linda Gray, OTR
S. Blaise Chromiak, MD

■ OUTLINE

KEY TERMS

Case coordinator
Case manager
Cultural competence
Fee for service (FFS)
Homebound status
Intermittent service
Medicaid
Medical necessity
Medicare

Occupational performance areas
Occupational performance
  components
Outcome and Assessment
  Information Set (OASIS)
Prospective payment system
  (PPS)
Skilled service

LEARNING OBJECTIVES

This chapter is designed to enable the reader to:
- Discuss the factors that have contributed to the recent growth in home health care.
- Describe the personal characteristics of the home-care occupational therapy practitioner that enhance the ability to deliver effective home health services.
- Describe the characteristics that make delivery of home health therapy services different from therapy services delivered in institution-based settings.
- Explain the roles of each member of the home health-care team.
- Identify important occupational performance areas and components for evaluation and intervention in the home health setting.
- List essential equipment and supplies that are needed for providing home-based occupational therapy.
- Describe proper procedures and circumstances for planning discharge of home therapy services.
- Identify the documentation skills needed to effectively satisfy third-party payers and meet quality standards for home health practice.

 ## INTRODUCTION

The word "home" conjures up images of comfort, security, familiarity, and escape from the world. It is more than just the physical structure and the place for everyday events. The home is part of a person's identity. Thus, the importance of the home cannot be understated, including its potential as a therapeutic setting (Opacich, 1997).

The home has many advantages as a therapeutic environment. For example, the client can be directly observed performing activities in his or her everyday environment, and the therapist can assess the support systems available. However, it also presents some unique situations and demands. The therapist in home health care must be an independent practitioner and feel comfortable and confident in situations that require spontaneous decision making. Home-based health-care delivery is currently experiencing a resurgence and growth that is predicted to continue. As a result, health-care providers in the home are faced with new and ever-changing challenges affecting the client's care.

The occupational therapy practitioner's role is to return people to functional independence and reclaim their identity. Doing so allows them to remain at home, an especially important and meaningful personal goal for the client (Atchison et al., 1997). For occupational therapy, providing care to persons in real environments, where many of the occupations of self-care, work, and leisure naturally occur, is optimal. Occupational therapy practitioners, who consistently have emphasized the impact of physical, social, and cultural environmental contexts on human performance, are natural providers of services in this community-based setting. As home-based therapy delivery grows, occupational therapy practitioners must be able to adapt to meet the needs of the population and also comply with ever-changing policy revisions that affect funding and reimbursement.

This chapter provides an overview of the historical events and factors impacting home-based occupational therapy and describes the personal qualities of the practitioner, safety, and family as unique aspects of home-based care. The chapter also presents information about the provision of home-based services, including the team members involved, referrals, reimbursement sources, and the requirements for service. Specific functions of occupational therapy in home health, such as evaluation, intervention, discharge planning, and documentation, are addressed to prepare practitioners to meet the challenges of the 21st century. The chapter concludes with a case study that highlights the use of occupational therapy in home health.

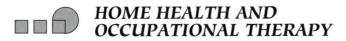

HOME HEALTH AND OCCUPATIONAL THERAPY

HISTORICAL OVERVIEW

Before the creation of the large health-care industry produced by the enormous growth in health-care technology of the 1960s, providing health care in the home was the norm. Voluntary nongovernmental agencies, such as Visiting Nurse Associations (VNAs), provided care in the home. These agencies, originally beginning in the late 1800s, continued to grow and expand, eventually including occupational therapy as a service (Youngstrom, 1997). Cases were recorded in the 1920s mentioning home occupational therapy services. The first article mentioning occupational therapy in connection with a home health-care agency was documented in 1949 (Youngstrom, 1997).

Many occupational therapy practitioners of today may be unaware that only 50 years ago, health-care delivery in the home was commonplace and natural. Home was where health care began, providing services such as births assisted by uncertified midwives, home visits by physicians, and palliative care for the terminally ill. Since those beginnings, home health as a service delivery system has experienced a rise, fall, and re-emergence. Although the advent of high-tech health care may make the home environment seem less appropriate for care, a major need for services in the home continues. However, much of the future growth of home health will be dependent on changes in health-care policy and its effect on reimbursement and referrals. The future offers many opportunities for occupational therapy practitioners to expand services and develop skills to meet health needs now and in the years ahead (Navarra and Ferrer, 1997).

FACTORS IMPACTING HOME HEALTH

The largest growth in home health to date occurred in the mid- to late 1960s, with the passage of **Medicare** (Title XVIII of the Social Security Act) and **Medicaid** (Title XIX of the Social Security Act). This legislation provided Medicare reimbursement for home health care of the elderly and Medicaid funding to states for care of the indigent. Later, in the early 1980s, the introduction of diagnosis-related groups (DRGs) for Medicare payments to hospitals significantly influenced the growth and expansion of home health agencies and services to its present level. With DRGs, hospitals are paid a predetermined amount per case, based on the diagnosis rather than on costs reported. As a result, the incentives for providing care for all of the clients' medical problems, typical prior to the introduction of DRGs, were lessened, leading to shorter hospital stays and the discharge of "sicker" clients in an effort to decrease costs and increase profits.

Today, earlier discharge of "sicker" patients to be cared for by families, friends, group homes, and other care providers continues to contribute to the growth of home health services (Youngstrom, 1997). Statistics also show that the rate of growth in Medicare utilization alone in home health care increased from 726,000 persons served in 1980 to an estimated 3.2 million in 1994 (Agency for Health Care Policy and Research, 1996). Similarly, the number of home health visits per capita rose from 22.5 per person in 1980 to an estimated 65.0 visits in 1994. Occupational therapy participation in home health has also increased. An increase of 106.2 percent in the number of occupational therapists declaring home health to be the primary employment setting was reported from 1990 to 1995. Plus, home health is also the most frequently listed setting for therapists working a second job (American Occupational Therapy Association, 1990). These data support the impression that home health services have increased significantly over the past ten to 15 years.

Future Growth

Several factors play a role in predicting future growth of home health care. One factor is a general trend toward deinstitutionalization of care. Currently, care is moving in the direction away from hospitals and into the local community environments.

Also impacting the future of home health is the projected increase in the elderly population as a result of the post-World War II baby boom. The percentage of elderly over age 65 in the U.S. population will increase from 12 percent in 1998 to 15 percent in 2016. In the year 2030, the number of elderly will be one in five, or 20 percent, of the total population (U.S. Bureau of the Census, 2000). Additionally, the numbers of "old-old" persons (those 85 years and older) will experience the greatest increase. Preventing fragile elderly from becoming dependent, thus necessitating institutionalization, will increase the demand for all skilled services to assist and support persons within their homes.

The case load of today's home health practitioner has also changed dramatically to include new and widely diverse client populations such as persons with mental illness, high-risk pregnancies, ill and developmentally delayed infants, and a variety of age groups with physical disabilities. And as medical technology evolves, more persons in the community are in need of skilled services. For example, ventilator-dependent persons and those requiring renal dialysis, who were previously confined to institutionalized care, are now residing in their homes and communities with supportive services. Treatments involving chemotherapy, pain control, and intravenous drug therapies, once only administered in an acute care facility, are now available in the home.

Additionally, concerns about funding for home health services abound as state and federal regulators plan spending cuts precisely because of an overwhelming growth in utilization and expenditures by Medicaid and Medicare (Joe, 1997). Changes in the Medicare reimbursement system are under way. A bundled payment system for home-care services similar to the Medicare DRG prospective payments is being implemented. Data are being collected by the Health Care Financing Administration (HCFA) of Medicare to help determine the appropriate level of reimbursement in a prospective payment system based on the patient's condition, functional level, and several other factors. The **prospective payment system (PPS)** reimbursement method uses a fixed, predetermined amount allocated for treating a patient and is based on rates set for an agency rather than payment based on actual cost reports. Future issues and growth trends will be impacted largely by the outcome of these funding changes (Marrelli and Krulish, 1999).

In response to these issues, which affect the future of home health, occupational therapy practitioners, like those in other disciplines, have expanded their traditional roles to include areas of prevention and embrace philosophies addressing the needs of the whole person. Rapid changes in client population and needs combined with changes in health-care policy, funding, and role changes impact the skills and competencies needed to thrive in the home health environment of the future.

UNIQUE ASPECTS OF HOME-BASED CARE

For most occupational therapy practitioners, career training usually begins within the security and structure of a health-care institution such as a nursing home, hospital, or clinic. Often, practitioners seek out these facilities as future employment settings. For many occupational therapy practitioners, serving people within their communities and particularly in their homes is a new environment presenting different challenges and rewards.

Although home has strong meaning and significance to the client, providing care in the home requires a shift in control and the power structure. In institutions the staff is in control. Rules and routines, such as visiting hours, therapy and meal times, and medication intervals, to which all must adhere, are set. The physical environment, such as overhead paging systems, antiseptic odors, shiny floors, and equipment, including intravenous infusion pumps and electric beds, is foreign to the client. Health-care personnel, including occupational therapy practitioners, know this environment well. The client is the outsider, often feeling like an anxious guest.

However, when the practitioner enters a client's home, the roles are reversed. The health-care professional is the stranger, encountering the unknown or unfamiliar, for example, interruptions by family members, the smell of food cooking, or floors that may be in need of repair. Sometimes the only available seating choice may be the bedside commode. The care receivers, not the practitioner, direct everything from the scheduling of therapy visits to the temperature in the room.

Whatever the conditions, the occupational therapy practitioner is a guest in the client's home. In most situations, clients and their families tend to be very grateful for the therapist's expertise. They often view the practitioner as a friend as well as a professional helper.

Personal Qualities of the Practitioner

Many occupational therapy practitioners find satisfaction in home care because the setting is less formal and the opportunity to develop a closer relationship with the client is enhanced. However, to be effective and successful in the home environment, certain personal qualities are beneficial for the practitioner to possess or develop.

FLEXIBILITY. Because the locus of control in the home environment is client and family centered, the occupational therapy practitioner must be flexible and creative in scheduling and developing treatment sessions. Clients and families are faced with adjusting to strangers coming into their home at frequent intervals, possibly even daily or several times a day. Discussing the expectations with the families and clients is helpful. Some clients may need to maintain more rigid control of their time and therapy sessions than others. Every attempt must be made to accommodate the family and the client.

Occupational therapy practitioners must also adjust to the schedules of other disciplines involved in the client's care, the geographical location of the client's residence, weather conditions, and the natural order of daily events in the person's life. For example, the practitioner who plans to work with a client on morning self-care routines skills should attempt to schedule therapy sessions in the morning and coordinate his or her visits with the home health aide to assist the person with self-care tasks. At times, scheduling joint visits with other disciplines to coordinate treatment approaches may be necessary. Also, in some situations, the client may not be able to tolerate multiple visits from therapists and other home health providers in one day due to fatigue or to disruptions to the daily activities and routines of the family unit. Individual and family preferences for scheduling must be respected whenever possible.

INDEPENDENCE. Occupational therapy practitioners working in home health settings must be able to work independently. Scheduling, modifying treatment, responding to emergencies, and independent problem-solving skills are all required because there is no peer or supervisor support available on site in the client's home.

In the home, some concerns require an immediate response. For example, if the occupational therapy practitioner finds the client having acute changes in medical condition, the therapist must use clinical judgment to decide the best course of action, such as calling 911 (emergency), notifying the physician or home health nurse, or another alternative action. Some situations in home health require an urgent response, but the opportunities for immediate consultation are unavailable. For example, when a client recovering from a hip fracture falls during a treatment session, the therapist must decide the best course of action. The options may include simply assisting the person to a chair or bed and then recommending that he or she see a physician or not moving the person for fear of causing further damage and calling for an ambulance. Even situations that are not urgent may present difficulty in obtaining a second opinion or consulting with a peer about a client's care. Therefore, the practitioner must have the confidence and clinical judgment to be able to respond to situations as they arise, without needing to rely on other professionals for assistance.

CULTURAL SENSITIVITY. Health care today is seeing an increase in the diversity of the client population with a wide range of cultures and customs that affect the way people relate to each other and carry out their daily lives. Culture is a shared and learned way of living that impacts a person's health and occupations. Cultural diversity is more apparent when working in the home. Cultural objects, foods, and clothing may be found in the home. In addition, there may be cultural customs or behaviors expected when one visits the home; for example, taking one's shoes off and leaving them at the door before entering. If the therapist is culturally unaware or not observant, he or she might unintentionally offend the client or misinterpret environmental cues for behavior. Therefore, the occupational therapy practitioner must be culturally sensitive to the client's needs to prevent interference with interpersonal interactions and treatments. Awareness is the first step in the development of cultural sensitivity and, ultimately, cultural competence (Box 11–1). **Cultural competence** can be defined as "a set of knowledge, skills, and attitudes that allows individuals, organizations and systems to work effectively with diverse racial, ethnic, religious and social groups" (Spector, 2000, p. 11). The practitioner must be aware of personal biases and examine the potential impact of these biases on the provision of care. In addition, the professional must learn about other cultures and be aware of the client's views and possible interpretations of the professional's interactions and methods.

Clients are a valuable source of information, providing teaching in many ways, often eager to explain their cultural beliefs and preferences. For example, cultures often vary in the expression of pain and discomfort. Persons raised in one culture, for ex-

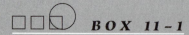

BOX 11–1

Developing Cultural Competence

The occupational therapy practitioner desiring to develop cultural competence should seek to achieve the following:

- Be willing to learn about another's culture.
- Acknowledge and value cultural diversity.
- Have specific and extensive knowledge of the language, values, and customs of particular cultures.
- Have a basic knowledge of human development as it relates to race, ethnicity, gender, disabling conditions, religion, sexual orientation, and lifestyle.
- Understand the influence of culture, gender, race/ethnicity, religion, disabling conditions, and sexual orientation on behaviors and needs.
- Understand that socioeconomic and political factors significantly impact the psychosocial, political, and economic development of ethnic and culturally diverse groups.
- Understand the impact of institutional and individual racism on the utilization of the health-care system by ethnic and culturally diverse groups.
- Understand professional values and codes of conduct as they relate to cultural interaction.
- Understand health-related values, perspectives, and behavior patterns of diverse populations.
- Avoid applying the "cookbook approach" to all people associated with a population or diverse group.
- Generate, modify, and adapt a variety of intervention strategies to accommodate the particular culture of a client.
- Use, send, and interpret a variety of communication skills—verbal and non-verbal—to facilitate the therapist/client interaction.
- Be creative and resourceful in identifying and utilizing cultural value systems on the behalf of the client.
- Help clients to understand, maintain, or resolve their own sociocultural identification.

Source: Wells, S.A. (1994). Cultural competency in occupational therapy. *A Multicultural Education and Resource Guide for Occupational Therapy Educators and Practitioners* (pp. 19–20). Rockville, MD: American Occupational Therapy Association. Copyright © 1994 by the American Occupational Therapy Association, Inc. Reprinted with permission.

ample, in Italian or Jewish families, may be emotionally expressive about pain, while others, for example, in Irish families, may be more stoic and ignore the pain (Spector, 2000). Beliefs about the meaning of pain may also vary. For the client believing that pain infers a problem, activities producing pain may cause the client concern. Through discussions with the client, the practitioner can learn about this belief and provide anticipatory explanation about the therapeutic aspects of the activity.

Occupational therapy practitioners must convey openness and acceptance of the uniqueness of the client's situation and lifestyle by seeking input and feedback from the client and family about their needs and reaction to the rehabilitation process. As a result, the client's culture becomes a source of pride during therapy, hopefully enhancing the client's self-esteem and also the therapeutic outcome. Demonstrating a respect for, and an understanding of, the implications of the client's culture is a major bridge toward building rapport.

ABILITY TO RELATE AND COMMUNICATE. To be effective, occupational therapy practitioners must be able to establish rapport easily and build a solid helping relationship while maintaining professional boundaries. In some cases, this may pose a difficulty because, frequently, the duration of home treatment is longer than it is in inpatient settings. Although this increased duration may attract a practitioner who enjoys a more enduring and deeper therapeutic relationship, the home health practitioner may become more emotionally connected with the client and his or her family. As a result, the practitioner may be more personally affected when a client's condition improves or deteriorates. Using peer support and "debriefing" may be helpful if the professional begins to feel overly attached.

Effective communication with the client and family are necessary as well. Active listening, speaking with clarity, and following up when necessary are essential for effectively communicating with clients and their families. Using therapeutic communication will likely improve overall client-centered care.

All professionals that provide home-based services are part of a multidisciplinary team, and intercommunication among team members is essential. Communication among team members is facilitated with the help of modern technology via cellular phones, pagers, voice mail, electronic mail, fax machines, and in-house communication systems.

Safety

Safety is an important aspect of care for any client, but it is especially significant for the home health practitioner. Two areas of safety are paramount: (1) infection control and (2) personal safety. Actions to secure the safety of the client and practitioner need to be consistently incorporated into daily behaviors so that these actions become habits (Law, 1997).

INFECTION CONTROL PRECAUTIONS. Awareness of infection control precautions is necessary due to the differences between an individual's home and a clinical environment. The typical hospital measures for cleaning and maintaining hygiene are usually not present in the home; for example, the use of special containers for disposal of contaminated waste. In addition, occupational therapy practitioners need to consider where to place their equipment and how to dispose of used materials. All equipment that may be reused with other clients must be properly and thoroughly cleaned with a diluted bleach solution to prevent cross-contamination and infection transmission (Atchison et al., 1997).

Occupational therapy practitioners also need to carry the necessary sanitary and protective devices for adhering to standard precautions, such as gloves, with them. To minimize trips to and from the practitioner's mode of transportation, most commonly a car, all needed devices and supplies, including an appropriate disposal system, should be brought into the home by the occupational therapy practitioner. An instant, no-water-required hand sanitizer is a must in some homes where soap, running water, and disposable towels are not available. Routine hand washing both before and after contact with each client is essential every time to prevent the spread of infection.

PERSONAL SAFETY. In hospital environments, therapists often take their safety for granted. The hospital provides a known and secure environment. However, this is often not the case when working in home health settings. Each home and neighborhood are new and unfamiliar environments. The community members and families are often strangers to the therapist and vice versa. As a result, the therapist must attend to some basic personal safety issues.

Because a majority of home health practitioners use a car for transportation and storage of equipment and supplies, safety measures related to vehicle safety and driving apply. To organize and transport treatment supplies, equipment, and office supplies, such as client records, progress notes, and plans of care, lightweight plastic crates are invaluable and are easy to remove when not needed. Keeping all personal items, client records, and valuables locked in the vehicle, out of view, is recommended. During the visit, placing vehicle keys in a pocket and keeping a spare key readily available, either on the person or in a wallet, helps to prevent being locked out of the vehicle. Only essential items required for evaluation and treatment should be brought into the home. Other safety measures related to the vehicle and driving include:

● Keeping windows up and doors locked
● Driving out of the neighborhood to the nearest phone or using a cellular phone to call for directions if lost, rather than driving around the neighborhood
● Driving to a public place, such as a service station or restaurant, and asking for directions if in an isolated or threatening area

Being prepared is essential. Detailed maps of the area are helpful. Occupational therapy practitioners must also be aware of weather conditions and plan accordingly. Common events, such as heavy rainstorms, can be problematic when clients live off paved roads or in flood-prone areas. The home-care provider should be informed on evacuation and disaster plans for the home health agency and area. Natural disasters can occur rapidly in some areas. Knowledge of the warning signs and safety precautions (or disaster plans) with each weather situation common to the area is important. The local radio setting of the weather station helps the practitioner to stay apprised of changing weather conditions during the day. Tuning in to traffic reports in metropolitan areas may help to avoid traffic jams and dangerous road hazards. Additionally, having the following supplies readily available in the vehicle are important: a shovel; sand, salt, and gravel; de-icer; tire chains; batteries for flashlights and cell phone; extra food and water; extra clothes; gear for cold and rain; phone numbers of towing services in the area; and a full tank of gas. In some areas, a four-wheel drive vehicle may be needed for traveling in hazardous weather and over hazardous terrain.

Daytime visits are recommended whenever possible to reduce the risk of dangers associated with night hours. Occasionally, joint visits can be scheduled with another staff member. Sometimes opening the door in a timely manner is a problem for the family or client. In these situations, calling ahead may be helpful. The client and family can watch for the occupational therapy practitioner and be ready to open the door or provide a hidden key for use by the therapist.

Dressing professionally or wearing a uniform accompanied by a name badge with minimal jewelry is important to help observers recognize the occupational therapy practitioner as a professional who is there to provide services to the community. Comfortable but appropriate clothing is the rule because therapists typically see a wide variety of clients, and services may require awkward positions or sitting on the floor to adjust equipment or take measurements of doorways. For these reasons and others, such as infection control, many home-care practitioners choose scrub suits because of their durability and recognition as a uniform of health-care workers. Clothing should be appropriate for the weather, allowing for flexibility such as in moving from overheated apartments in the winter to the chilly outdoors or in going to homes with no air conditioning in the summer.

Because the home health practitioner often travels alone, leaving a schedule with someone in the home health agency and checking in two or three times a day is advised. A cellular phone is an invaluable tool, especially in an emergency. Spare batteries and a jack that plugs into the cigarette lighter are good backups for use if a cellular phone loses its charge.

Occupational therapy practitioners should not hesitate to report any suspicious activity to the authorities when it is safe to do so. Leaving the area immediately is advised if personal safety is being threatened. Precautionary measures such as those listed earlier and common sense will help to reduce the chances of becoming stranded or a victim of crime.

Family as the Caregiver

Currently, health care focuses on including the family in most aspects of the client's care. Unlike institutional environments, in the home the family is usually the full-time caregiver. In the past, social programs and formal support groups were widely available. However, as funding for these programs decreased due to cost-cutting measures, informal networks are now stressed to fill the void.

The typical caregiver in the home, based on research on care for the elderly, is either a spouse or a female caring for a mother or mother-in-law (Stone, Cafferata, and Sangl, 1987). Often, a daughter or daughter-in-law provides home-management support such as laundry, grocery shopping, and meal preparation for aging parents. When the client is in a different age range, the profile of the caretaker differs. For example, when the client is a physically disabled child or teen, the caregiver would most likely be a young or middle-aged adult parent.

Once in the client's home, occupational therapy practitioners may be introduced to many family members. Assessment of the family must focus on the abilities of the caregivers to provide for the physical needs of the client, his or her support system, and ability to cope with the physical and emotional burdens of caregiving. Caregiver burnout is a very real phenomenon. Options for respite care should be discussed.

Occupational therapy practitioners play an important role in validating the feelings and new responsibilities of the caregiver. Often, the client comes home from a health-care facility where most of the needs were met by the staff. Plus, it may be the first time in the client's lifetime that this family member was dependent on other family members for care. In conjunction with the client's feelings, the family also is dealing with the loss of role fulfillment by the client. For example, the client may be a male who is not working or able to maintain care of the yard and family vehicles at the present time and unable to complete these tasks temporarily or permanently following his illness and disability. The loss of this role has a profound effect on the client's family as well as on his self-image and self-esteem. In addition to dealing with these losses, the caretaker may have to acquire the skills to assume the responsibilities of the client, in addition to the new role of being a caregiver for someone who formerly was independent. These changes can be very stressful and difficult for the caregiver to manage. The practitioner's role in these situations includes providing support, problem solving, and making suggestions for coping with the new demands.

Regardless of the adaptations required, many families will go to great lengths to keep a family member at home, preventing the need for institutional care. Many personal sacrifices may be made, including quitting a job, changing work schedules, and using family leave or vacation time to shoulder this burden. Often feelings of isolation, guilt, resentment, and anger, along with increased daily exhaustion, are connected with these sacrifices.

Caregivers commonly are required to perform a multitude of tasks, often leading to feelings of being overwhelmed by their responsibilities. Examples of some of these tasks are listed in Box 11–2. Support groups may assist in alleviating these feelings so that the caregiver is aware that he or she is not the only person dealing with such problems. Although organized support groups have a role in helping family members through dif-

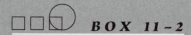

BOX 11-2

Caregiving Tasks

- Be available when (or if) needed.
- Supervise prescribed treatment and general recommendations.
- Evaluate options for treatment and/or services.
- Monitor course of condition and evaluate significance of changes.
- Evaluate strengths/resources of care receiver.
- Anticipate needs for future assistance and services.
- Provide structure for care receiver's daily activities.
- "Run interference" for care receiver in social and community settings.
- "Normalize" care receiver's routine, within bounds of the impairment(s).
- Supervise/directly manage care receiver's resources.
- Cope with difficult or upsetting behavior of the care receiver.
- Maintain adequate communication with care receiver.
- Perform basic ADL for the care receiver.
- Satisfy need for creative/originality to offset tedious routines.

Source: Clark, N.M., and Rakowski, W. (1983). Family caregiving of older adults: Improving helping skills. *The Gerontologist, 23*(6), p. 638. With permission.

---

ficult times, the occupational therapy practitioner also can build a relationship with the caregiver to provide support and allow him or her to express feelings and seek solutions to problems. Asking how the caregiver is doing and actively listening to the replies help to build rapport. Validation of the frustrations, offering suggestions that other families use with success, and referral to community agencies may help. This form of communication acknowledges the burden of caring and opens the door for the home-care provider to be of therapeutic assistance to the family and the client.

TEAM MEMBERS

Numerous disciplines may be involved in the care of the client at home. However, the client and family are the center of the team. One of the professional disciplines assumes the role of the coordinator. Additionally, individual team members assume responsibility for coordinating their care with that of other team members. Interdisciplinary team case conferences and informal mechanisms facilitate this process.

Case Coordinator

Typically, a registered nurse functions as the coordinator of care. In some situations, other disciplines, such as physical or occupational therapists, speech pathologists, or social workers, may fulfill this role. The **case coordinator** (the person making the initial visit to determine the home health needs of the client) is aware of all disciplines providing care to the client and is able to discuss the overall plan of care with the physician and the client/family members when needed. Responsibilities of the case coordinator include communicating changes in status, such as a client's change of residence or changes in medical status, to the team members. Often, the case coordinator also is responsible for informing the team of funding issues and coverage for a particular client. Finally, the coordinator oversees all of the services provided to ensure the client's needs are met while avoiding duplication of services.

The team members also are responsible for informing the case coordinator of pertinent information about the client's case. The occupational therapy practitioner should inform the case coordinator of changes in the client's rehabilitation potential or caregiver situation, impending discharge, or any unusual circumstances.

Registered Nurse

The registered nurse (RN) performs the initial assessment of the client prior to any other disciplines by making visits to the home. Currently, the **Outcome and Assessment Information Set (OASIS),** a standardized and federally mandated format for data collection, is being used to collect data during the initial evaluation to comply with Medicare changes pursuant to the Balanced Budget Act of 1997. OASIS is discussed in more detail later in this chapter.

The RN provides necessary skilled nursing visits. Skilled services provided by home health nurses (in compliance with applicable state laws) include, but are not limited to:

- Monitoring of compliance with medication regimens
- Skilled observation and assessment for drug interactions and side effects
- Wound dressing changes
- Catheter changes
- Monitoring of blood sugars, preparation of insulin, and/or administration of insulin injections
- Monitoring of general medical status, including vital signs
- Performance of intermittent supervisory visits for all licensed practical nurse (LPN) and certified nursing aide (CNA) services
- Education of client and family

A licensed practical nurse (LPN) may be involved in the care by seeing the client between visits by the RN. The LPN provides care similar to that of the RN, under the RN's supervision. However, some agencies do not employ LPNs. The care provided by LPNs must also comply with state practice acts and the duties assigned vary from agency to agency.

Mental Health Nurse

To deliver more comprehensive care, a trend is evolving to include a nurse whose specialty is mental health care. In addition to mental health issues inherent in any physical disability, a growing number of persons with mental illness as a primary diagnosis are being referred to home health agencies for care. Mental health nurses can develop and oversee the services provided for clients in need of mental health interventions. The mental health nurse may also be involved in the completion of the OASIS data initially and intermittently through the client's course of care in Medicare cases.

Home Health Aide

One of the primary needs of clients referred for home health care is that of assistance with activities of daily living (ADLs). While the home health aide (HHA) can provide needed assistance for the client to complete self-care routines, the occupational therapy practitioner must work collaboratively with the HHA, providing the HHA with information about adaptive techniques or equipment being used by the client. Client independence and compliance is reinforced through this instruction.

It is important to explain to the client and family that the occupational therapy practitioner will work toward client/family autonomy and independence so that when the aide services are no longer available, the family and/or client is able to manage daily living tasks. This helps the family and client to realize that the HHA services are temporary in most cases, reinforcing the need for them to work toward achieving self-sufficiency with the therapist's direction.

In most cases, the RN supervises HHAs. However, a therapist can supervise the HHA when the client is being seen by a therapist but does not require a skilled nursing service. Current Medicare regulations state that HHA services will not be reimbursed unless the client requires another service that is considered skilled under the Medicare definition. However, other payment sources, for example, private insurance, may cover these expenses.

Homemaker/Sitter

Although not routinely part of home health care, some agencies offer homemakers and sitters. Medicare does not reimburse these services, but other reimbursement sources may pay for some or all of the service. Additionally, special grant programs, other community agencies, or special Medicaid programs may pay for homemakers and sitters. Homemakers provide services such as housekeeping, meal preparation, errands, and laundry. Sitters provide supervision and companionship and perhaps some light care duties, but these care duties are very limited when compared to those of HHAs.

Occupational Therapy Personnel

The registered occupational therapist (OTR) evaluates and designs a treatment plan to address deficits in the performance areas of work, self-care, and leisure. During the evaluation, which may include items from the OASIS, deficits in **occupational performance components** (sensory, neuromusculoskeletal, motor, cognitive, and psychosocial), **occupational performance areas** (activities of daily living, work and productive activities, and play or leisure activities), and/or prevention issues may be identified. Since performance can be assessed in the home context, important issues such as family support and home accessibility can be evaluated. The therapist gains valuable insights about what tools are available and the lifestyle of the family. This information can be advantageous in designing effective home programs and suggestions for adaptations. Additionally, the family can receive instructions in routine tasks that reinforce the client's achievement of therapy goals.

CERTIFIED OCCUPATIONAL THERAPY ASSISTANT. The primary role of the certified occupational therapy assistant (COTA) is to carry out the treatment as planned and supervised by the OTR following completion of the evaluation. Although routine visits by the COTA can be carried out independently, supervision patterns are established and documented. The frequency of supervisory contact varies with the situation, but most agencies will have guidelines stating the frequency of covisits to be made by the COTA/OTR team. Factors that help to determine the frequency of supervisory contacts needed include competence and experience of both practitioners in the home health practice area, client-specific factors, and requirements of regulatory bodies. Covisits can be used to problem solve issues and modify goals and activities to ensure the effectiveness of the treatment plan. In addition, regular documented contact between the COTA and OTR is essential.

Some insurance payers may require the OTR to cosign the COTA's notes. Although a recommended practice, cosigning does not take the place of covisits and verbal supervisory exchanges.

Physical Therapy Personnel

The physical therapist (PT) evaluates and treats problems in mobility, including gait, transfers, muscle strength, general endurance, and balance. In home health settings, the PT also may be involved in completing the OASIS assessment. Physical therapists also assess and treat musculoskeletal pain. Similar to the role of the COTA, licensed physical therapy assistants (LPTAs) may deliver home health physical therapy services under the supervision of a PT.

Often the PT and the OTR may visit together or confer with each other to share observations and strategies concerning a client/family care issue. This is natural given the relationship of the two professions' contributions in total client care. Sometimes a joint visit allows the therapists to utilize a treatment technique not possible without the skills of both.

Speech Language Pathologist

The speech language pathologist (SLP) on the home health-care team is responsible for evaluating and treating communication deficits, hearing loss, and dysphagia. As skilled clinicians, the SLPs may collect data needed to complete the OASIS. Occupational therapists may also be involved in managing and treating dysphagia, with or without the speech pathologist.

Social Worker

The social worker (SW) is a resource person for the staff, client, and family. The OTR may call upon the SW to assist in obtaining resources in the community, including financial resources for adaptive equipment needs, transportation for physician appointments, respite services, and alternative housing that the client might need. Counseling on funding issues or advising families and clients in ways to meet their psychosocial needs are other important functions of the SW.

Physician

Home health agencies receive referrals from physicians. Some primary-care physicians make house calls, but most only provide care at office visits. The physician makes the initial referral, certifies or recertifies the plan of care, and helps to problem solve for urgent changes and daily concerns. The therapist and staff should report any changes in the client's medical condition to the physician and implement any physician orders affecting the care plan. Likewise, the occupational therapy practitioner provides feedback to the physician after care plan changes.

Occasionally, physicians who are specialists are involved for managing complicated problems, such as pain, or high-tech therapies, such as ventilators or dialysis. Their expertise in these areas provides the knowledge and competence to care for these complicated medical problems at home with greater safety.

Other Health-Care Professionals

In some situations the services of other professionals and allied health practitioners may be needed and provided. These may include:

1. Diet and nutritional counseling by a registered dietitian (RD)
2. Enterostomal therapy and wound care by a trained nurse specialist
3. Dental services (DDS or DMD)
4. Podiatry services (DPM)
5. Orthotics and prosthetics specialists (COP)
6. Nontraditional practitioners such as acupuncture and chiropractic medicine

Medicare or private insurance may or may not cover some of these services.

Family

The family is an integral part of the home-care delivery team, assuming responsibility for monitoring the client's condition and follow-through of all care routines. The therapists and other staff must be aware of the family's needs for education and also include the family in all decisions made regarding the case.

Client/Patient

Home health practice is client centered. Thus, the client is the heart of the home-care team. His or her needs are central to all activities. Incorporation of the client's goals and desires should be the focus of the team. All team members must emphasize empowering and enabling the client to reach personal, as well as health-care, goals.

REFERRALS FOR SERVICE

The occupational therapist may receive referrals from numerous sources. For example, a client may have been recently discharged from a rehabilitation or general hospital where he or she received occupational therapy services. The therapist working in that facility may have recommended a continuation of occupational therapy services to be provided in the home during discharge planning. This led to the person being admitted to the home health agency with orders for occupational therapy.

Another source of referral may be the case coordinator in home health, usually a nurse making the initial visit to assess the home health needs of the client. A need for occupational therapy may have been identified by the nurse or by a physician's order to initiate occupational therapy services. Similarly, the physical therapist or speech pathologist may request an occupational therapy consult for problems in activities of daily living or other functional deficits.

Occupational therapy practitioners may receive referrals when a client relocates. Occupational therapy services that are provided prior to the move are deemed necessary to be continued. As a result, the home health agency may receive a referral to continue occupational therapy services.

A home health agency routes the referrals to individual therapists. When more than one occupational therapy employee/contractor is involved, geographic location most commonly determines who gets the referral. Territories are usually established by the agency, and new referrals are routed to the person covering that territory. This, however, does not always work out equitably. Sometimes one therapist has an abundance of clients in one area, while another therapist's territory is low on referrals. Clients needing special expertise, such as clients with mental health problems or pediatric clients, may influence case assignments. Therefore, the person handling the routing of referrals needs updated information on the current caseload of each therapist to distribute the work as evenly as possible.

The use of contractors may be helpful in allowing the agency to utilize a person who lives near the client to cover a case if the number of full-time therapists is small. Use of contractors may be more efficient and productive than sending one or two employees to all coverage areas of the agency. The use of contractors may be helpful in allowing the agency to utilize a person who lives near the client to cover a case, if the number of full-time therapists is small. Use of contractors may be more efficient and productive than sending one or two employees to all coverage areas of the agency. However, due to the recent tightening of the definitions of independent contractor status by the Internal Revenue Service (IRS), most individuals are classified as employees for IRS purposes. Regardless of whether the individual is an employee or contractor, some written agreement stating the nature of the relationship and the expectations of both parties is necessary.

Another consideration in routing referrals relates to the supervision of therapy assistants. Occupational (and physical) therapists must perform intermittent supervisory visits with COTAs and LPTAs, respectively, when involved with treating the client.

This usually does not require a permanent change in the assignment of the case. Instead, the therapist can switch visits with the assistant to see the client who has been assigned to the assistant on an as-needed basis. As a result, the therapist may need to travel to another territory to make supervisory visits as needed. Another consideration relates to how many assistants one therapist can reasonably supervise. In some states, licensure laws limit the number of assistants a therapist can supervise. Therapists should be aware of and comply with the laws in the state(s) in which they are practicing.

Once the routing decision is made, the therapist may receive a phone call, a page, a fax, or written memo notifying him or her of the new referral. Most agencies have a time limit for addressing new referrals, usually within 48 hours. Sometimes the routing of a referral is determined by which therapist can address the referral within the required time frame.

In some situations, the family may be overwhelmed with the adjustment to the client's homecoming and may request a later time for the first visit. This request may be honored. However, the therapist must document the initial contact and the request of the client and/or family members for delaying the initial visit.

REIMBURSEMENT

Various sources of payment for home health services are available and often differ from those for inpatient and other outpatient settings. Due to the recent growth in home health utilization and the skyrocketing costs of health care in general, plans are currently under way to change the reimbursement systems that pay for home health services.

Government Funding Sources

Two major sources of government funding are Medicare and Medicaid. Medicare is a federally funded insurance program for the elderly (those over 65 years of age) that pays for nearly 50 percent of all home health services provided (Agency for Health Care Policy and Research, 1996). Medicaid, a program for indigent children and adults, is administered and regulated by state governments with some federal funding. Medicaid programs vary in their policies. Coverage of OT services varies from state to state. Medicaid programs also do not have the same stringent requirements, such as for being homebound, found in Medicare policy. Because Medicaid is a program for indigent children and adults, many of the clients seen by occupational therapy practitioners in home health may be disabled children and mentally ill adults rather than the elderly. The primary services that qualify a person for skilled intervention are not defined as they are in Medicare regulations. Therapists should be aware of the Medicaid policies and reimbursement rules that apply to the state(s) in which they practice.

Because payment systems change over time, the discussion on reimbursement will begin with the recent retrospective payment system, followed by the current interim payment system, and future plans for a prospective payment system. Until as recently as 1997, in most cases, Medicare Parts A and B paid providers of home health services *retrospectively* on a **fee-for-service (FFS)** basis. This means that agencies submitted bills for services provided and were then reimbursed for these services. The reimbursement was based on actual costs as long as the amount did not exceed a limit that was based on a calculated mean for the geographic region. This ceiling was established to prevent exorbitant charges. A Health Maintenance Organization (HMO) option available to Medicare subscribers (sometimes known as Medicare Complete or C Plus) includes incentives to encourage subscribers to sign up for this option. The HMO option of Medicare coverage includes the same services as those covered by Medicare Parts A and B. It also includes coverage for many preventative services and some durable medical equipment (DME), such as bathroom equipment, not typically covered by Medicare Parts A and B. The lack of Medicare coverage for adaptive bathroom equipment has long been an obstacle for both occupational therapy practitioners and clients.

The Medicare HMO reimburses for services on either a discounted fee schedule or a capitated rate. The least common type of reimbursement is when an HMO is the service provider. Usually, this happens in large HMOs with the ability to have a home health agency within the network owned and operated by the HMO (Schlenker and Shaughnessey, 1992).

The Balanced Budget Act of 1997 created the interim payment system to reduce Medicare costs until a prospective payment system could be developed. The interim system states that the home health agency will be paid the lesser of:

● Actual allowable costs
● Per-visit cost limits reduced to 105 percent of the national median
● A new agency specific, per beneficiary annual limit (Siebert, 1998)

This system is not radically different from the former system, in that the amount an agency can be reimbursed is near its present costs if the costs are kept within reasonable limits.

Because the advent of diagnostic-related groups (DRGs) and prospective payment was so successful in reducing the costs of hospitalization to Medicare in the 1980s, the concept was destined to pervade reimbursement in other treatment settings. The new payment system for home health services will be a prospective payment system. Currently, reimbursement in long-term care facilities is undergoing a change from a cost-reporting system (retrospective payment) to a type of prospective payment system based on the acuity level of the client. Similarly, cuts in funding and changes in reimbursement methods are occurring for outpatient settings. However, the details of how rates per case will be determined for home health-care providers is yet to be determined.

Several systems have been proposed and field-tested. The three prominent systems are: (1) bundled payment, (2) prospective per-visit payment, and (3) prospective per-episode payment. In the bundled payment system, a predetermined amount of money would be shared between acute and long-term care providers such as hospitals, skilled nursing homes, and home health agencies. The networking effect could allow HMO-owned home health agencies to reduce their costs by providing lower-cost services in the home instead of services in higher-priced settings.

If the home health agency is paid per visit prospectively, the incentive for the agency is to keep costs reasonable and provide maximum services. The incentive for the HMO is to minimize use of home health services. In the prospective payment per episode, a contract between the HMO and the home health agency provides a financial incentive for the HMO to keep visits to a minimum. In contrast, the incentive for the home health agency is to keep visits high. In the payment per-episode arrangement, the incentive for home health agencies is to keep visits low while the HMOs incentive is to keep numbers of home health admissions low but the amount of service per beneficiary high (McQuire, 1997).

The type of system that eventually will be in place will impact occupational therapy utilization. In some situations, competition among disciplines is a possibility. Perhaps a case manager will decide which disciplines to consult for a client and which services will not be used. The home health agency may be financially rewarded for providing less, rather than more, service. In this situation, occupational therapy must be recognized by the agency management, the rehabilitation team, and, in particular, the case manager as a cost-effective service that will speed the discharge of the client from the case load at a higher level of functioning.

Private Insurance Funding

Private insurance policies may offer similar coverage to that provided by government-funded plans. Fee-for-service (FFS) plans are dwindling in prevalence. Managed care plans are becoming more commonplace.

Currently, most private HMO insurance plans have a case management system, and it is likely that a case manager will approve a limited number of visits prospectively. A **case manager** is the person responsible for obtaining the services a patient or client needs by linking with service providers. The purpose of a case management system is to increase quality and continuity of care while simultaneously reducing health-care costs. This system requires the occupational therapist to contact the case manager following the initial visit with the client to discuss the plan of care, including the short-term and long-term goals, approaches, frequency, and duration. If the case manager approves the plan, the therapist will have authorization for a specified number of visits. When the number of approved visits has expired and the therapist determines more visits are necessary, approval for more visits must be requested, and the rationale for continued treatment, the requested frequency and duration of treatment, and the anticipated outcome of therapy must be provided. A well-prepared therapist is more likely to provide objective information that will result in continuation of services. Optimally, the details of this approval should be recorded in writing. These records may be placed in the practitioner's files but should never be part of the client's medical record. When the maximum benefit has been reached, approval for further visits will likely be denied.

Employer-Funded Programs

The incidence of worker compensation cases in home health is relatively low. Worker compensation programs are state regulated. In many states, the regulations require services for injured workers to be provided in comprehensive outpatient facilities or inpatient rehabilitation units. A worker's compensation case referred to a home health agency would likely be assigned a case manager from a private agency.

Typically, worker compensation organizations have their own case managers with the responsibility for approving expenditures on therapy services and equipment needed by the client related to his or her injury. The case manager functions as a liaison between service providers and the worker compensation board, assuring that all services recommended and provided are reasonable and necessary for the client's well-being and functioning. The primary focus of any services should be directed toward returning the injured worker to work when and where possible. The occupational therapist must be aware of the differences in worker compensation programs, as compared to other payers, in terms of their purpose and methods of operation.

REQUIREMENTS FOR SERVICE

Specific requirements must be met for an individual to receive home-based services. Medicare requires the strict adherence to these requirements for reimbursement. Because Medicare is a federally funded program, many other insurers also use the Medicare guidelines for reimbursement. To qualify for reimbursement, most funding agencies use the following as criteria:

1. Homebound status (a Medicare definition)
2. Intermittent service
3. Medical necessity
4. Skilled service
5. Physician care and treatment

Homebound Status

When Medicare Part A is the payer (Medicare, 1996, Chapter 2, Section 204.1, Subsection A, Transmittal A), **homebound status** is defined as:

> a normal inability to leave home and consequently leaving home would require a considerable and taxing effort. If the patient does in fact leave the home, the patient may nevertheless be considered homebound if the absences from the home are infrequent, or for periods of relatively short duration, or are attributable to the need to receive medical treatment. Absences attributable to the need to receive medical treatment include attendance at adult day care centers to receive medical care, ongoing receipt of outpatient kidney dialysis, and the receipt of outpatient chemotherapy or radiation therapy. It is expected that in most instances absences from the home that occur will be for the purpose of receiving medical treatment. However, occasional absences from the home for non-medical purposes (e.g., an occasional trip to the barber, or walk around the block or drive) would not necessitate a finding that the individual is not homebound so long as the absences are undertaken on an infrequent basis or are of relatively short duration and do not indicate the patient has the capacity to obtain health care provided outside rather than at home.

Although severe physical limitations may not be present, individuals with mental illness may qualify for homebound status. Major cognitive deficits may make an individual unsafe to leave home alone or may prevent leaving home at all. The presence of bizarre and socially inappropriate behaviors, dementia, hallucinations, delusions, reclusive behavior, suicidal ideation or attempts, and/or severe anxiety may qualify the individual for homebound status. The presence and severity of these problems must be documented as justification. A description of the reasons why the person is unable to leave home unaccompanied is important for obtaining reimbursement (Harper, 1989).

The current definition of homebound status is being challenged. One group challenging this definition consists of individuals with spinal cord injury because an interpretation of the current definition promotes being confined to home to receive needed services (Steib, 1998). A person with a chronic disability who is able to leave home intermittently to engage in social and health services is denied coverage of other home-based services he or she may need. A new definition of homebound is being studied due to problems identified by Medicare's fraud and abuse department. It is anticipated that the new definition will be *more* restrictive than the current one.

Intermittent Service

Home health services are, by nature, intermittent. Medicare (Health Care Financing Administration, 1989, Chapter 2, Section 206.7, Subsection B, Transmittal 222) defines **intermittent service** as:

- Up to and including 28 hours per week of skilled nursing and home health aide services combined provided on a less than daily basis;
- Up to 35 hours per week of skilled nursing and home aide services combined that are provided on a less than daily basis, subject to review by fiscal intermediaries on a case by case basis, based upon documentation justifying the need for and reasonableness of such additional care; or
- Up to and including full-time (i.e., 8 hours per day) skilled nursing and home health aide services combined, which are provided and needed 7 days per week for temporary, but not indefinite, periods of time up to 21 days with allowances for extensions in exceptional circumstances where need for care in excess of 21 days is finite and predictable.

Home health staff should make clients and their families aware of the implications of these rules. Home health services are not a reasonable substitute for full-time care needs.

Medical Necessity

Home services provided must be medically necessary and reasonable. **Medical necessity** means (Trufant, 1994):

● The service must be of a level of complexity and skill such that only a therapist can perform the service safely and effectively or the general supervision of a therapist is required.
● The service must be reasonable and necessary to the treatment of the illness/injury.
● The person's condition requires the involvement of a skilled therapist to meet his or her needs, promote recovery, and ensure medical safety.
● Regardless of the medical condition, the therapist's skills are needed to treat the injury/illness.
● The service provision must be reasonable and necessary for the condition being treated. Additionally, the frequency and duration of the treatment must be reasonable.
● The treatment must be effective and specific to the condition.
● There must be a reasonable expectation that the treatment will result in improvement of the patient's condition within a predictable amount of time. When the services are needed to establish a maintenance program, the program must be effective and necessary for the safety of the patient.
● Services to teach patients/caretakers must be reasonable and necessary to treat the condition.

Skilled Service

In addition to meeting the preceding requirements for medical necessity, currently occupational therapy services alone do not qualify toward attaining skilled status under Medicare Part A benefits. Individuals can qualify for **skilled service** status if they are receiving or have received at least one visit from physical therapy, skilled nursing, or speech-language pathology. However, if the person has already been receiving occupational therapy, and other disciplines that were treating the client have discontinued their visits, the occupational therapist may continue visits with documentation of need until discharge occurs.

This limitation is not true for visits billed under Medicare Part B (and other private insurance) benefits where occupational therapy can be reimbursed even if it is the only discipline in the home. These services are reimbursed at the rate of 80 percent of allowable charges, possibly leaving the client responsible for payment of the remaining 20 percent, unless he or she has supplementary insurance to cover the balance. In this case, the "homebound requirement" of Medicare Part A benefits also does not apply.

Physician's Care and Treatment

In addition to the four previously mentioned requirements, Medicare also requires that home health services be prescribed by a physician who has established and approved the plan of care. The physician must certify that the individual requires "skilled services." The person must be "under the care of" that physician for the duration of the home health services.

 ## OCCUPATIONAL THERAPY FUNCTIONS IN HOME HEALTH

Because of rapid changes in the health-care environment, more and more individuals who have a physical disability are being referred to occupational therapy in home health settings. A list of physical conditions commonly treated in home health is provided in Table 11–1. Although this list is not all-inclusive, it may be helpful to the new home health therapist to assist in screening appropriate clients for occupational therapy treatment.

Many individuals prefer to remain in their home environment for treatment after a physical illness or injury. If a person has adequate abilities to take care of basic needs with the intermittent support of home health staff or the financial resources to hire help, he or she may resume and/or continue living at home and receive the needed services via home health.

Sometimes family, friends, or neighbors can provide additional help to meet the needs of the client while convalescing. When the condition is chronic or progressive in nature, the occupational therapy practitioner aids the client/family in considering whether it is reasonable and safe for family members and friends to continue to provide care for the person.

TABLE 11–1

CONDITIONS COMMONLY TREATED IN HOME HEALTH

Conditions	Examples
Neurological conditions	Cerebral palsy Traumatic brain injury Spinal cord injury Cerebrovascular accident Guillain Barré syndrome
Progressive neurological dysfunctions	Parkinson's disease Multiple sclerosis Amyotrophic lateral sclerosis
Orthopedic conditions	Knee replacement Hip fracture and/or replacement Arthritis Multiple fractures Spinal fractures Complications of osteoporosis Surgeries requiring prolonged, severely limiting immobilization procedures Amputations Surgeries related to back conditions
General medical conditions	Chronic obstructive pulmonary disease Congestive heart failure Coronary artery disease and bypass surgery Visual loss related to retinopathy or macular degeneration General medical debility secondary to prolonged illness/hospitalization

EVALUATION/ASSESSMENT

A major concern for the home health occupational therapist is the safety and accessibility of the home environment and the safety and adequacy of the care given by others (employees, friends, and family). Because there are many areas to assess in the home environment, the therapist may need to prioritize only the most important issues initially, addressing other issues later as the situation requires.

Interviewing the client and family member(s) during the initial visit is useful for gaining information. This interview also begins the process of establishing rapport. Listening carefully and observing the nonverbal responses of the client and family members provide important information. As with any client/family, the home-care provider should begin by explaining the goals of occupational therapy, including specifics on the role the therapist will play in this particular case. The family and client need to be made aware of the intermittent nature of intervention, meaning that the aide or the family members will need to provide for the client's therapeutic needs when the therapist and other staff are not present. Occupational therapy focuses on returning the individual to self-sufficiency rather than providing custodial care for a dependent client.

During the initial evaluation, the therapist should observe all areas of the home that the client uses in his or her daily living routines. Thorough assessment of the bathroom area is necessary in almost all cases. Accessibility and safety concerns in the kitchen may be another area needing assessment, depending on the roles and tasks of the client. In cases where the person lives alone, entrances to the home, laundry and storage areas, and access to cabinet space are key assessment areas.

The ability to evaluate the clients' abilities in the natural environment where these activities occur in daily routines is a major advantage of working in a home health setting. Often, any enhancements or constraints of client performance by the environment will be more apparent. Plus, the feasibility of implementing solutions will be more obvious. The practitioner can problem solve and try out solutions to assess their effectiveness. The family's and client's responses to the suggestions and observation of them using the methods also can be assessed. For example, measurements and drawings of the floor space in the bathroom provided to the OTR or COTA in the clinic may be insufficient for understanding wheelchair accessibility in the bathroom area.

The home-care provider's presence in the real environment facilitates more accurate determinations of the needs of the client/family. In addition, because the family is likely to be assuming the role of caregiver, the therapist is in an excellent position to assess the family's coping abilities and provide education and support based on the family's needs, level of comprehension, and acceptance. The caregiver and client are likely to be establishing their own methods of accomplishing daily living in new and different ways than previously. The occupational therapy practitioner can be of great assistance to the person in establishing adaptive methods that prevent further disability and assist him or her in achieving independence.

In most situations, immediately following the onset of the condition and up until returning home, members of the health-care staff were the caregivers who assumed the primary responsibility for attending to the client's needs. In the home, the occupational therapy practitioner will focus on the abilities of the client and caregiver to establish effective routines such as medication management, dysphagia management, and bowel and bladder management.

Caregivers may be new to this role, requiring some guidance regarding expectations for the future. Most families think in terms of full recovery for the client and, therefore, eventual return to life as it was before the incident. In most cases, this is not true. The grief of the family and client is a natural sequela. Thus, the professional must assist the client and family to cope with this change. The impetus for coming to terms may be most obvious when the family is thrust into the caregiver role, resulting more fully in a realization of the implications of the newly acquired functional problems and limitations of the client.

Additionally, caregivers also need relief from caregiving duties (preferably at regular intervals) to preserve their health and complete their own self-care and self-maintenance tasks. Assuming that a caregiver is ready and able to provide 24-hour care on a daily basis with no relief from these duties is unrealistic. The practitioner needs to help the family identify this need and be able to provide suggestions for resources and training of relief workers. Respite care could be provided through formal networks, such as a sitter hired through a sitter service, or through informal networks, such as family and friends. Validation and support for respite care may be one of the most important interventions that the professional provides to the family.

Anticipating the duration of the client's care needs and dealing with these issues early on in treatment can possibly avert problematic situations. For example, if the caretaker becomes ill, in part from the stresses of caregiving, making plans for placement of the person outside the home is appropriate. Prevention of the placement of an individual into a long-term care facility is not always possible, however. The evaluation summary should include a statement of the family's ability to provide for the client's needs and address the family's coping skills/resources.

Assessment of activities of daily living (ADLs), such as feeding, dressing, grooming, bathing, and toileting, is a primary focus of evaluation in the home health setting. In addition, assessment of other performance areas, such as functional communication, emergency response, and sexual expression, also may be appropriate. Additionally, in depending on the role of the client in the home, home management skills may need to be addressed. For other clients, care of others and leisure pursuits are areas of need that require evaluation and possible intervention. When Medicare is paying for the client's treatment, completion or contributing to the OASIS data is necessary. Much of the routine assessment data collected by the OTR is addressed by completing the OASIS.

In the professional literature, there has been discussion about the "top-down" versus the "bottom-up" approach to evaluation (Trombly, 1993). In the *bottom-up* approach, the therapist focuses on the occupational performance component deficits as they relate to occupational performance area deficits. The assumption is that by addressing deficits in performance components, occupational functioning will be enhanced. In the *top-down* approach, the therapist assesses occupational performance areas and contexts to ascertain deficits in occupational functioning. The top-down approach appears more beneficial in the home health practice setting. Assessment of all occupational performance components could be time consuming and may not yield information regarding the functional needs of the client/family unit requiring expedient intervention.

The choice of assessment tools the therapist uses is determined by the problems and needs of the client. Assessment tools similar to those used in rehabilitation settings may be used for home health OT evaluation. These may include: Assessment of Motor and Process Skills (AMPS), Routine Task Inventory (RTI-2), Canadian Occupational Performance Measure (COPM), Kohlman Evaluation of Living Skills (KELS), Milwaukee Evaluation of Daily Living Skills (MEDLS), and the Home Observation for Measurement of the Home Environment (HOME). Inexpensive, portable, minimal equipment assessment tools that focus on quantifying occupational performance deficits are essential in home-care practice.

OASIS is a tool that is being used to systematically evaluate outcomes in home health care. Similar to the Minimum Data Set (MDS) used in long-term care facilities, the OASIS addresses functional abilities. The instrument is used preintervention and postintervention and in some situations at other intervals to measure change, either progress or decline, in function. The areas addressed by OASIS are listed in Box 11–3.

The data collected from OASIS will allow the quantification of outcomes and com-

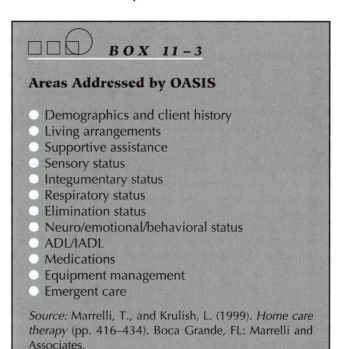

Source: Marrelli, T., and Krulish, L. (1999). *Home care therapy* (pp. 416–434). Boca Grande, FL: Marrelli and Associates.

parison of one agency to another, including nationwide comparisons. It is designed to increase the standardization of care. Since this tool is nondiscipline specific, any skilled professional team member can be responsible for completing the assessment in part or in its entirety. Usually, home health agencies decide, as a matter of policy, how it will be accomplished and which team members will be responsible for evaluating the client. It may seem natural to assign this duty to the nurse on the team. However, this practice may lead to unreimbursed visits by nursing personnel. In this scenario, clients who are seen for therapy services only would require a nurse to visit at intervals to complete the data set. Since the person does not require nursing services, the costs of these visits could not be recovered from Medicare.

Occupational therapists may use this tool to quantify performance levels at the onset of treatment and at discharge (Shaughnessy, Crisler, and Schlenker, 1995). Appropriate OT assessment tools would be used to evaluate the client; then the therapist would also score the performance based on the OASIS scale.

INTERVENTION

Upon completion of the evaluation data collection, the therapist must use clinical reasoning skills to plan the treatment course of the client. Numerous factors are included in the reasoning process leading to development of goals and interventions. These include the goals and priorities of the client and the family, the estimated treatment time that will be reimbursed, the course and progress expected according to the medical condition, and the person's prior level of function.

Collaboration with the client and family is necessary for determining the focus of intervention and the sequence of goals. For example, if the client is not independent in feeding, the therapist may explain the reasons for the person's difficulties in self-feeding. The occupational therapy practitioner may explain to the client and family that goals related to increased independence in a basic-level skill, such as self-feeding, are likely to precede achievement of more complex skills, such as bathing. This decision should be made considering the desires and values of the client and family, as well as other factors such as the person's prior level of function. For example, if the family says the client has not self-fed for three years but that he used to help his wife turn him from side to side in bed and is now unable to do so, the bed mobility problem may be addressed first.

The family and client must be given information at their level of understanding. This enables them to be a partner with the therapist in the treatment. Providing this information assists the family in feeling that the professional is helping them achieve their goals rather than imposing the therapist's agenda on them.

Although some of the approaches the home-care practitioner uses to address problems may be remedial in nature, meaning the therapist attempts to restore lost functions, other strategies are adaptive in nature. The real life environment creates a push for mastery of daily living tasks. Therefore, the client must be able to perform at the highest level achievable as soon as possible.

Skilled intervention approaches used by occupational therapists for clients in home health environments may include:

- Splint fabrication and/or modification
- Training of clients/caregivers in functional mobility and transfer techniques
- Recommendations for adaptive equipment for the home
- Client and family education in such areas as energy conservation/work simplification
- Home safety issues and home modification for accessibility
- Design and modification of home programs for use between therapy sessions
- Motor control techniques, strengthening, and facilitation of upper extremity function
- Cognitive and perceptual retraining and adaptive strategies
- Homemaking/home management training
- ADL retraining that may include the use of adaptive techniques and/or equipment
- Functional communication
- Facilitation of sexual expression
- Leisure skills and management of leisure time

The duration of OT intervention is based on the prognosis for functional gains, client motivation/compliance, prior level of function, and available funds. The intensity is somewhat dictated by the condition, the reimbursement, and the anticipated course of the condition. Some conditions will benefit most from intensive therapy at first, followed by a tapering frequency. For example, a client with a recent rotator cuff surgical repair will need more therapy initially. Typically, the person is in a shoulder immobilizer 23 hours a day, except during therapy. Intermittent range of motion within limitations, ordered by the physician, is necessary to prevent adhesions during early healing. Later in the treatment course, the restrictions on motion will be lessened, and the client may be instructed to actively exercise on his or her own between visits, thus requiring less intensive occupational therapy service.

As always, the home-care provider must do what is best for the client within the available resources and constraints. This means utilizing the resources the person has, including the social network, home environment, and finances, to best benefit by prioritizing services that would be beneficial.

Equipment and Supplies

When treating a client, a variety of equipment and supplies may be necessary. Size, weight, portability, and cost limit the treatment equipment that can be used by practitioners in the home. The equipment must fit into the vehicle and be easily carried or assembled. Often the professional is responsible for providing his or her own equipment and supplies. Although cost is always a consideration, access to the tools needed to provide adequate treatment is key. Most equipment and supplies for use in therapy sessions are routinely present in the client's home. Therefore, only a few are absolutely essential to purchase. Supplies already in the home may include dining utensils, clothing, toiletries, kitchen and cleaning utensils, art supplies, and craft materials. Some of the essential equipment and supplies, such as assistive devices, may need to be purchased from a local durable medical equipment (DME) company or catalog company (such as Fred Sammons or North Coast). In addition, the practitioner must transport all office supplies and consumable items for infection control.

Transmitting infectious diseases from one homebound client to another must be avoided at all costs. If materials and equipment are carried from one client to another for use, adherence to the Occupational Safety and Health Administration (OSHA) regulations for infection control is essential. These regulations include (Medcom, 1993):

- Using disposable equipment, when possible, and/or having a separate piece of equipment that is left at each client's home throughout the treatment period
- Wearing gloves, protective glasses, masks, and disposable gowns whenever there is the possibility of coming into contact with bodily fluids, such as during toileting and dressing changes, in the case of a client who is incontinent
- Washing hands before donning gloves and after removal, allowing soap to remain on the hands for at least 15 seconds
- Handling and disposing of hazardous materials, such as gloves, gowns, masks, soiled clothing, eating utensils, and bed linens, appropriately when necessary
- Sterilizing equipment according to the manufacturer's directions and in compliance with OSHA and the home health agency's policies and regulations (for example, allowing some objects to remain in a solution of diluted bleach for 10 to 15 minutes before removing and allowing objects to dry completely before storing after washing them) and using a disposable towel or newspaper under any equipment that must be carried from one client's house to another
- Acquiring infection-control packages (which comply with OSHA infection-control regulations) from the home health agency prior to the home visit

DISCHARGE FROM OCCUPATIONAL THERAPY SERVICES

Planned termination of OT services usually occurs for one of three reasons: (1) the goals of treatment have been met, (2) the client is no longer considered homebound, and/or (3) the therapist has made a clinical judgment that the goals cannot be met at this time. Reaching treatment plan goals may prove impossible within the time allotted to the therapist. The client may have reached a plateau in his or her progress or the therapist may feel that the person is still too "sick" to benefit from a strenuous therapeutic program at the present time. The professional may also believe that if the client is discharged, and the client and family diligently perform the home program for a period of time, occupational therapy can be resumed with a greater potential for achievement at a later date.

Unexpected termination of OT services may result from a variety of circumstances. Possible examples include:

- Denial of reimbursement for continued treatment by Medicare or the managed-care HMO provider, due to limited service benefits or failure to provide adequate documentation to justify continued treatment

- A need for the client to return to the hospital, nursing home, or other institution due to exacerbation of illness
- Current inability to meet the criteria for home-bound status
- Noncompliance of the client and/or family with the treatment program
- Persistent absences from the premises when home visits are scheduled
- A judgment by the therapist that the client is no longer safe in his or her present environment

Discharge planning usually occurs during a formal case conference at the home health agency. With the shortening of treatment periods allocated to each discipline due to Medicare regulations and managed care, the client may be discharged before a formal case conference can be convened. The formal case conference may evolve into informal communications among professionals to discuss the client's progress and proposed date of discharge.

If the termination of service or discharge is anticipated, the occupational therapy practitioner is responsible for:

- Preparing the client and family for discharge in advance.
- Notifying the client's case manager of the pending discharge.
- Providing the client with a recommended course of action: home program to perform; referral to community resources; and contact information for outpatient clinics to seek additional treatment as recommended.
- Discussing the client's occupational therapy home program with the physical therapist or speech pathologist, as appropriate (the therapist may request his or her assistance in encouraging client and family compliance with the home program).
- Requesting a social worker referral if transportation or financial problems arise when outpatient therapy is recommended.
- Notifying the home health aide in advance when occupational therapy is the last discipline to discharge the client. Home health aide services (a nonskilled service) will no longer be reimbursed under Medicare Part A after occupational therapy discharges the client.
- Advising the home health agency of the client's status prior to the discharge.
- Notifying the referring physician of the client's discharge as a courtesy.

At discharge, the occupational therapy practitioner may recommend additional treatment at an outpatient facility. Discussion with the client and family about the logistical issues concerning the transition to outpatient services is crucial. Issues as to ability to meet the costs, transportation needs, and physical assistance for mobility must be addressed. A referral to a social worker may be indicated for resource information to assist the client and family with logistical problems related to accessing outpatient treatment. The referring physician and/or home health agency will need to be contacted regarding processing the referrals.

The professional may determine that it is unsafe for the person to remain at home with the amount of supervision available, possibly recommending that a paid attendant be present during the daytime hours. If the family cannot afford this service or is unwilling or unable to provide it, placement in a nursing home, assisted living center, or group home could be recommended. An alternative is recommendation for placement at an adult day-care center for care and supervision when no one is home during the day.

Family Education

By using a combination of client- and family-centered approaches (Weinstein, 1997), the family is kept informed of OT intervention, adapted equipment, and activities as they are introduced. The many different types of family situations require the use of a variety of approaches. Practitioners must consider the cultural heritage, social structure, size, geographical location, and hierarchy of the family. For instance, there might be an extended family in a rural area whose members desire to assist in the client's care or an older husband and caretaker wife living in a low-income, urban high rise.

Due to the variety of family situations, different methods may be used to promote a smooth discharge. These might include techniques such as writing down specific dressing directions, making charts as a reminder to carry out certain activities, and drawing pictures of how the client should be positioned in the bed. In the final days of treatment, the client, the family, and the therapist should collaborate and write up a comprehensive home program. Then the program should be developed, demonstrated, and practiced by client, family, and therapist to ensure a smooth transition after home health services are discontinued. The occupational therapy practitioner must document the training and home programs provided, including the therapist's assessment of the client and family's ability to follow through on the recommendations.

DOCUMENTATION

Sound and complete documentation are critical for reimbursement. Documentation must be legible and complete, and must substantiate the course of action taken by the practitioner. Documenting fully *all* skilled care provided during each visit and noting the results in measurable terms are necessary to quantify progress made by the client. Failure to meet all of these criteria can lead to denial of payment by third-party payers.

Documentation provides an opportunity to educate others about occupational therapy and justify its existence as a skilled service. McQuire (1997) states that high-quality documentation:

● Focuses on function, underlying causes, progress, and safety
● States expectations of progress
● Explains slow progress or lack of progress
● Summarizes the skilled services delivered

Referrals

Orders must be signed by the referring physician who is coordinating the client's care and overseeing the plan of treatment. Frequently, the reason for referral to occupational therapy and any limitations will be stated. These may include physician's orders for weight-bearing restrictions, active or passive range of motion (ROM) limitations imposed due to the client's condition, or wearing instructions regarding immobilizers. Although not common, the referral may also specify the recommended duration of treatment. If not stated, the occupational therapist or funding source may determine the duration of therapy.

Evaluation

The evaluation data form may include identifying information, responsible party data, and caregiver information. A brief history of the current illness and any past medical history (PMH) significant to the current status of the client is elicited because the referral sheet may include only limited information. The therapist will need to ask questions of the client and/or family members during the interview portion of the evaluation to obtain a better picture of the past history. The OT evaluation should include assessment of occupational performance components and occupational performance areas affected by the client's condition. Additionally, addressing the performance contexts, particularly the cultural, social, and physical (home) environment, of the client is a crucial element of the home health assessment. The in-depth home assessment of these areas differs from that in institution-based care. With the advantage of observing the client in his or her home environment, problems that need to be addressed, such as safety and accessibility issues, may be discovered that were not detected in an inpatient evaluation. The primary focus of therapy in this setting is to increase independence and safety in performance of activities of daily living, home management, and leisure pursuits.

Various assessment tools may be used to collect data concerning the presence and nature of deficits in occupational performance components and occupational performance areas. Standardized tools should be used when possible and as appropriate for the condition and setting. Frequently, the treatment plan portion of documentation is combined with the evaluation data on the same form.

Intervention / Treatment Plan

Following completion of the evaluation, the treatment plan is formulated in collaboration with the client and family. Asking the person about his or her goals and assessing the needs of the family/caregiver guides the therapist in setting appropriate goals that meet the needs of the client.

After formulation of the problem list, which includes deficits to be addressed by the occupational therapist, short-term goals (STGs) are established. The time frame for achievement of short-term goals is usually approximately halfway through the anticipated course of therapy or one month from the initial evaluation, whichever is shorter. This is only a guideline for new practitioners to use because accurate estimation of time required for goal attainment can be difficult. More experienced therapists may use other determinants to guide their decisions about time frames for achievement of STGs.

Goals should be written to reflect the performance of the client rather than the therapist or family. Short-term goals should be measurable and functional, addressing the occupational performance deficits of the client. The conditions and performance levels should be specified. See Table 11–2 for examples.

Although a goal of increasing active range of motion (AROM) may be measurable because a goniometer can be used to measure increases in joint range of motion, this goal is not functional unless the therapist connects enhanced occupational performance with the increased AROM. Therefore, to clarify and reinforce the unique contribution of occupational therapy to the overall treatment of the client, an emphasis

 TABLE 11–2

DOCUMENTATION EXAMPLES

Poor Example	Reason	Good Example
Goal:		
Family will provide set-up assist for client to self-feed.	Not measurable.	Client will self-feed 75% of lunch with set-up assist.
Client will self-feed.	No conditions or performance level specified.	Client will self-feed using built-up handle spoon (conditions) with min (A) (performance level).
Progress Note:		
Client requires mod (A) with LE dressing.	Does not describe the nature of the client's difficulties.	Client requires mod (A) with LE dressing due to poor standing balance.

on restoring the person to his or her occupations must be the focus of treatment goals and outcomes.

Long-term goals (LTGs) focus on increasing independence in occupational performance areas. From the client's initial status, the therapist projects and determines the functional gains to be attained by the end of the therapy course. For example, if the initial evaluation reveals the family is unable to transfer the client safely, perhaps safe transfer of the client will be one of the outcomes of therapy. The time frame for achievement of the LTG may be several months or just a few weeks, depending on the circumstances. When projecting long-term goals, the certification period for Medicare patients of 60 days must be kept in mind. Some home health-care recipients will require a longer duration of care (beyond the 60 days), while others will need a shorter duration.

The case manager will usually notify the occupational therapist of an impending recertification deadline. At this time, the OTR determines if continued therapy is needed. The need for continued therapy would necessitate recertification by the physician that the client/patient: (1) continues to require skilled care and (2) remains homebound. If these two criteria are not met, discontinuation of all home health services may be necessary. Again, new goals should be stated in measurable terms and focused on improving the occupational performance level of the client.

The intervention/treatment plan indicates to third-party payers what types of treatment approaches will be used. Reimbursable services must always be "skilled," defined as those that require the knowledge and skills of an occupational therapist or occupational therapy assistant.

When establishing the frequency of visits, the occupational therapy practitioner must remember that home health services are less intense and less acute than inpatient services. A typical initial visit frequency may be three times per week. The decision on the frequency and duration may be recommended by the occupational therapist, but the actual number of visits reimbursed by the client's insurance provider may be set by a case manager. In this case, the company representative will give authorization for a stated number of visits, and the therapist will determine the number of visits per week that would be most advantageous for the client's condition. Visit frequencies are rarely the extremes of five times per week or one time per week, although exceptions are possible. Five visits per week are generally considered too intense for a homebound client, while one visit per week is considered too intermittent to merit skilled service status. Therefore, the typical frequency will be either two or three times per week. Some therapists initially treat the client three times per week, then taper the frequency to two times per week or less as the client progresses to being more self-sufficient and able to carry out a home exercise program between visits or as the client nears discharge.

Interdisciplinary Plan of Care

Most home health agencies have some form of interdisciplinary plan on the client's chart that states the total care plan with input from all disciplines involved in the person's care. The occupational therapist may be required to include goals of therapy in the appropriate section of the document, or the OT goals will be integrated into the problem list of the client. The latter is the case with a problem-oriented medical record (POMR) system where all problems of the client are listed on an integrated list and disciplines share responsibility for addressing the goals based on their area of expertise. For example, in a POMR system, the nursing staff and the occupational therapist may share the role of helping the client to achieve the goal "client will dress UE with min (A) using hemitechnique." The therapist will train the client in hemitechniques and inform the staff of any particular adaptations required by the client, and the nursing staff will assist in achieving this goal by coaching the client to follow through using hemitechniques whenever they assist him or her with ADLs.

Some home health agencies may utilize the case manager to compile the goals of each discipline into one plan of care. In this situation, the case manager will write the integrated plan after reviewing the individual plans of each of the rehabilitation team members. In both the POMR system and the multidisciplinary model, there is an integrated approach to the client's needs in one central location on the chart.

Progress Notes

In home health care, a separate note must document each visit. Although the format used in note writing varies with agency policy, the basic content does not. The note indicates any pertinent information given to the therapist by the client and family. This may include comments regarding their general health and well-being on that day, their responses to the home program given by the therapist, and/or the effectiveness of adaptive equipment or techniques recommended and taught by the occupational therapy provider. The therapist should include a statement that includes all skilled services provided that day and the response of the client and family in factual, objective, and measurable terms. Documenting the client's response includes the conditions under which the client was able to perform. This may include the use of adaptive techniques and/or equipment, a special set-up, environmental adaptations, or the need for verbal cues (which usually points to the presence of a cognitive deficit). The therapist's note should explain the relationship between a performance area deficit and the underlying occupational performance component. Inclusion of the occupational performance component deficit that interferes with functioning explains why other parts of the therapy session were focused on particular performance components. See Table 11–2 for examples.

Including a statement regarding progress toward treatment goals and remaining problems that will be addressed in the coming visits also is recommended. Any modifications to the stated therapy goals, treatment approaches, duration, or frequency of visits should be recorded on the progress note. The therapist may focus on the progress of the client in the note and fail to document continuing problems that justify the need for continued therapy. Documenting the entire picture of the client's abilities *and* difficulties makes a denial of payment less likely.

Additionally, initial visits should involve assessing the deficits in occupational performance and underlying causes *and* at least one skilled treatment intervention. This requirement for Medicare Part A services is somewhat unusual and unique to the home health setting. The intervention noted may involve family education, instruction in a home program, or teaching an adaptive technique.

Missed Visits

Because documentation is required for all visits in home health, the reason for any missed visits must be documented. The occupational therapy practitioner may arrive for a scheduled visit to find the person not home due to hospitalization, the family may call to cancel a visit because the client is not feeling well, or the client may be refusing treatment that day. The therapist should be aware that multiple missed visits may raise questions as to whether the client/patient meets the criteria for homebound services.

Case Communication

Any communication regarding the client's care that is not specifically documented in progress notes must be noted on the agency's interstaff communication form. For example, if the client experiences a decline in health during treatment, the therapist should notify the case manager of this change. Communication with the case manager or nurse describing specific changes observed should be written as a case communication, providing a written record of the person informed, the concerns, and the date/time. Another example would be a piece of durable medical equipment (DME) that is malfunctioning or unsafe and posing a safety hazard. An appropriate action would be to notify the DME company of the problem and then to document on the case communication form the date and time of the call, the person spoken to, and the company's verbal response. This results in a paper trail that may be important if the company fails to respond in a timely manner to the faulty equipment, and accidental injury to the client and/or family member occurs. Keeping a copy of the communication form for one's personal records also is a good practice.

Summaries

Some agencies may require the therapist to complete a summary of a client's progress after one month of treatment. The data included summarize the client's initial functional status (or status at the beginning of the month) and his or her status at the end of the month. Any skilled interventions being performed and identification of any remaining needs/deficits of the client that subsequent treatments will address need to be included. Frequency and duration of continued therapy should be specified.

Discharge summaries should be completed by the therapist on all clients at the conclusion of the therapy course. Statements of the client's level of functioning on admission, the services provided, and the current functional level are all components of the discharge summary. The conclusion should state the reason for discharge and any recommendations for care following discharge. The therapist may recommend continued therapy on an outpatient basis, a home exercise program, or OT services at a later date, and mention the conditions under which each option should be considered.

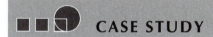 **CASE STUDY**

MAGGIE

Maggie is a 65-year-old African-American female who suffered a cerebrovascular accident 10 weeks ago. She has right hemiplegia, dysphagia and aphasia, is incontinent of bowel and bladder, and has a history of non-insulin-dependent diabetes mellitus (NIDDM) and hypertension. She was receiving a 1500-calorie pureed diet with thickened liquids and has a PEG tube used only for supplemental feedings at this time. She was placed in a skilled nursing facility for rehabilitation following her stroke. Home health care for continued therapy was recommended by the occupational therapist in the nursing home after her family brought her home. She is also receiving home health speech and physical therapies. Her current home equipment includes a wheelchair that is inappropriate for her needs, a semielectric hospital bed, and a bedside commode. She was right-hand dominant prior to her stroke.

Maggie has an extended family living nearby. The daughters rotate shifts to provide care for their mother, with one of her daughters staying with her at all times. Sandy is the primary caregiver, spending most days with Maggie. The other family members provide weekend relief and help with transportation for doctor visits. Frequently, grandchildren are present in the home, with the older ones helping out with the client's daily care needs.

When the occupational therapist evaluated Maggie, she found the family's greatest physical burden in caring for the client was related to her bowel and bladder incontinence and the amount of assistance the client required to transfer to the bedside commode and back to her wheelchair. Her bed mobility skills were dependent, and she was unable to maintain her static sitting balance. When transferring, she had poor standing balance. She was unable to propel her wheelchair throughout the house. Part of her difficulty with wheelchair mobility was due to apraxia.

She required maximum physical assistance to complete her bath and dress. She was unable to comb, style, or care for her hair. She required supervision in feeding due to impulsive behaviors that led to pocketing of food and overloading her mouth.

Maggie is able to greet people with socially appropriate automatic speech. She demonstrated verbal perseveration. Her replies to personal questions are "no" appropriate; however, "yes" replies are not reliable. She also demonstrates a significant delay in response time.

Initially, the therapist focused on basic needs of the client such as justifying and obtaining an appropriate wheelchair and seat cushion. Since the client had a painful right shoulder and less than one finger's breadth subluxation at the glenohumeral joint, the therapist instructed the family in appropriate handling and positioning of the affected extremities in the wheelchair and bed. To prevent undue stress on the client and family during transfers, the therapist recommended that the family purchase a gait belt. To improve the client's position in the wheelchair, the therapist recommended the purchase of a lap tray. The family was compliant with these recommendations. Maggie discovered she could move her wheelchair throughout the home by pulling on the furniture.

The therapist began instructing the family members in the set-up and best cues to help the client during transfers. Maggie was not cooperative during visits from the physical therapist and, after approximately three weeks, she was discharged from physical therapy services because it was unlikely she would be functional in ambulation even with assistive devices. The family and client felt quite disappointed when the physical therapist discontinued visits because it seemed to indicate to them that Maggie would never walk again. She complained frequently of joint pain in her knees and shoulders. The occupational therapist requested the client be medicated with simple analgesics prior to therapy to help with this problem.

Maggie was very motivated to dress herself and would practice one-handed techniques for dressing with the therapist each visit. Her apraxia made new learning difficult, but she could problem solve well on her own to complete the tasks. Maggie was tearful at times during therapy but seemed pleased when she completed tasks independently.

The family began to notice that Maggie would let them know when she was already soiled or wet. The therapist suggested a toileting schedule for providing opportunities for her to void before an accident occurred while simultaneously working to improve her transfer skills.

The family was instructed and practiced transfer techniques. The family was also taught a technique for helping the client to initiate sit-to-stand by helping her maintain a forward head position. With this technique, Maggie could initiate sit-to-stand for transfers with minimal assistance.

At the time of discharge, after 11 weeks of occupational therapy, Maggie was requiring verbal and gestural cues to set up her wheelchair for transfers. She moved sit-to-stand with only contact guard and required moderate assistance to pivot during stand-pivot transfers. She put on her housedress with moderate assistance and was able to snap it independently. She could put on her socks and sneakers after set-up. She would bathe her upper body in bed after set-up. She propelled her wheelchair throughout the house with occasional assist due to her right-sided neglect. She had 90° of pain-free passive range of motion in her right shoulder for flexion and external rotation. She did not experience any return of active movement. Her physician wanted her to begin outpatient therapy. When the family was trained in how to transfer the client to the car, she was discharged from home health for continued therapy as an outpatient.

 ## CONCLUSION

Home health is a vital area of practice for occupational therapy and offers many unique opportunities and challenges. The home offers a rich environment for learning about client needs and daily concerns in real-life situations. Occupational therapy's focus on activities of daily living makes it very natural for practitioners to provide services in the home environment.

Focusing not only on the client's needs and the family's concerns but also on the social and physical environment of the home make it a challenging setting in which to practice. The rewards, however, are numerous. Home health care allows the practitioner to become part of the "family," develop relationships with caregivers, and sometimes even establish rapport with the household pet. It provides the therapist with a sense of gratification and reward knowing the services provided have direct applicability to the client's daily life at home.

It is anticipated that home health-care services will continue to expand over the coming decades as the U.S. population ages. Individual practitioners and the profession as a whole share the responsibility to educate and train future occupational therapy professionals to participate fully in this community practice setting.

 STUDY QUESTIONS

1. Compare and contrast the role of occupational therapy in home health care with typical inpatient rehabilitation services.
2. Describe the roles of home health-care team members.
3. Identify the components of high-quality home health-care documentation.
4. Discuss how legislation and reimbursement mechanisms have impacted home health services.
5. Describe the characteristics of effective home health-care practitioners and assess your readiness to work in this community-based setting.

REFERENCES

Agency for Health Care Policy and Research. (1996). Health care and market reform: Workforce implications for occupational therapy. Washington, DC: Author. (A report prepared for the American Occupational Therapy Association.)

American Occupational Therapy Association. (1990). AOTA member data survey. Bethesda, MD: Author.

Atchison, B., Youngstrom, M., Dylla, L., Oates-Schuster, E., Anderson, K., O'Sullivan, A., and Livingston, S. (1997). Establishing a frame of reference for occupational therapy in home health care practice. In M. Youngstrom and M. Steinhauer (Eds.), *Occupational therapy in home health: Preparing for best practice (module 2)*. Bethesda, MD: American Occupational Therapy Association.

Center for Health Services and Policy Research. (1998). Outcome and assessment information set (OASIS-B1). In T. Marrelli and L. Krulish. (1999). *Home care therapy* (pp. 416–434). Boca Grande, FL: Marrelli and Associates.

Clark, N.M., and Rakowski, W. (1983). Family caregiving of older adults: Improving helping skills. *The Gerontologist, 23*, 637–642.

Harper, M.S. (1989). Providing mental health services in homes of the elderly: A public policy perspective. *Caring, 8*(6), 5–9, 52–53.

Health Care Financing Administration. (1989). *Medicare home health agency manual.* Washington, DC: Author.

Joe, B. (1997). Coaxing Congress on home health care. *OT Week, 11*(27), 16.

Law, J. (1997). Ethical concerns in home health care. *Home and Community Health Special Interest Section Quarterly, 4*(1), 2–3.

Marrelli, T., and Krulish, L. (1999). *Home care therapy.* Boca Grande, FL: Marrelli and Associates.

Medcom. (1993). *Universal precautions: AIDS and hepatitis B prevention for health care workers.* Garden Grove, CA: Author.

McQuire, M.J. (1997). Documenting progress in home care. *American Journal of Occupational Therapy, 51*(6), 437–445.

Medicare. (1996). *Home health agency manual.* Washington, DC: Health Care Financing Administration.

Navarra, T., and Ferrer, M. (1997). *An insider's guide to home health care.* Thorofare, NJ: Slack.

Opacich, K. (1997). Moral tensions and obligations of occupational therapy practitioners providing home care. *American Journal of Occupational Therapy, 51*(6), 430–435.

Schlenker, R., and Shaughnessy, P. (1992). Medicare home health reimbursement alternatives: Access, quality and cost incentives. *Home Health Care Services Quarterly, 13*(1/2), 91–115.

Shaughnessy, P., Crisler, K., and Schlenker, R. (1995). *Medicare's OASIS: Standardized outcome and assessment information set for home health care.* Denver: Center for Health Policy Research.

Siebert, C. (1998, June). Guide to changes in home health care mandated by the Balanced Budget Act. *Home and Community Health Special Interest Section Quarterly, 5*(2).

Spector, R.E. (2000). *Cultural diversity in health and illness.* Upper Saddle River, NJ: Prentice Hall.

Steib, P. (1998, July). Can home health be healed? *OT Week, 12*(27), 13.

Stone, R., Cafferata, G., and Sangl, J. (1987). Caregivers of the frail elderly: A national profile. *The Gerontologist, 27,* 616–626.

Trombly, C. (1993). Anticipating the future: Assessment of occupational function. *American Journal of Occupational Therapy, 47,* 253–257.

Trufant, D. (1994). Home health skilled therapy services. Medicare Medimessage, June 9.

U.S. Bureau of the Census. (2000). *www.census.gov/population/projections/nation*

Weinstein, M. (1997). Bringing family centered practices into home health. *Occupational Therapy Practice, 2*(7), 35–38.

Youngstrom, M. (1997). Occupational therapy in the home health care setting: An introduction. In M. Youngstrom and M. Steinhauer (Eds.), *Occupational therapy in home health: Preparing for best practice (module 1)* (pp. 1–11). Bethesda, MD: American Occupational Therapy Association.

12

CHAPTER

Specialized Practice in Home Health

Donna A. Wooster, MS, OTR, BCP
Linda Gray, OTR
Kathy G. Lemcool, MA, OTR

■ OUTLINE

Antepartum
Consumer model
Family-centered care
Least restrictive environment

Parenting skill training
Perinatal services
Postpartum
Preconception

LEARNING OBJECTIVES

This chapter is designed to enable the reader to:
- Describe the major psychiatric diagnoses seen in home health, including the reasons for occupational therapy referral.
- Describe appropriate occupational therapy assessments and interventions in psychiatric home health care.
- Discuss the potential range of perinatal occupational therapy home health services.
- Identify the types of children who may need occupational therapy home-care services.
- Describe the concept of family-centered care.
- Identify potential sources of financial support for pediatric home health-care services.
- Describe appropriate occupational therapy assessments and interventions in pediatric home health care.

INTRODUCTION

In the 21st century, the concepts of wellness, health promotion, and family-centered care will dominate (Frieda, 1994). Models of health services will continue to evolve with increased availability of affordable technology, increased accountability for health-care services, expected cultural competency for health-care professionals, and overall improved community accessibility for clients. This will bring a greater challenge for improved quality and quantity of community-based services.

Home health care is moving from the medical model approach to the consumer model approach, with the medical model being reserved for the hospital setting and the consumer model for community settings. In the medical model, the physician directs the patient's treatment. In the **consumer model,** the team, which includes the physician, other health-care professionals, the consumer, and the consumer's family, determines the goals of treatment. This movement from the medical model to the consumer model is due to two major factors: (1) the consumer's desire to take a more active role in his or her health care and (2) the necessity of the family and consumer to become involved much earlier in the treatment after illness or accident due to shorter hospital stays and less home health coverage.

The occupational therapist's role is as a "hands-on" consultant to the consumer and family. The consumer and family collaborate with the occupational therapist in setting up long- and short-term goals of treatment. These goals are accomplished using the team approach, with the consumer, the family, and the therapist as intervention agents.

During the past several years, advances in the medical field have impacted the scope of practice in home health. More than ever, people are surviving illnesses and living with disabilities. The typical caseload for a home health therapist has expanded to include an array of patient/client populations not seen previously by the home health practitioner.

Most likely, the trend of increasing numbers of client groups with diagnoses rarely seen before by home health services will continue to grow. At least two factors can be identified that contribute to this. First is the extension of the life span. More and more fragile babies survive infancy. On the other end of the age continuum, the life expectancy of older adults continues to rise. Institution-based care is decreasing while community-based options, especially in the area of mental health, are on the rise. Chapter 11 presents information regarding traditional home health practice.

This chapter focuses on some of the emerging populations with special needs that may be a part of everyday practice for some practitioners or may be populations that are underserved but who could benefit from occupational therapy delivered in the home setting. This chapter contains information that may be helpful in treating clients with primary or secondary diagnoses of mental illness, high-risk pregnancies, and infants and children with disabilities that may require preventative care. In all probability, the types and numbers of "nontraditional" client groups will continue to increase in the coming years as the population's needs change in response to advances in medical science.

 ## EVALUATION AND INTERVENTION WITH MENTAL ILLNESS

TRENDS

Trends in the treatment of persons with mental illness in the home are similar to trends shaping the treatment of other home health diagnoses. Hospital stays are shorter now, and the person is sicker when he or she arrives home.

Coverage for home health expenses is being reduced so the occupational therapist now primarily fills the role of consultant to the family while continuing to function, to a lesser degree, as a provider of services to the consumer. Treatment in the home will be family centered, with the therapist recommending treatment to address the family's and the consumer's needs. The family, the consumer, and the therapist will collaborate and work together as a team to set up long- and short-term goals that are possible to attain during the future home health sessions (Weinstein, 1997).

Adjustments will need to be made in the approach to devising a home program for the homebound mentally ill consumer. The home health client will need to be evaluated as quickly and efficiently as possible so treatment can begin immediately. Short, yet effective, assessments are necessary. As the health-care dollars continue to shrink, technology used inventively can help "pick up the slack." For example, a money management video can be left for the consumer to view at home to help prepare him or her for the next therapy visit, thus allowing the therapist to make more efficient use of treatment time by building on information that has already been presented to the consumer. The family will need to be persistent in encouraging the consumer to do his or her homework before the next therapy visit.

Reimbursement will likely become more limited, so the therapist will need to look to other sources besides Medicare, Medicaid, and private insurance for funding. The possibilities of raising money through writing grants and developing home health programs funded by charitable organizations represent two future opportunities that could be explored (Ramsey and Auerbach, 1997).

EVALUATION

A theoretical frame of reference provides the framework for use by the occupational therapist. Around this framework, the assessment instruments are chosen, the goals of treatment are written, the methods of intervention are determined, and the documentation is organized. A holistic way of approaching the consumer's dysfunction is developed. Many theoretical frames of reference have been developed for working with the mentally ill. These include sensory integration (SI), cognitive-perceptual (CP), the model of human occupation (MOHO), and occupational adaptation (OA). It is not within the scope or purpose of this book to discuss each individually, but only to refer to the importance each holds in providing a framework from which to design therapeutic programs.

Occupation and environment are two key words in home health assessment and intervention. According to theorists such as Fidler, Reilly, Kielhofner, and Yerxa, activity performance (or occupation) is a basic instinct of human nature. Occupation is necessary for health and can be used for intervention in the treatment of mental illness. Environment, which equally affects health, refers to the physical, social, cultural, and emotional milieu of the consumer. The person-environment-occupation model (Law et al., 1996) embodies all three elements to be considered in the occupational therapy home health assessment and intervention. This model implies their interconnectedness. An example of this three-part scenario might be a consumer who is referred to occupational therapy because he or she has recently lost a lifelong mate and is depressed. He or she will be adjusting to the loss, loneliness, and living alone and will need to develop new hobbies, activities, and friends to continue to function in society. The consumer is the person; recently acquired widower- or widowhood and solo living arrangements are the environment; and hobbies, activities, and family and friends are the occupation.

A recommendation for an occupational therapy consult to evaluate a consumer with mental illness may come from the primary-care physician, a psychiatrist, the home health agency's admission nurse, or from some other health-care professional who feels that occupational therapy would benefit the consumer. A written or verbal order is needed from the consumer's physician.

A primary reason for a referral for occupational therapy is the inability of the consumer to perform a task/activity independently, safely, adequately, or efficiently (Holm, Rogers, and Stone, 1997). The dysfunction may be due to a recently diagnosed mental illness, an exacerbation of a mental illness, or a mental illness secondary to a physical condition. However, another reason for a referral may be so the occupational therapist can monitor the effects of a medication on activity performance. For instance, as the physician attempts to improve the consumer's behavior at home, his or her medication may need to be changed. If the therapist is working with the consumer in the area of activity performance, the therapist will be aware of any beneficial or adverse affects the new medication may have on the consumer. A third reason for referral may be so the occupational therapist can determine the least restrictive environment in which the consumer can safely live. **Least restrictive environment** refers to the setting that provides the appropriate level of support for the individual and imposes the fewest limitations on personal autonomy. If the person is a threat to self and/or the community, he or she may need additional supervision. This will become apparent, for instance, as the occupational therapist works with the consumer in performing activities of daily living.

The occupational therapist's initial contact with the consumer is usually a phone call to the home to provide an introduction, answer any questions about occupational therapy, secure permission to come for the visit, get directions to the home, and begin establishing a rapport with the consumer and family. During this call, the therapist may be able to gain information about the consumer's physical, social, cultural, and emotional environment. The subsequent initial assessment is improved by allowing the therapist advanced preparation for the first visit, including which supplies, materials, and equipment will be needed.

The first visit is spent evaluating the consumer. An integrative approach to assessment is recommended to provide a more holistic view of the consumer (Hemphill-Pearson, 1999). The initial interview, whether standardized, for example, the Occupational Case Analysis Interview and Rating Scale (OCAIRS), or informal in nature is an opportunity for the therapist to learn personal details about the consumer and to establish rapport with the consumer and his or her family (Kaplan and Kielhofner, 1989). In the treatment of mental illness in the home, the following tools are recommended:

1. The Allen Cognitive Levels (ACL) test
2. The Role Checklist
3. The Canadian Occupational Performance Measure (COPM)
4. The Comprehensive Occupational Therapy Evaluation (COTE)
5. The Kohlman Evaluation of Living Skills (KELS) or the Bay Area Functional Performance Evaluation (BaFPE)
6. Certain assessments for evaluating specific diagnoses such as:
   a. The Self-Rating Depression Scale by William W.K. Zung, MD
   b. The State Trait Anxiety Inventory by James L. Jacobson, MD, and Alan M. Jacobson, MD

All of these assessments, performed in a short period of time, require very little equipment to be purchased and carried into the home. The ACL is a good, short screening tool to determine the consumer's present cognitive level of functioning (Allen, 1985). The Role Checklist is used for role identification and values verification. It helps the therapist determine which roles the consumer has performed and which are valued by the consumer at the present time (Oakley, Kielhofner, Barris, and Reichler, 1986). The Canadian Occupational Performance Measure (COPM) is designed to identify and prioritize occupational performance problems from a consumer or client-centered perspective. The COPM addresses all performance areas, including activities of daily living, work and productive activities, and play or leisure activities, and incorporates the roles and role expectations of the client (Law et al., 1994). The COTE can be used during the performance of a daily living task, thus beginning an ADL assessment while gathering valuable information about how the consumer approaches task performance (Brayman and Kirby, 1976). The KELS or BaFPE are excellent measures of functional performance and basic living skills (Bloomer and Williams, 1982; Kohlman-Thomson, 1992).

With the interview to gain personal information and establish rapport; the ACL for the cognitive level; the Role Checklist for values verification; the COPM to identify and prioritize problems from the client's perspective; and the COTE, KELS, or BaFPE for actual functional level of task performance, the therapist obtains a great wealth of information to use in working with the family and consumer in establishing goals. As mentioned previously, the method of reaching those goals is determined by the theoretical frame of reference and should be incorporated into the treatment plan along with the long- and short-term goals and frequency and duration of proposed treatment.

INTERVENTION

The major diagnoses treated by the home mental health occupational therapist include depression, anxiety, schizophrenia, schizoaffective disorder, Alzheimer's disease, bipolar disorder, and substance use. If the mental illness is accompanied by a physical condition, the therapist may treat the consumer for both the mental illness and the physical condition.

Three to five types of intervention are available, depending on which author's work is cited. Holm et al. (1997) state that intervention is in the form of remediation/restoration, compensation, and education. An example of education as a type of intervention would be for the therapist to take appropriate books, tapes, and other media related to the diagnosis into the home for the consumer to use. For a consumer diagnosed with anxiety, the therapist may give a tape on relaxation for the consumer to listen to prior to the next visit, when the consumer and therapist may practice the relaxation techniques described on the tape. A book on self-awareness may be given to the consumer to read prior to playing a table game. The information in the book may enhance the consumer's understanding of his or her approach to problem solving while playing the game that may then be projected into his or her problem solving in everyday life experiences. Atchison et al. (1997) describe five types of intervention: (1) establish or restore, (2) adapt, (3) alter, (4) prevent, and (5) create. This last intervention approach incorporates the environment into the intervention plan as an area of change to bring about improved function. One example of this environmental intervention is altering the social environment by having the family allow the consumer diagnosed with anxiety to dine alone in a quiet location in contrast to dining with boisterous siblings.

Occupational therapy intervention addresses three performance areas: (1) activities of daily living, (2) work and productive activities, and (3) play or leisure activities. The performance components affected by the mental illness diagnoses are from all three major areas—sensorimotor, cognitive integration, and psychosocial. Psychotropic medications may affect certain sensorimotor components such as vision, reflexes, and motor control. The Shroeder-Block-Campbell Adult Psychiatric Sensory Integration Evaluation is used to detect dysfunction in the sensorimotor area (Hamada and Schroeder, 1988). Dysfunction in cognitive integration and psychosocial components is usually obvious. The initial interview, the ACL, the COTE, and the Role Checklist should readily demonstrate dysfunction in these areas. For instance, during the interview, dysfunction will become obvious in the cognitive components of level of arousal, orientation, attention span, and memory. The ACL will allow the therapist to observe the consumer's problem-solving abilities, and the Role Checklist will identify roles and consumer values.

Table 12–1 provides examples of various mental health diagnoses, evaluative findings, and intervention approaches. For treatment, a variety of useful supplies can be brought into the home by the therapist. Examples may include:

  TABLE 12–1

EXAMPLES OF MENTAL HEALTH INTERVENTIONS

Diagnosis	Performance Component Dysfunction	Example of Intervention
Depression	Initiation of activity	Hourly time log Interest checklist
	Attention span	Graded activity from interest checklist
Anxiety	Coping skills	Relaxation exercises and guided imagery tapes
Schizophrenia	Money management	Budgeting assistance Table games such as Life and Monopoly
Alzheimer's disease	Memory	Task organization, Reminders, such as 3 × 5 cards, taped on wall

- A tape recorder
- Audiotapes (relaxation tapes and various types of music)
- Art supplies such as pen and pencil, colored pens, white lined and plain paper, colored paper, glue, and blunt-tipped scissors
- Small decorative art projects
- Table games such as playing cards, dominoes, and checkers
- Games dealing with money management such as Monopoly and Life
- Games that develop socialization skills such as Charades and Pictionary
- A small library of paperback books, booklets, and/or brochures on a variety of topics
- Gardening supplies such as paper cups, potting soil, seeds, and small gardening tools
- Donated cosmetic samples, brushes, nail file, and nail polish and remover

As goals are met, the consumer and family will be prepared for discharge. A home program of activities will be developed, practiced, and written down for the consumer along with recommendations for community resource involvement.

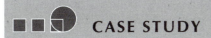 **CASE STUDY**

JEREMY

Jeremy is a 33-year-old male with a history of schizophrenia. His first psychotic episode occurred at age 19 while he was attending a university several hours' drive from his hometown. His illness forced him to withdraw from school and return to his parents' home.

Jeremy was hospitalized for three weeks and was treated with thiothixene. At admission, he complained of insomnia, anxiety, and thought disturbance. He was convinced that the alcohol and marijuana he had ingested had poisoned him.

After discharge, Jeremy registered for classes at a local community college, worked part-time, and lived at home. After four years, upon completion of an associate of arts degree, he accepted an entry-level management position in retail sales, and his parents encouraged him to find his own apartment. Within six months of moving out of his parents' home, he was rejected by a coworker in whom he expressed interest, and his ability to function in the areas of self-care and work became impaired.

Subsequently, he was hospitalized a second time with auditory hallucinations, irritability, paranoid delusions, and withdrawn behavior. During this five-week hospitalization a variety of antipsychotic medications were tried. He returned to his parents' home and remained unemployed for several months.

Jeremy's father worked for an express delivery service and was eventually able to get a low-paying position for his son on the loading dock. Jeremy did well at this job and enjoyed the work. His supervisor gradually increased his responsibilities, and at the end of one year, Jeremy was offered a supervisory position in the company. He was uncertain about whether he wanted to accept this promotion, but his parents encouraged him saying that he would again be able to afford his own apartment.

Jeremy took the supervisory position and once again moved out of his parents' home. The job was demanding, forcing Jeremy to work 50 to 60 hours per week. He began drinking and displayed inappropriate behavior toward female subordinates. He quickly decompensated and had to be rehospitalized.

After restabilization on antipsychotic medications, he was discharged to a partial hospitalization program (PHP). He became withdrawn, had blunted and inappropriate affect, and developed unusual postures and staring spells. He rarely attended the PHP. The psychiatrist ordered home health services, including occupational therapy.

A home health occupational therapy evaluation revealed occupational performance deficits in cognitive integration, level of arousal, attention span, initiation of activity, problem solving, and stress management that resulted in limited ability to participate effectively in self-care, work, and leisure activities. Jeremy described a variety of symptoms, including auditory hallucinations, paranoid delusions, insomnia, anxiety, and agitation, which worsened in response to stress. Jeremy's parents were angry about his illness and blamed his current situation on his adolescent drug use. They both wanted Jeremy to continue working but disagreed about whether he should continue to live in their home.

The priorities established by Jeremy in consultation with the occupational therapist included managing stress, finding a part-time job that he enjoyed, developing leisure interests, and moving out of his parents' home. Initially, the occupational therapist worked with Jeremy on stress-management techniques, including diaphragmatic breathing, imagery, and the use of positive self-talk and humor. Jeremy indicated an interest in physical fitness, chess, religious activities, and dating. The occupational therapist recommended that he begin his fitness program by taking a daily walk and following a videotape exercise program. In addition, Jeremy began attending church services with his parents and learned to play chess with the help of a friend.

Eventually, with the coaching of the occupational therapist, Jeremy learned how to use public transportation, joined the local YMCA, found a part-time job, and moved into a supervised apartment with a roommate.

 ## *EVALUATION AND INTERVENTION WITH PREGNANT WOMEN*

PERINATAL HOME HEALTH CARE

Perinatal services in the home will be one trend that occupational therapy should plan to be deeply involved in for prevention, wellness, and postpartum care. Perinatal care can include **preconception** (before becoming pregnant) care, low- and high-risk **antepartum** (during pregnancy) care, home birth, and **postpartum** (after giving birth) care. Perinatal services in the home will be reinforced by societal acceptance of natural childbirth, shortened hospital stays, cost effectiveness, and improved technology and monitoring (Association of Women's Health, Obstetric and Neonatal Nurses, 1994).

Although some home health perinatal services are currently practiced, most of them have been after a child with special needs is born. Nursing has been the primary provider thus far in home visits during pregnancy (Smith and Hanks, 1994). Brooten et al. (1984) studied women after cesarean births who received transitional care from a clinical nurse specialist. Findings indicated that women went home 30 hours earlier, had greater satisfaction with care, and had a 29 percent reduction in health-care charges. Brooten et al. (1986) evaluated low-birth-weight infants who received clinical nurse specialist follow-up care in the home environment and found that these infants were discharged 11 days earlier from the neonatal intensive care unit (NICU), saving thousands of dollars. The nurses providing these services required advanced training to be qualified to provide this level of services. Some even served as exercise therapists. Services have consisted of physical and psychosocial assessments of the mother and physical assessment of the newborn. A complete list of recommended assessments is available from research done by Kemp and Hatmaker (1996). Occupational therapists can provide health education for wellness of both the mother and the child before and after the birth.

Preconception Home Health Care

When planning a pregnancy, much thought goes into the timing, resources, health, and financial needs of the family. Most women desire and strive to have a healthy baby. Families may need to assess their genetic risks, the safety on the job of the pregnant woman, the resources available to them if complications should occur, and the health-care options for the delivery process.

Much research has been done to confirm the risks of certain behaviors during pregnancy. Women should be alerted to this information and encouraged to make healthy choices for themselves and their child. Occupational therapists study normal development from conception forward and are aware of these health risks. Counseling to promote optimal health during pregnancy should be a vital role. Involvement in a women's health clinic to provide some information should be considered. Also, many women seek information from adult education classes, attend health/fitness clubs, and are involved in civic organizations.

When pregnancy results without planning, often the woman may not recognize she is pregnant during some of the critical times of development (Craig, 1992). This means that her behaviors and health habits may be affecting the fetus before she even knows about the pregnancy. This poses greater risks for any woman who may not understand the consequences of behaviors and may not confirm the pregnancy to well into the fourth month or beyond. Teenagers are vulnerable to this situation. Occupational therapists who work in public schools or health clinics should become involved with ensuring that women of child-bearing age understand the signs of pregnancy, the consequences of behaviors, and the importance of seeking medical attention early. An unplanned or unwanted pregnancy may also cause greater stress and anxiety as the woman copes with her decisions and future plans. Women over 35 years of age who are experiencing pregnancy are informed of the increased risk of specific conditions by their physician and undergo tests specific to detect possible problems in the fetus.

Occupational therapists may contribute to preconception care in the following ways:

- Exercise programs for prepregnancy optimal health
- Smoking, alcohol, and substance abuse cessation
- Nutrition (team approach with a registered dietitian)
- Monitoring of blood pressure, blood sugar/diabetes, and environmental risks
- Education about pregnancy issues
- Stress reduction
- Family planning

Antepartum Home Health Care

Antepartum care is care of the family experiencing pregnancy. Pregnancy brings about inevitable physical changes for the expectant mother. Preparing for these changes and adapting a healthy lifestyle (specific to the pregnancy demands) can significantly improve the outcome for mother and infant. Women are increasingly conscious of their habits during pregnancy and seek information to aid them in decision making about exercise, nutrition, work environments, daily routines, and activities that may place them at risk. Teenage girls may not be psychologically prepared for the changes and may try to avoid the impending physical changes. Some teenagers may not eat well due to adolescent habits, and some may limit the food intake to decrease normal weight gain associated with pregnancy. Some pregnant teenagers may try to hide the pregnancy for as long as possible and not seek medical attention. These women need information to guide healthier decision making for themselves and their fetus.

The most frequent maternal health problems include preterm labor, pregnancy-induced hypertension, teenage pregnancy, nutritional risk, gestational diabetes, hyperemesis gravidarum, and substance abuse (Association of Women's Health, Obstetric and Neonatal Nurses, 1994). Premature birth is the major cause of neonatal morbidity and mortality, with 83 percent of deaths occurring between 22 and 37 weeks gestation (Creasy, 1993). Preventing these problems and premature delivery should be the primary emphasis of an antepartum program. Providing health education about signs of early labor and identification of risk factors also is important.

Barlow (1994) promotes a model antepartum program designed to meet the needs of the pregnant woman. The program consists of therapy services for the prevention of low back pain and carpal tunnel syndrome and the provision of environmental modifications and adaptive equipment as needed. Physical and occupational therapists work to address these needs. This program utilizes an obstetric back brace to provide abdominal muscle support and minimize low back pain. Health promotion and education are key components of the program.

Another need to be considered is on-site job modifications. Women continue to be a major part of the work force in the United States, and many continue to work as long as possible during their pregnancy to continue their health-care coverage and allow them more time off after the birth of their infant. Although pregnancy is not a condition that qualifies a person under the Americans with Disabilities Act, some employers or some women may be willing to pay privately for occupational therapy services. This could prove to be cost effective to the individual and the employer. A small amount of money paid for a few short visits may allow a pregnant woman to remain on the job for several more months. Simple modifications may be all that is needed, but sometimes the therapist may need to identify the risks of a particular job and provide information to the individual and the employer. Table 12–2 lists some examples.

The occupational therapist must be knowledgeable about the recommendations from the American College of Obstetrics and Gynecology for appropriate exercise and health standards. A woman should be encouraged to exercise properly throughout the pregnancy unless instructed otherwise by her physician. Classes, including follow-up classes after delivery, could be offered for pregnant women. Individualized programs may need to be developed to meet the needs of a particular client. Occupational therapists have much to offer women in antepartum care (Box 12–1).

Marmer (1995) promoted an antepartum home-care program that proved to be cost effective. This program primarily served women discharged home and placed on bed rest for the remainder of their pregnancy. In-home services included social services, occupational therapy, and nursing. Any woman who required bed rest for more than four weeks received occupational therapy. Occupational therapy treatment consisted of activities for building strength and endurance; increasing control over the environment; minimizing psychosocial complications of depression, anxiety, and boredom; promoting relaxation; increasing bed mobility; and adapting the environment to promote independence and engagement in meaningful, purposeful occupations. Crafts were used as a purposeful activity. The therapists also stressed the importance of compliance with the bed rest protocol to avoid injury or harm to the developing fetus. Marmer's (1995) results indicated better outcomes for mother and infant and reduced costs with fewer hospital admissions.

The rise of HIV infection is another factor that may contribute to the use of occupational therapy services in perinatal home health care. Many women may be too ill or reluctant to seek medical attention in a clinic-based program. Mothers need to be informed of the advances of the use of zidovudine (AZT) to reduce transmission of HIV from mother to fetus/infant (Advance for Occupational Therapists, 1997). When both mother and infant have HIV, occupational therapy should be a primary service. Occupational therapists can assess the mother and infant and make recommendations for adapted child-care techniques. Many infants with HIV have feeding and developmental issues that occupational therapy could address with the parent. Working with the parents to promote child development and make informed decisions for

TABLE 12–2

ANTEPARTUM MODIFICATIONS TO HOME/WORK ENVIRONMENTS

Problem	Solution
Change in size of abdomen	Modify work surface shape/height. Adjust chair height/depth. Use back support pillows.
Carpal tunnel syndrome	Use wrist supports. Limit repetitive motion. Consider alternative input device for computer if needed. Purchase precut vegetables. Limit salt intake and decrease fluid retention.
Low back pain	Use abdominal support brace.
Limited flexibility or bending ability	Use back support pillows. Change positions frequently. Limit unsupported standing. Use antifatigue mats. Use wheeled stool to minimize standing unsupported. Limit lifting loads. Teach proper lifting techniques. Use reacher and other aids for self-care.
Limited endurance	Teach energy conservation/pacing techniques. Place commonly used items within easy reach.
MD-ordered bed rest	Teach about adaptations for independence. Encourage purposeful activity. Perform exercises for strengthening in bed. Use table side cart with supplies. Use bedside phone/computer/books. Give decision-making/control ability.

themselves and their child would be a necessary component. Additionally, if the advances in medicine allow parents and children to live longer with HIV infection, then more long-term care will need to be provided.

Research on antepartum services for high-risk mothers reveal that 98 percent were satisfied with the physical and emotional care they received at home in specific programs (Goodwin, 1994).

Postpartum Home Health Care

The cost containment trends of the health-care business will increase the role of professionals in postpartum home health care. Women and infants come home sooner after birth. Some women may opt to have in-home deliveries. Hospitals compete to provide a comfortable environment for this population because most stays are relatively short and uncomplicated.

Societal influences that may contribute to the increases in postpartum referrals include the increases in multiple births from fertility techniques, family-centered services as mandated under the Individuals with Disabilities Education Act Part H, the number of children born with HIV, and foster home placements for children. Additionally, the number of grandparents acting as primary caregivers has increased for a

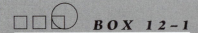

BOX 12-1

Role of Occupational Therapy in Antepartum Care

- Safe home exercise program
- Home-safety checklist
- On-the-job evaluations
- Assessment of potential risk factors
- Treatment for low back pain, carpal tunnel syndrome, depression
- Prevention of infectious disease
- Treatment for women placed on bed-rest precautions
- Adaptations for changes in body size/proportions
- Treatment for modifications to chores, child-care, and household responsibilities
- Preparation for birth experience
- Developmental screening for other children
- Preparation for parenting role

variety of reasons. These grandparents may not have been prepared for this responsibility. Plus, they may have medical needs of their own. Children born with special health-care needs may require services in the home. The emphasis will be on teaching caretakers to be able to provide the needed care to their child.

Caretakers who may be most in need of in-home occupational therapy services are parents who are young or immature, who are substance abusers, who have HIV, who are raising children born with HIV, or who are disabled or have special needs and are living with their parents, with both their parents and themselves contributing to the care of the child. Also, when a child is born with special needs such as cerebral palsy, Down's syndrome, congenital abnormalities, prematurity, or chronic illness, caregivers will need guidance and instruction.

The role of occupational therapy will be primarily to assess family needs and provide caregiver education to promote child development. Developmental assessments of infants will be essential. Occupational therapists should be the primary providers when the child has a known difficulty with feeding, poor sensory processing, abnormal muscle tone, impaired vision or hearing, or impaired motor development. Children with cognitive deficits also may need occupational therapy to establish a self-care program with parents.

Encouraging parental involvement is important for bonding and confidence/competence building. When the infant was hospitalized, the medical staff may have been the primary caretaker, allowing the parent to visit with the child. This does little to prepare parents for the responsibilities they will encounter at home. Additionally, even when parents are taught procedures in the hospital, many feel insecure without the primary medical team immediately available. Although many parents are glad to be home, at the same time, they are also nervous and fearful.

Many theories about family coping with and response to the diagnosis of a child with special needs exist. Occupational therapists need to understand these theories and models. Anger may be the primary emotional reaction that limits involvement with the child with special needs. Feelings of inadequacy in providing care also may occur, resulting from the restriction in early caregiving opportunities, ongoing medical complications, parental substance abuse, financial concerns, need for education and instruction, and the need for mentoring from an experienced caregiver (Alfonso et al., 1992). Some theories do not agree that all families go through defined stages. Research has shown that some feelings and behaviors will distance parents from involvement with their child. Careful observation and sensitive discussion of these ideas with family members is important. Early involvement in the caregiving process is necessary. Infants and toddlers whose parents are included in the intervention process demonstrate greater developmental change than those whose parents are not participating in the process (Dunst, Trivette, and Deal, 1988).

Other family members may be willing to participate in the care of the infant but may not have been taught the "how-to's," with the result that they watch and feel re-

 TABLE 12–3

EXAMPLES OF POSTPARTUM INTERVENTIONS

Problem	Solution
Increased numbers of children born with special needs	Caregiver education Education about diagnosis Developmental assessments Direct home assessment and intervention Stress management Coping skills Parental engagement in caregiving tasks immediately after birth
Caregivers with physical or psychological illnesses or limited parenting abilities	Environmental adaptations to ease demands of child care and ensure safety Task modification Recognition of changes in themselves to seek medical attention Utilization of community resources Parental education for understanding nonverbal communication of the infant's signals of sensory overload Instruction on calming strategies to aid infant in sleeping better Education about age appropriate expectations of the child Equipment adaptation as needed
Children with severe medical needs	Education of family members in care of equipment and safety issues Parental assistance with recording valuable information about health issues as way to monitor child's condition Instructions to parents about when to contact MD or emergency services
Families with limited financial and people resources	Utilization of community resources Support groups with focus Teaching of child-care skills to interested significant others

luctant to assume responsibility. This can limit the resources and respite care available to the family. The parents should be encouraged to invite those persons possibly willing to learn to bathe, feed, or care for the child to the next therapy session to learn.

Another option for occupational therapists will be to get involved in parenting skill training. Many model programs include alternatives to keep pregnant teenagers in school. In some programs, the teenage mothers attend an alternative school program or the same school program for a specific amount of time during and immediately after pregnancy. The infants attend school with the mothers. Care of the infants is provided by high school students in child development classes or by adult paid or volunteer grandparents. Some schools have certified day-care centers in the school. The school nurse provides instruction in planning for birth and postpartum changes. For example, **parenting skill training** provided by occupational therapists may include classes on the following topics: reading your child's signals, using calming techniques for the infant, performing infant massage, preparing the home environment for your child, and using proper feeding techniques. The topic of sensory overstimulation has proved to be a valuable lesson for teenage parents whose lifestyle may increase the child's irritability at a time when they want the child to sleep. A variety of potential postpartum interventions are listed in Table 12–3. More information about the role of occupational therapy in pediatric home health services is available later in this chapter.

Occupational therapists should begin to prepare themselves to be more assertive in the health and wellness component of perinatal care. Occupational therapists should be a primary team member with defined roles along with nursing, social services, registered dietitians, and physical therapists.

The future could find occupational therapists working more in health promotion and wellness and in community outreach facilities. Preparing to expand one's knowledge base and recognizing the valuable information and contributions of occupational therapy to home health makes the future challenging and exciting.

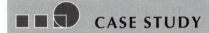 CASE STUDY

MARY

Mary is a pregnant 38-year-old at 19 weeks gestation. Ultrasound indicates twins, and bed rest is ordered. Mary has a 3-year-old daughter and, until two weeks ago, worked full time as a registered nurse supervisor at the local nursing home.

The in-home interview indicates that the client is usually a very active person and is having a difficult time adjusting to the bed rest. Family supports are available to assist with the care of the 3-year-old child while the husband is at work. The client expresses concern about the many things she should be doing and about the lack of preparations for the twins.

Physical findings reveal a relatively healthy woman with some edema in her lower extremities. Intermittent spotting is noted but controlled with positioning. Upper-body strength is normal at the present time. An environmental assessment indicates that there is little within the mother's reach except the remote control for the television. An examination of the nursery indicates that clothing needs to be sorted by sizes and organized in preparation for the twins. Family members are doing all of the chores and not allowing Mary to participate in any tasks. She is feeling useless and depressed about the future.

Occupational therapy services were provided to Mary twice weekly for six weeks. The primary goal was to adapt the environment and assist Mary to engage in meaningful occupation while still maintaining her bed-rest precautions. Mary needed to feel that she was contributing to her family's care, which would improve her self-esteem. She and the occupational therapist identified some household chores that Mary could do. She and family members were educated in the appropriate set-up for these chores.

A small table was provided at bedside, with a lazy Susan that contained many needed items. The chores that were set up in bed or at bedside for Mary included folding laundry, cutting/peeling vegetables for meals, choosing her daughter's clothing for the day, styling her daughter's hair in the morning, paying bills, mending clothing, writing grocery lists, and organizing coupons for shopping. Also, the baby clothes were brought in for Mary to sort and organize by sizes in preparation for the twins. Mary wrote out lists of chores that needed to be done by others and encouraged family and friends to assist. This eased the responsibilities placed on her husband and allowed those who wanted to help to choose a task they wanted to do. This list included tasks involving setting up the nursery, getting bassinets ready for when she first came home from the hospital, packing her suitcase for the hospital, and purchasing and organizing all of the additional baby items. Mail-order catalogs were obtained to allow Mary to select and price items that were needed. A telephone at bedside allowed her to contact friends at work and keep in touch with her colleagues and patients.

Mary was allowed out of bed for showering and toileting. At evaluation, the occupational therapist determined that Mary needed moderate physical assist to get in and out of the bathtub. A tub seat and a hand-held shower allowed her to sit and shower more easily and safely. Elastic shoelaces were not useful with the varying degrees of edema she experienced. Thus, slip-on shoes were recommended to eliminate the bending required for shoe tying. A reacher was provided to help Mary reach the blankets at the foot of the bed, items on the floor, and objects in the room. Mary missed having family meals together with her husband and daughter. A small table was placed in the bedroom to allow the family to eat together.

An interest checklist revealed that Mary had many interests but limited time to pursue her hobbies prior to bedrest. She had several projects that she started but not yet finished. Mary's leisure activities included reading, sewing, cross-stitching, swimming, biking, and planting flowers. The occupational therapy practitioner helped Mary to determine which projects she could complete while on bed rest. She had several books for reading. She finished a cross-stitching project and started some new ones. Mary also expressed interest in learning to make hair bows and ribbons for her daughter. The occupational therapy practitioner provided her with instructions and materials to start this project as well.

A list of books about rearing twins was provided to help her prepare for this new role. She was connected with a local support group for parents with twins. An in-bed exercise and positioning program was implemented to maintain strength and provide relief from back pressure. In summary, Mary reported that she felt much more in control of her life, was more connected with her family roles, and was able to remain active and healthy despite the bed-rest precautions.

 ## EVALUATION AND INTERVENTION WITH CHILDREN

The future for pediatric home health care is unclear at this time. The need for home services, including occupational therapy, is expected to increase, but the availability, supplier, and payer of these services are uncertain. Many changes contribute to the need and support for in-home services for children, including family structure, the health needs of children, reimbursement options, and the law. Attempting to meet the needs of families, the development of statewide early intervention programs, and the provision of supportive family-centered services rather than institutionalization have proven cost effective and useful.

Occupational therapists must prepare themselves for these changes by developing the ability to provide "best practice" intervention in a variety of home environments. Occupational therapists will work with teams to reach out to rural communities to establish health care and support systems with culturally diverse families. The primary goal will be mentoring families to care for their children in healthier ways. Failure to meet these goals could result in increased morbidity, mortality, and developmental delay secondary to abuse, neglect, malnutrition, dehydration, and decreased quality of life.

Pediatric home health care is different from adult home health care. First, children do not need to meet the Medicare definition of "homebound" to be eligible for services in the home. Also, different reimbursement options are available, such as early intervention funds, Medicaid, private insurance options, private funding by the family, and payment through a written individualized education plan (IEP) through the public school system. The payer of the service will impact the role of occupational therapy with the family and child. The payer and the agency will determine the required documentation. This variety may make documentation cumbersome, confusing, and frustrating to the therapist. Many agencies hire staff that is experienced with the adult population. A therapist may be asked to treat a small number of children and will need to determine his or her comfort level in working with this medically fragile population.

Pediatric home health services may be provided as part of a continuum of services. A child may move from inpatient acute hospitalization to a rehabilitation hospital to home health services. Later the child may return to school and possibly to outpatient services. The home health occupational therapist will need to consult the previous team members to provide the most effective treatment program (Austill-Claussen, 1995).

AREAS IMPACTING CHILDREN'S HEALTH

Much research has been done to document the health changes in children. Research has identified the major risk factors affecting morbidity and mortality (Hogue, Buehler, Strauss, and Smith, 1987). The health and age of the mother and the birth weight of the infant are very important factors. As medical knowledge continues to increase and more children survive serious medical conditions, many may have some residual developmental delay (Goldson, 1996). The population of children who require medical in-home intervention has changed also. Many of these children have combined biological and environmental risk factors that may promote or impede their outcomes. Children may qualify for in-home therapy services for a variety of reasons; for example, difficulty with endurance and tolerance to get to outpatient services or a weakened immune system that requires them to stay home. Or it may be too taxing for the parent to bring the child in to a clinic (Adams, 1996). Availability of services is a major problem for rural communities where services are not offered and public transportation systems are poorly developed or nonexistent.

CHILDREN WITH ACUTE MEDICAL NEEDS. Some children will qualify for home health services and only need a specific course of medical intervention for defined amounts of time. These children are easily identified by their primary physician. Eventually, the children will no longer need in-home services and may transition to an outpatient clinic or the school system. For example, a child recovering from surgery for scoliosis may be out of school for some time and require adaptations to function at home. Eventually, the child is expected to return to school and be able to function normally. However, outpatient services may be initiated to continue the rehabilitation process after the child is discharged from home health services.

CHILDREN WITH CHRONIC ILLNESS. This population has ongoing or recurrent medical needs. Often, these children have multiple problems that affect many systems and functional skills, most in need of a continuum of services that changes with their health-care needs (MacQueen and Gittler, 1997). The most involved may require extended or recurrent hospitalizations. Their health problems may strain family resources and create emotional turmoil and long-term exhaustion for caregivers. Multiple family members must be encouraged to get involved in the child's care (Bailey et al., 1986). As the child grows and survives into adolescence, the physical assistance requirements may change due to the child's size. Established routines may be disrupted. Hormonal changes may make verbal exchanges more frequent, causing different behaviors to emerge. As previous techniques fail, modifications and adaptations must be made.

Children with chronic illness also face biological and environmental issues that affect their outcomes. Poverty, limited resources, inadequate transportation, and prior poor role modeling of parenting skills place these children at greater risk and more in need of in-home therapy services.

CHILDREN REQUIRING TECHNOLOGICAL ASSISTANCE. Improved life-saving techniques at birth and afterward have resulted in better health outcomes with more children's lives being saved. Some of these children will need assistance with life functions such as breathing, dialysis, feeding, elimination, and others, requiring temporary or permanent dependence on machines to sustain life. Parents and caretakers must learn to provide this medical care; for example, to use sterile techniques to prevent infections and identify changes in health status that warrant notification of the medical system, in addition to the normal demands of parenting. The severity of the problems and the intensity of care required place demands and significant responsibilities on families (Kohrman, 1991). When the need for care is longer, typically the family disruption and burden are greater. Families have the best outcomes when technology is required for two years or less (Quint, Chesterman, Crain, Winkleby, and Boyce, 1990).

Families are faced with financial concerns, fatigue, fear, lack of privacy, and health-care changes that may affect the assistance available to them (Levy and Pilmer, 1992). Some families may even have exhausted their lifetime maximum (cap) available through their health insurance. Sullivan-Belyai (1990) states that the best outcome results when the discharge plan includes a well-organized, interdisciplinary team with a designated case manager.

CHILDREN WITH HIV/AIDS. HIV infection is one of the leading causes of morbidity and mortality among children. Ninety percent of the cases are attributed to perinatal transmission from infected mother to fetus (Centers for Disease Control, 1995). The rise of HIV infection in women will likely be accompanied by a rise of HIV infection in children. Research supports that 76 to 90 percent of all children with HIV demonstrate neurodevelopmental delays as infants and neuropsychological deficits as older children. Advances in medical treatment, especially AZT and protease inhibitors, may result in children living longer with HIV infection. Some of these children may outlive their parents, requiring the children to be placed with other family members, in foster care, or in extended care facilities, adding stress to an already burdened social services and health-care system.

CHILDREN BORN PREMATURELY WITH LOW BIRTH WEIGHT AND COMPLICATIONS. The science of neonatology has made tremendous advances. Although more infants are surviving, their medical problems and complications make them more fragile, often with life-long disability. Birth weight is one of the most important predictors of positive outcomes (Hogue, Buehler, Strauss, and Smith, 1987). Any very low-birth-weight infant will have the potential for long-term problems. Klepitsch (1995) writes from personal experience about the emotional "roller coaster" for these parents.

CHILDREN BORN TO SUBSTANCE-ABUSING PARENTS. As drug use continues to be prevalent in our society, some expectant mothers continue to abuse drugs, causing harm to the fetus. Additional maternal risks of undernutrition, sexually transmitted diseases, and inadequate prenatal care further compound the problem (Batshaw and Conlon, 1997). Drug abuse often occurs in the midst of poverty and family instability (Bauman and Daugherty, 1983). Infants born to substance-abusing mothers have an increased risk of prematurity, lower birth weight, irritability, and poor skills for attachment. Substance-abusing parents may not have learned or developed effective parenting skills. Some parents have unrealistic behavioral expectations of their children, resulting in negative reinforcement, inappropriate punishment, or abuse of the child. Other parents may not provide the care or the structure the child needs, so the child is neglected, possibly roaming about and hungry. Even though some children will have normal IQ's, the combination of medical problems and negative environmental effects on development may have serious consequences for these children.

CHILDREN BORN TO TEENAGE MOTHERS. As the incidence of teenage pregnancy rises, the risk of prematurity, low birth weight, complications, and mortality continues to rise. Many expectant teenagers do not seek timely medical attention because they lack an awareness of their condition or attempt to hide it. Most are unmarried, with limited financial resources. Many are from families burdened by the addition of another child. The fate of these children born to children will be compounded if their needs are not met. Many children of teenage mothers suffer poor health and demonstrate poorer school performance (Brooks-Gunn and Fustenberg, 1986). Much of the social stigma previously attached to teenage pregnancy has abated. However, now the expectation is for teenage mothers to raise their child instead of considering adoption. Some teenagers may feel pressure to keep a child despite their lack of parenting skills and experience.

Changes in the Family

FAMILY STRUCTURE. The typical American family has undergone many changes during the last 30 years. There are more extended families, blended families, single-parent families, teenage parents, grandparents as primary caretakers, joint custody situations, and foster parents. Some of these changes can strengthen families and provide more parental and financial resources for the children. However, some parents are left isolated and alone to care for a child. Family supports may be minimal or lacking due to separation or relocation. Because of the changes, some families will be more vulnerable, needing additional support to survive and endure.

FAMILY RESPONSIBILITY. Despite changes in family structure, families continue to be the primary caretakers of children with special health-care needs. Families are the primary source of nurturance and survival. Additionally, the responsibility to the child becomes life long, with new demands and challenges over time. Women continue to be the primary caretakers, with responsibility shifting from mother or grandmother down the generations. With increasing age, this responsibility may shift to the eldest nondisabled female sibling (Erickson and Upshur, 1989).

FAMILY RESOURCES. Families living in rural poverty do not have access to the same level of care as families with greater financial means (St. Peter, Newacheck, and Halton, 1992). For example, transportation may be a serious problem for the family. Often, children with disabilities belong to poor or dysfunctional families living in disadvantaged communities with fewer opportunities for a high quality of life (Thompson, 1992).

Changes in Medical Reimbursement

Traditionally, private insurance has paid for home health occupational therapy services for children. The rates paid to the agency varied, depending on the policy. Often multiple payers were involved, and each policy had to be studied to clearly understand the coverage and limitations. Now insurance coverage is a complex maze of options with deductibles, copayments, pre-existing conditions, waiting periods, capitation, and strict limitations for types of benefits and lifetime limits. The extent of coverage available to the child depends solely on insurance coverage. Some plans limit the number of visits while others limit the total money spent per illness. Some plans refuse to provide services to children with chronic illness. Some managed-care options may result in financial incentives and utilization controls, making it difficult or impossible for children to get the specialized care that they need (Berman, Gross, and Lewak, 1995; Freund and Lewitt, 1993).

A continuum of health-care services that is cost effective is proposed (MacQueen and Gittler, 1997). At the primary level, each child would have a primary physician acting as the coordinator and gatekeeper of the child's health care. This concept may be new for families that utilize the emergency room for routine care. At the secondary level, specialized consultants and direct services, such as therapeutic interventions, are utilized for unusual or severe problems. This requires a referral from the primary physician. At the tertiary level, highly specialized consultants and direct services are provided. Examples of these are the services of children's hospitals and specialists such as neonatologists or cardiac surgeons. At higher levels of treatment, the care is more expensive. The primary physician's role is to refer only as necessary and to coordinate all services provided to the child.

State-run Medicaid programs have become the largest payer for health services for the poor in this country (Fleming, 1993). Each state has control over the extent of services, eligibility criteria, and regulations. Most states provide some provision for coverage of occupational therapy services in the home. Reimbursement for therapy services from Medicaid is considerably lower than that from private insurance or Medicare. Each state is required to conduct early periodic screening and diagnosis treatment (EPSDT) to screen for disability and chronic illness and to provide services as early as possible. This screening can include occupational therapy evaluation to determine if a developmental delay or other health problem warrants services. Diminished access to service from limitations in insurance coverage is a key factor in the relationship between low socioeconomic status and disability (Halfon and Newacheck, 1993). Unless reimbursement changes occur, it is unrealistic for the competitive home health agencies to strive to service this Medicaid population. Some states are modeling their Medicaid program on HMOs. All families select primary physicians who must authorize all admissions and specialized services. The concept is to save money by decreasing the use of emergency room services for routine problems, thus providing better coordinated care through a primary physician.

Each state receives block grant money for maternal and child health services. Each state is also required to match part of the funding. Since 1990, 30 percent of this money provided to each state is targeted for children with special health-care needs (Hutchins and Hutchins, 1997). The lead agency is usually the state health agency that allocates and disburses money as appropriate.

Some children with chronic illness have no insurance coverage. Parents may have to sell possessions to pay medical bills. Once parents have spent most of their assets for medical costs, the child or family may qualify for Medicaid coverage. Presently our society has a two-tiered health system, one for children with private insurance and one for poor children.

Families must learn to be advocates so their children receive needed services. Parents must appeal inappropriate denials from insurance companies and continue to pursue payment. Managed-care systems force professionals to be accountable and make the most of every minute with patients. Therapists are forced to do more in less time with better outcomes. These quick outcomes and improvements may be unrealistic for children with chronic illness, thus increasing the likelihood for denial of services.

Social Security income (SSI) was extended in the 1980s to include children with chronic illnesses. More liberal income criteria were used to help families to care for their child at home. Recent criteria are stricter because of reported fraud and abuse in the system. Families often use this supplemental income to purchase extra electricity for technology-assisted children, supplemental nutrition, larger-sized diapers, or a large piece of equipment such as a stander or stroller. Also, eligibility for SSI funding was linked to eligibility for Medicaid funding, enabling families to obtain health insurance (Hutchins and Hutchins).

The early intervention system provides services to children from "birth through 2" or "birth to 3" who are developmentally delayed or at risk for delay. This system is mandated to include family support and in-home services. Occupational therapy is a primary service provider in this system, which is more of a combination medical/educational model. Please refer to Chapter 14 for more details on early intervention.

As a society, we need to make commitments to provide quality in-home services to families, guarding against the isolation, neglect, or abuse of these children (Thompson, 1992). Services that strengthen the family and necessary community resources must be a priority. Albrecht and Higgins (1977) found that the rehabilitation success of children and adolescents depends largely on family support. This includes returning the children to safe environments and teaching family members how to promote independence in daily functioning in each child. Mothers function better with disabled children when the mothers are provided resources and consistent social supports (Anderson and Telleen, 1992).

Needs of Families

CURRENT AND RELEVANT INFORMATION. Families need to understand the diagnosis and its implications to form a plan for intervention. They can formulate relevant questions and prioritize tasks. Families want education to be customized and tailored for them, preferring personalized instruction and reinforcement for completion of specific skills. Families reported that they appreciated information in a variety of forms, including written handouts, pictures, and diagrams.

Families want information to help them make informed decisions about their child's health. This includes information about surgical procedures, such as rhizotomies and spinal fixation surgery, and current treatment methods, such as botox (botulinum toxin) injections or a diet to prevent seizures. The occupational therapist may be able to provide resources to allow the family to access the needed information. The family should know the positives and negatives of each procedure to make an informed choice for their child.

In the **family-centered care** model, the needs of the family are the primary concern for the health-care team member. The family is treated as an equal partner in decision making, viewed as a resource on the daily abilities of their child and valued in their ability to care for their child. The health-care team members support and nurture the family in the role of caretaker. The natural home and community are felt to be the best environments for children with disabilities (Brewer, McPherson, Magrab, and Hutchins, 1989).

EMPOWERMENT. Parents want service providers to offer information and encouragement for them to seek information and make decisions based on their family needs. They want to be the decision makers for their child. They want to raise their child in a safe environment that is compatible with their cultural and religious beliefs. Understanding their culture is the responsibility of the service providers.

The birth of a child with a disability has different meanings in various societies and families. Cultural values and beliefs shape the family perspective on medical interventions, acceptance of the child, responsibilities in family roles, and religious significance. Societal perspectives change over time. The standard philosophical view in this country of what is best for a child with mental retardation was very different 25 years ago than it is today. All these variables will shape the perspectives of different family members.

In the United States, with its mixture of ethnic groups, the occupational therapist must be knowledgeable about the communities he or she serves. Food is very much part of cultural and regional upbringing. Regional foods, such as red beans and rice in Alabama, gumbo in New Orleans, bagels in New York, and baked beans in Boston, may or may not be representative of this individual family culture. Some suggestions to guide health-care professionals in their cultural understanding are listed here:

- Encourage the family to discuss their perspectives and definitions of the situations and needs. This will allow the therapist to hear the family's viewpoint, which may be very different from the therapist's.
- Attempt to learn the native language and, at least, to have an interpreter available as needed for communication. Selecting someone well respected and trusted in the community as an interpreter can make a significant difference in how families view the therapist's intentions and services.
- Avoid making assumptions. Respect the family's home and personal belongings.
- Be tolerant of unfamiliar customs. Pay attention to how the family establishes duties/chores/responsibilities of various family members. Families may not want to change. This may be an important constant in their lives.
- Attempt to learn and understand more about the culture, ask parents how they want to be addressed, and speak succinctly to avoid confusing parents or other family members (Roelse, 1996).
- Be aware of cultural differences that may include avoidance of direct eye contact and speaking only to the father or only to the mother when the father has left the room.
- Remember that gender-specific expectations are relevant within cultures and that traditions are sacred.

Referral Sources

The home health agency may not be aware of the need for pediatric home health occupational therapy services. Often, in-home occupational therapy services are the best choice. Box 12–2 lists some of the factors that promote the need for home health occupational therapy services. In-service training to develop this awareness may help the staff identify the role for pediatric home health, thus making appropriate referrals to occupational therapy. The agency may also begin to prepare to have nursing staff available with expertise in pediatrics such as wound care, tracheotomy care, gastrostomy tube care, and other pediatric needs, depending on potential referrals.

Other referring agencies may not be aware that the home health agency is accepting pediatric referrals. A one-page handout that identifies the services the agency can provide to children, with the phone number and the name of the contact person for referrals, will be very helpful. Contacting local children's hospitals, rehabilitation facilities, trauma centers, acute-care hospitals, and local early intervention staff provides a good beginning for a referral base.

ASSESSMENT TOOLS

Most often, the evaluation process, including choosing the most appropriate assessment tool, is determined by the occupational therapist. Therefore, the occupational

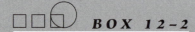

BOX 12-2

Factors that Promote the Use of Home Health OT Services

- Lack of or difficulty with transportation to outpatient centers
- Child with weakened immune system
- Precautions needed to minimize infection risk
- Belief that child does best in natural environments
- Family attempting outpatient services but missing many visits
- Mandates in early intervention laws encouraging this choice
- Increased stress on all family members when child is hospitalized
- Beneficial effect of spending some time at home

therapist must choose an assessment tool best suited for the child and context. Many home health-care agencies have their own generic occupational therapy evaluation form, which may or may not be appropriate for use with the pediatric population. Adaptation may be necessary. Information is gathered from chart review and contact with the parent by telephone before choosing an assessment tool. Doing so may help to enhance the interaction and improve the initial visit. The questions listed here can serve as a guide:

1. What fine-motor, self-help, and cognitive skills would be considered age appropriate? It is important to understand "normal" child development. For example, what can a 2-year-old be expected to do in terms of self-care skills?
2. How does the referring diagnosis affect functional performance in terms of performance areas and components? For example, for a referring diagnosis of cerebral palsy, all performance areas (self-care, play, and work) are affected.

SENSORIMOTOR ASSESSMENT. Movement and postural control must be evaluated, including abnormal muscle tone, contractures, and coordination. Is there any history of seizures, especially with the spastic form of cerebral palsy (CP) and is the child taking seizure medication? The child may have visual and cognitive impairments. Is any information about glasses, eye muscle control, and eye doctor available? What about the child's cognitive status, ability to communicate, indicate needs, and follow directions? Has any previous testing been done?

DEVELOPMENTAL ASSESSMENT. Most pediatric referrals to occupational therapy in home health will be for feeding, generalized developmental delay, and significant health impairments. Purchasing a variety of assessment tools is an expensive investment. Instead, choosing tools that can be used with a variety of ages is advisable and allows information to be organized for a variety of developmental skills. Generally, at least one type of developmental checklist that allows for parental involvement is useful and less expense. Examples include the following (refer to chart in the Appendix for specifics about ages and ordering information):

- Hawaii Early Learning Profile
- Hawaii Early Learning Profile for Special Preschoolers
- Carolina Curriculum for Infants and Toddlers
- Carolina Curriculum for Preschoolers with Special Needs

- Early Learning Accomplishment Profile
- Learning Accomplishment Profile-D

FINE-MOTOR ASSESSMENT. The Peabody, a versatile assessment tool for birth to 83 months, is especially valuable in evaluating gross and fine-motor skills. The tool is both standardized and criterion referenced. Although the tool needs to be supplemented with a checklist for a closer look at adaptive skills, it provides a good baseline of information.

The Bruninks-Oseretsky Test of Motor Proficiency is often at too high a level for use with most of the children seen in home health settings. It may be appropriate if referrals will be for school-aged children with mild to moderate motor impairments. The information is standardized by age groups but is not relevant to functioning in the home environment.

SELF-CARE ASSESSMENT. The Pediatric Evaluation of Disability Inventory (PEDI) allows for age flexibility. Therapists are able to rate the amount of assistance required for the child to complete daily tasks. This may be very helpful for assessing children with motor impairments from CP, muscular dystrophy (MD), and traumatic brain injury (TBI).

FEEDING ASSESSMENT. Many commercially available feeding assessment tools are available. The Oral Motor Feeder Rating Scale is applicable to a variety of children. Usually a very detailed understanding of the normal developmental sequence of oral motor skills is necessary to appropriately interpret the results and develop optimal interventions. Some key points to remember when conducting a feeding assessment are listed in Box 12–3.

When conducting a feeding assessment, a travel feeding kit is recommended for use. Useful supplies include consumable items that may be given to parents such as a variety of nipple types, cups with and without covers, pediatric-sized adaptive utensils, a squeeze bottle (for cleft palate), bottle handles, Nuk brush sets, infadents, straws, scoop dish, and plate guard. Positioning devices include the back jack, an infant head support, small wedges, and aids for positioning in infant seats, car seats, and high chairs. Since every family requires a car seat, this can be the best place to begin the feeding assessment, allowing instant evaluation of some items that may be left with the family for immediate implementation of feeding recommendations.

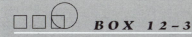 **BOX 12–3**

Key Points in Feeding

- Prefeeding programs are necessary—"use it or lose it" philosophy.
- Positioning is an essential prerequisite.
- Normalizing tone is necessary to facilitate better motor control.
- Feeding should be done in natural environments and at normal eating times when other family members are eating.
- Feeding is an interactive process and communication is essential.
- Sensory defensiveness must be remediated if it is present.
- Feeding is very much a cultural activity—awareness is important.

For safety reasons, children transitioning from tube feedings to oral feedings may need evaluation by an expert feeding team at the nearest children's hospital. The team has suctioning, videofluoroscopy, and medical intervention available on site. These specialists can conduct the feeding evaluation and provide useful suggestions for home implementation. Good judgment with pediatric feeding problems is necessary.

OTHER ASSESSMENTS. If referrals for older children who are leaving rehabilitation are anticipated, the therapist may need other assessment tools. These would be useful for evaluation of motor coordination, visual perceptual skills, visual motor skills, self-care, and higher-level occupational tasks. Assessment tools may be selected based on potential referrals.

INITIAL VISIT AND PARENT INTERVIEW

As a guest in the family's home, the therapist must request permission to see, hold, and treat the child. During the initial interview, the child should be allowed to stay in the arms of the parent to provide time for the child, parents, and therapists to become comfortable with each other. Eliciting information, especially about parental concerns, such as those listed here, is important:

- Contextual effects on this family/child.
- Influence of culture/beliefs on issues of health, child development, feeding, dressing, and discipline.
- Family hopes for desired outcomes.
- Acceptable range of toys, equipment, daily routines, expectations of siblings, and tolerance for loud play in the home environment.
- Safe outdoor play area or a nearby park.
- Family members actively involved in child care. Are others willing but unsure or afraid due to the child's needs?

Explanation of the assessment to the parent, involving them in the assessment, using care not to offend them, and mentioning at the start the reasons that coaxing the child's performance is not recommended will improve the success of the evaluation.

The type of assessment utilized discovers the baseline abilities of the child. This information is essential and impacts all future decisions about interventions. It must be as accurate a picture as possible of the child's true abilities at the current time, so every effort must be made to obtain good, reliable information. Some important points to consider when assessing a child and planning intervention are listed in Box 12–4.

Few parents can, or should, spend hours exercising a child. Appropriate positioning for routines at bath time, meal times, during diaper changing or bathroom time, and during car rides is necessary. Safe positioning of the child is incorporated into the routine of the caregivers, including self-care and work-at-home times, to provide them with more control in their life.

Before leaving from the first visit, typically the next visit is scheduled. The therapist and family also decide how the family would notify the therapist of changes in schedule. Providing a business card with phone numbers is helpful.

INTERVENTION

Occupational therapists must adhere to state laws regarding home health practice, which may require different continuing education competencies, documentation, and

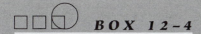

BOX 12–4

Considerations in Evaluation and Intervention with Children

- Children should be safe in their own home and should have as much freedom of movement as possible.
- Recommendations should fit the lifestyle and daily routine of the parents.
- Assessments should provide accurate, current, and reliable information.
- Parents should be involved in the evaluation process.
- Children generally perform better on assessments in natural environments.
- While assessing the child, careful observation is important for developing potential intervention strategies.

referral procedures. Most states and insurance companies will require a physician order for occupational therapy evaluation and treatment. Some acute diagnostic conditions may come with very specific orders for completion of specific types of testing, splinting, positioning, or intervention.

Intervention at home can be most functional and allow for optimum communication with parents. Children will be practicing skills, especially self-care skills, in the environment where they use them. This is a great advantage and should be capitalized on when choosing skills to address. Allowing the child to develop self-feeding and self-toileting skills is very important due to the frequency and time demands placed on caregivers. Occupational therapists must carefully select self-care activities that fit the routines of the family (Hinojosa and Anderson, 1991).

Actively listening to parental concerns for the first five to ten minutes of each visit may provide information that may change the focus of treatment for that day. Changes in medical status and new problems must be communicated and addressed. Explaining the focus for that day's visit, obtaining parental permission, and being open to suggestions enhance the effectiveness of the visit.

Another advantage of home health intervention may be the availability of previously enjoyed games, sports, and hobbies that can facilitate the child's ability to return to purposeful leisure and play activities. Although the previous daily routines may need some alteration, the key is allowing for leisure/play. Siblings and friends may be willing to get involved with some of these activities, possibly promoting friendly relationships with peers while allowing parents time off from routine care.

The factors that affect the child's ability to transition to school-based or outpatient therapy, and the goals for transition back to the community as soon as able, are the focus of the treatment plan. Insurance will mandate that these factors be addressed and goals accomplished early in treatment whenever possible. In preparation for the transition, areas that include the child's ability to maneuver outside of the home, transfer to and from the family vehicle and the school bus, and age-appropriate social and cognitive skills in the classroom environment are addressed.

At the end of the visit, the family is thanked for their cooperation and provided with a verbal summary of the progress noted on that day. The next visit also is scheduled. This interaction increases the opportunity to blend with family routines and optimize their skills in learning to manage the child's disabilities.

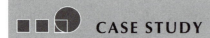 **CASE STUDY**

TOMMY

Tommy is a 9-month-old who is HIV positive and receiving occupational therapy for developmental delay and feeding problems. The child presents with slightly low tone, poor endurance, and poor head and trunk control against gravity. The infant, receiving Isomil for higher-caloric intake, drinks 7 ounces in 20 minutes. Tommy is living in a foster home and the foster parents want to introduce spoon feeding with infant cereal and fruits.

Occupational therapy evaluation reveals slightly low tone in the face and trunk, poor lip closure on nipple, poor endurance, and difficulty with head and trunk control against gravity. Development according to the Early Learning Accomplish Profile (ELAP) indicates the following:

1. Gross-motor skills at 4 months
2. Fine-motor skills at 3 months
3. Cognitive skills at 5 months
4. Language skills at 4 months
5. Self-help skills at 3 months
6. Social/emotional skills at 4 months

Occupational therapy services were provided in the foster home. The home trainer attended some of the sessions with the occupational therapist to assist with carry-over. Therapy was provided twice weekly for the first three months, reduced to once weekly for the next three months, and then to once monthly for the rest of the year.

The therapist worked cooperatively with the foster parents to establish a feeding routine. Feeding was a major concern for this infant and family, and standard precautions were necessary. The program included a prefeeding routine with tone-building and sensory stimulation activities. This prepared the infant for the feeding process. The best positioning for feeding was found to be in an infant seat with a slight recline. The therapist worked with the family to gradually introduce infant rice cereal and fruits. The cereal was mixed with the infant's formula to the consistency of apple sauce. Lower-lip support was provided to help with lip closure. Wiping of the mouth was done by wiping up on the bottom lip and down on the top lip, always toward lip closure. One food was introduced at a time and responses were recorded. The infant was monitored closely in case of allergic reactions but none were identified.

Once the feeding program was established, the amount of food intake was recorded and the family was instructed to weigh the baby regularly. The oral intake of food and formula resulted in weight gain. The occupational therapist monitored the feeding program and made suggestions/changes as appropriate.

Tommy needed to be placed in a variety of positions daily. Varying positions would allow him to develop different muscle groups, obtain multiple sensory experiences, and manipulate toys to build cause-and-effect relationships. The positioning/play program was developed around family routines. Safe positions (lying on the side, prone over a small chest roll, and supine) on a mat on the floor, within eyesight of the mother, were used at times when she needed to be cooking, cleaning, and tending other children. Supported sitting positions in a stroller and infant car seat were used when going to the bus stop with the other children, out in the community for errands, and in other areas of the home. Toys with multisensory feedback and some with switch activation were chosen and adapted for different positions. Specific techniques to address head and trunk control were demonstrated for each transition. This included when changing positions, changing diapers, dressing, bathing, and carrying the infant.

The concept of partial participation was utilized to build some self-care routines. Both parents were shown how to provide tactile and verbal cues to the infant and wait for an appropriate response (initiating movement of the arm/leg toward the clothing, for example). The therapist suggested slow, gradual changes in expectations as Tommy became more responsive and able to participate. The occupational therapist also role modeled for the foster parents how to involve the other children in Tommy's daily routines and play. The children provided excellent role models for Tommy, who showed increased arousal and vocalization when the other children were playing with him. This provided positive feedback to the children for their efforts.

In summary, occupational therapy allowed this foster family to provide the needed care for Tommy while maintaining their daily routines and other responsibilities. Tommy gained weight, was able to hold his head in alignment when sitting upright, move his extremities to partially participate in dressing tasks, and activate a variety of toys. He progressed to being able to hold his own bottle, and drinking from a cup was gradually introduced.

 ## CONCLUSION

Although home health has been established as a practice area of occupational therapy for many years, the parameters of the practice area are constantly changing. New patient groups emerge with needs that are best met by the skills of an occupational therapist. Several of these emerging client groups are discussed in this chapter.

Since the onset of deinstitutionalization of persons with mental illness, the healthcare system has been attempting to find appropriate delivery systems for identifying and meeting their needs including via home services. Special considerations are necessary to adapt mental health services to the home health setting. Issues, such as limited reimbursement and the need to document functional deficits and outcomes, must be considered.

A second group that has recently been evolving as a part of home health practice consists of women and children with special needs. As medical science advances, more children with special needs survive and methods of prevention for at-risk mothers are identified. With this progress comes opportunities for occupational therapists to be a service provider in meeting these needs.

Since one occupational therapist may receive referrals to address all types of client problems and the variety of clients who present for care is ever increasing, the need for continuing competency is apparent. Updating one's skills and understanding the health-care environment and the needs of special populations is an ongoing task.

 ## STUDY QUESTIONS

1. Explain the role of occupational therapy theory in assessment and intervention for persons with mental illness.
2. Describe the components of an antepartum occupational therapy home health program.
3. Discuss the role of occupational therapy in parenting skill training.
4. What do families with special needs children report that they want from health-care providers?
5. Describe the characteristics of a culturally competent therapist.

6. Discuss the types of assessments used in home health for persons with mental illness, pregnant women, and children.

7. Describe potential home health interventions for persons with mental illness, pregnant women, and children.

REFERENCES

Adams, R. (1996). Pediatric home care. *Advance for Occupational Therapists, 12*(28), 18.

Advance for Occupational Therapists. (1997). Increase in prenatal care would cut perinatal HIV transmission. *Advance for Occupational Therapists, 13*(14), 24.

Albrecht, J., and Higgins, P. (1977). Rehabilitation success: The interrelationships of multiple criteria. *Journal of Health and Social Behaviors, 18,* 36–45.

Alfonso, D., Hurst, L., Mayberry, L., Haller, L., Yost, K., and Lynch, M. (1992). Stressors reported by mothers of hospitalized premature infants. *Neonatal Network, 11,* 63–72.

Allen, C.K. (1985). *Occupational therapy for psychiatric diseases: Measurement and management of cognitive disabilities.* Boston: Little Brown.

Anderson, P.A., and Telleen, S.L. (1991). The relationship between social support and maternal behavior and attitudes: A meta-analytic review. *Journal of Community Mental Health 20*(6), 753–774.

Association of Women's Health, Obstetric and Neonatal Nurses. (1994). *Didactic content and clinical skills verification for professional nurse providers of perinatal home care.* Washington, DC: Association of Women's Health, Obstetric and Neonatal Nurses.

Atchison, B., Youngstrom, M.J., Dylla, L.R., Oates-Schuster, E., Anderson, K., O'Sullivan, A., and Livingston, S. (1997). Establishing a frame of reference for occupational therapy in home health care practice. In M.J. Steinhauer and M.J. Youngstrom (Eds.), *Occupational therapy in home health: Preparing for best practice.* Bethesda, MD: American Occupational Therapy Association.

Austill-Clausen, R. (1995). Pediatric services in the home. In *AOTA's guidelines for occupational therapy practice in home health.* Bethesda, MD: American Occupational Therapy Association.

Bailey, D., Simeonsson, R., Winton, P., Huntington, G., Comfort, M., Isbell, P., O'Donnell, K., and Helms, J. (1986). Family-focused intervention: A functional model for planning, implementing, and evaluation of individualized family services in early intervention. *Journal of the Division of Early Childhood, 10,* 156–171.

Barlow, C. (1994). OT intervention reduces pregnancy aches and pains. *Advance for Occupational Therapists, 10*(26), 18.

Batshaw, M., and Conlon, C. (1997). Substance abuse. In M. Batshaw (Ed.), *Children with disabilities* (4th ed.). Baltimore, MD: Paul H. Brookes.

Bauman, P., and Daugherty, F. (1983). Drug addicted mothers' parenting and their children's development. *International Journal of Addiction, 18,* 291–302.

Berman, S., Gross, R.D., and Lewak, N. (1995). *A pediatrician's guide to managed care.* Elk Grove Village, IL: American Academy of Pediatrics.

Bloomer, J., and Williams, S.K. (1982). The Bay area functional performance evaluation. In B. Hemphill (Ed.), *The evaluative process in psychiatric occupational therapy* (pp. 255–308). Thorofare, NJ: Slack.

Brayman, S.J., and Kirby, T. (1976). Comprehensive occupational therapy evaluation. *American Journal of Occupational Therapy, 30*(2), 94–100.

Brewer, E.J., McPherson, M., Magrab, P.R., and Hutchins, V.C. (1989). Family centered, community based, coordinated care for children with special health care needs. *Pediatrics, 83,* 1055–1060.

Brooks-Gunn, J., and Furstenberg, F. (1986). The children of adolescent mothers: Physical, academic and psychological outcomes. *Developmental Review, 6,* 224–251.

Brooten, D., Kamar, S., Brown, L., Butts, S., Finkler, S., Bakewell-Sachs, S., Gibbons, A., and Delivoria-Papadoupoulus, M. (1986). A randomized trial of early hospital discharge and home follow up of very low birth weight infants. *New England Journal of Medicine, 315,* 934–939.

Brooten, D., Ronceli, M., Finkler, S., Arnold, L., Cohen, A., and Mennuti, M. (1984). A randomized trial of early hospital discharge and home follow-up of women having cesarean births. *Obstetrics/Gynecology, 84*(5), 832–838.

Centers for Disease Control (1995). U.S. Public Health Services recommendations for human immunodeficiency virus counseling and voluntary testing for pregnant women. *Morbidity and Mortality Weekly Report, 44*(7), 2–3.

Craig, G. (1992). *Human development* (6th ed.). Englewood Cliffs, NJ: Prentice Hall.

Creasy, R. (1993). Preterm birth prevention: Where are we? *American Journal of Obstetrics and Gynecology, 168*(4), 1223–1230.

Dunst, C., Trivette, C., and Deal, A. (1988). *Enabling and empowering families: Principles and guidelines for practice.* Cambridge, MA: Brookline Books.

Erickson, M.E., and Upshur, C.C. (1989). Caretaking burden and social support: Comparison of mothers with infants with and without disabilities. *American Journal of Mental Retardation, 94,* 250–256.

Fleming, G. (1993). *The health insurance status of children: 1990–1992.* Elk Grove Village, IL: American Academy of Pediatrics.

Frieda, M. (1994). Childbearing, reproductive control, aging women and healthcare: The projected ethical debates. *Journal of Obstetrical, Gynecological and Neonatal Nursing, 23,* 144–152.

Freund, D.A., and Lewitt, E.M. (1993). Managed care for children and pregnant women: Promises and pitfalls. *The Future of Children, 3*(91), 109–111.

Goldson, E. (1996). The micropremie: Infants with birth weight less than 800 grams. *Infants and Young Children, 8*(3), 1–10.

Goodwin, L. (1994). Essential program components for perinatal home care. *Journal of Obstetrics, Gynecology and Neonatal Nursing, 23,* 667–674.

Halfon, N., and Newacheck, P. (1993). Childhood asthma and poverty: Differential impacts and utilization of health services. *Pediatrics, 91,* 56–61.

Hamada, R., and Schroeder, C. (1988). Schroeder-Block-Campbell adult psychiatric sensory integration evaluation: Concurrent validity and clinical utility. *Occupational Therapy Journal of Research 8*(2), 75–88.

Hemphill-Pearson, B.J. (1999). *Assessments in occupational therapy mental health: An integrative approach.* Thorofare, NJ: Slack.

Hinojosa, J., and Anderson, J. (1991). Mothers' perceptions of home treatment programs for their preschool children with cerebral palsy. *American Journal of Occupational Therapy, 45,* 273–279.

Hogue, C., Buehler, J., Strauss, L., and Smith, J. (1987). Overview of national infant mortality surveillances (NIMS) projects: Design, methods, results. *Public Health Reports, 102,* 44–152.

Holm, M.B., Rogers, J.C., and Stone, R.G. (1997). Referral, evaluation and intervention. In M. Steinhauer and M.J. Youngstrom (Eds.), *Occupational therapy in home health: Preparing for best practice.* Bethesda, MD: American Occupational Therapy Association.

Hutchins, V., and Hutchins, J. (1997). Public sector health services for children with special health care needs. In H. Wallace, R. Biehl, J. MacQueen, and J. Blackman (Eds.), *Mosby's resource guide to children with disabilities and chronic illness* (pp. 30–41). St. Louis, MO: Mosby.

Kaplan, K.L., and Kielhofner, G. (1989). *Occupational case analysis interview and rating scale.* Thorofare, NJ: Slack.

Kemp, V., and Hatmaker, D. (1996). Perinatal home care. *Family and Community Health, 18*(4), 40–48.

Klepitsch, L. (1995). Having a premie changed my outlook as a therapist. *Occupational Therapy Forum,* July, 4–6.

Kohlman-Thomson, L. (1992). *The Kohlman evaluation of living skills.* Bethesda, MD: American Occupational Therapy Association.

Kohrman, A. (1991). Psychological issues. In M. Mehlman and S. Young (Eds.), *Delivering high technology home care.* New York: Springer.

Law, M., Baptiste, S., Carswell, A., McColl, M.A., Polatajko, H., and Pollock, N. (1994). *Canadian occupational performance measure.* Toronto, Canada: Canadian Association of Occupational Therapists.

Law, M., Cooper, B., Strong, S., Stewart, S., Rigby, P., and Letts, L. (1996). The person/environment/occupation model: A transactive approach to occupational performance. *Canadian Journal of Occupational Therapy, 63,* 9–23.

Levy, S., and Pilmer, S. (1992). The technology-assisted child. In M. Batshaw and Y. Perret (Eds.), *Children with disabilities: A medical primer* (pp. 137–157). Baltimore, MD: Paul H. Brookes.

MacQueen, J., and Gittler, J. (1997). Future directions of community based service system for children with special health care needs and their families. In H. Wallace, R. Biehl, J. MacQueen, and J. Blackman (Eds.), *Mosby's resource guide to children with chronic illness* (pp. 57–71). St. Louis, MO: Mosby.

Marmer, L. (1995). How managed care is changing home health. *Advance for Occupational Therapists, 12*(28), 19.

Oakley, F., Kielhofner, G., Barris, R., and Reichler, R.K. (1986). The role checklist: Development and empirical assessment of reliability. *Occupational Therapy Journal of Research, 6*(3), 157–169.

Quint, R., Chesterman, E., Crain, L., Winkleby, M., and Boyce, W. (1990). Home care for ventilator-dependent children: Psychosocial impact on the family. *American Journal of Diseases of Children, 144*(11), 1238–1241.

Ramsey, R.M., and Auerbach, E. (1997). Forms follow function: Documentation for reimbursement in mental health OT. *Occupational Therapy Practice, 2*(8), 20–23.

Roelse, T. (1996). Cultural issues of patient care in home health. *Home and Community Health. Special Interest Section Newsletter, 3,* 4. Bethesda, MD: American Occupational Therapy Association.

Smith, J., and Hanks, C. (1994). Reaching out to mothers at risk. *RN, 57*(10), 42–46.

St. Peter, R.F., Newacheck, P.W., and Halton, N. (1992). Access to care for poor children. *Journal of the American Medical Association, 267,* 2760.

Sullivan-Belyai, S. (1990). All better: Preparing parents to take their medically complex children home. *Continuing Care, 9,* 24.

Thompson, T. (1992). For the sake of our children. In T. Thompson and S. Hupp (Eds.), *Saving our children at risk: Poverty and disabilities.* Newburg Park, CA: Sage.

Weinstein, M. (1997). Bring family-centered practices into home health. *Occupational Therapy Practice, 2*(7), 35–38.

13 CHAPTER

Hospice

Michael Pizzi, MS, OTR, CHES, FAOTA
S. Blaise Chromiak, MD

■ OUTLINE

Adaptation

Bereavement

Client-centered care

Death with dignity

Family-centered care

Grief

Hospice

Hospice Assessment of
   Occupational Function (HAOF)

Market segmentation

Marketing

Meaningfulness

Spirituality

Stages of dying

Symbolic loss

Terminal diagnosis

LEARNING OBJECTIVES

This chapter is designed to enable the reader to:
- Describe the history and philosophy of hospice care.
- Discuss the roles and functions of each of the members of the hospice team.
- Describe the themes in hospice care relevant to occupational therapy practice.
- Explain the key principles of occupational therapy intervention in hospice.
- Describe the role of the occupational therapy practitioner in the grieving and bereavement process.
- Explain the process for developing a proposal and marketing occupational therapy services to hospice providers.
- Compare and contrast the direct treatment approach with the consultation model.

 INTRODUCTION

Hospice care and philosophy are unique, transcending the use of standard medical models that focus on disease. The underlying concepts of hospice care are derived from the perspective of the dying person's individual needs rather than from a biomedical knowledge base (Agich, 1978). These needs, in contrast to the usual focus on body system function and treatment, are the impetus for the client's care. The client's interests, values, goals, roles, and abilities are primary. Within this context, occupational therapy facilitates purposeful activities and meaningful occupations. A respectful consideration of the developmental, temporal, social, cultural, and environmental contexts of the client's life is vital to the hospice-based therapist's holistic evaluation and intervention.

Capra (1982) identified the need for a paradigm shift in thinking on health and healing from a biomedical model to a systems perspective. True healing requires abandoning a "reductionist" focus on mechanical functioning and incorporating the total human being, including the "complex interplay among the physical, psychological, social and environmental aspects of the human condition" (Capra, pp. 123–124). With this in mind, occupational therapists have a vital role in community-based hospice care.

This chapter presents a concise overview of the history and philosophy of the hospice, including the idea of the hospice as a concept of care and as an environment for community-based occupational therapy practice. The chapter also discusses the interplay of occupational therapy theory, evaluation, and intervention within the context of the hospice and discusses reimbursement and documentation issues. Basic guidelines for developing a community-based hospice clientele and strategies for implementing a program are proposed. Finally, case studies are used to highlight the integration of these concepts.

 ## CONCEPTS OF HOSPICE CARE

The concepts of hospice care evolved from concerns about easing the dying process. Western cultures believe that people need to master their environment. In the field of medicine, control over disease and death is desired. When illness is incurable, the hospice provides an alternative system of providing care to persons who are dying.

HISTORICAL OVERVIEW

The term "hospice" (from the same linguistic root as "hospitality") can be traced back to early western civilization when it was used to describe a place of shelter and rest for the weary and sick traveler. In eleventh-century Europe, monastery-based hospices were established. With their later decline, the concept of hospice in the modern age was transformed by the pioneering work of Dr. Cicely Saunders. At St. Joseph's in London in the early 1950s, she developed pain-control techniques and a system of total care for dying persons which has become commonplace worldwide (Corless, 1983). Dr. Saunders used a grant from a patient and fellow visionary to create St. Christopher's Hospice in 1967. This center combined **spirituality** (a sense of connection with a life force or deity) with knowledge in the fields of medicine, nursing, and allied health to pioneer optimal care for persons who were dying, along with teaching the concepts of the hospice. Today, the term **hospice** stands for a steadily expanding concept of humane and compassionate care that can be implemented in a variety of settings.

PHILOSOPHY

In 1965, Dame Cicely M. Saunders stated (p. 70):

> It seems to me that the way to find a philosophy that gives confidence and permits a positive approach to death and dying is to look continuously at the patients; not at their need but at their courage; not at their dependence but at their dignity.

As a result of her influence, hospice philosophy is holistic and client-centered. The National Hospice Organization (NHO) (1979) states:

> Dying is a normal process whether or not resulting from disease. Hospice exists neither to hasten nor to postpone death. Rather, Hospice exists to affirm "life"—by providing support and care for those in the last phases of incurable disease so that they can live as fully and comfortably as possible. Hospice promotes the formation of caring communities that are sensitive to the needs of patients and their families at this time in their lives so that they may be free to obtain that degree of mental and spiritual preparation for death that is satisfactory to them.

The standards for hospice care that define a hospice program, and 22 standards and supporting principles for the programs, enable program evaluation and comparison (National Hospice Organization, 1979). The clarity of these standards enhances their relevance to and application in occupational therapy.

The American Occupational Therapy Association (AOTA) *Guidelines for Occupational Therapy Services in Hospice* (1987) document applies NHO standards and principles to the occupational therapy process. These include holistic and health- and occupation-centered caring and provide a framework for hospice-based practitioners.

 ## OCCUPATIONAL THERAPY AND HOSPICE: PARALLELS IN PHILOSOPHY AND PRACTICE

The philosophy and goals of the hospice—providing life-affirming, client-centered services through which the dying person can live with maximum dignity and function—parallel the philosophy and principles of occupational therapy. As a profession with a humanitarian focus since the early 1900s, occupational therapy assists people in discovering new purpose through participation in self-directed, meaningful *occupation*.

The philosophy of hospice incorporates basic values of **client-centered** and **family-centered care,** which include the following:

1. The basic regard for the recipient of care
2. Acceptance of death as a natural part of living
3. Consideration of the entire family as the unit of care
4. Maintenance of the patient at home for as long as possible
5. Assistance for the patient attempting to assume control over his or her own life
6. Instructions for patient self-care
7. Reduction or removal of pain and other distressing symptoms
8. Total, not fragmented, care
9. Comprehensive provision of services by an interdisciplinary team
10. Continuity of services after death (Koff, 1980, pp. 18–19).

The community-based hospice allows care of the dying to move from an institutional setting to a homelike environment, where the dying person can surround him- or herself with family, friends, and comforting possessions. Due to consideration of the importance of the sociocultural and environmental aspects of care, and occupation and adaptation, occupational therapy is an ideal match for hospice care.

The interface between the principles, values, and philosophy of hospice and occupational therapy seem obvious. A person with a terminal illness experiences occupational performance deficits, loss of control of environmental mastery, difficulty with the "doing" process, and degeneration of habits and skills. With a **terminal diagnosis** (defined as life expectancy of six months or less), fluctuations between occupational function and dysfunction are common, as are fluctuations between **adaptation,** or the ability to respond effectively to new situations, and maladaptation. Kubler-Ross (1969) identified five **stages of dying:** (1) denial, (2) anger, (3) bargaining, (4) depression, and (5) acceptance. The terminally ill person can remain in, or alternate among, any of the stages at any given time. If maladaptive occupational behaviors develop in interactions with human and nonhuman environments, these may impede the dying process unless positive adaptations can be promoted.

In practice, using occupational behavior theory may enhance these adaptations. Gammage, McMahon, and Shanahan (1976), in their study of occupational therapy in terminal care, suggest that flexibility and the ability to change roles are important for the dying person to effectively respond to environmental demands. Pizzi (1984) supports the principles of occupation and adaptation. These enhance the client's sense of control and quality of life. Several authors (Flanigan, 1982; Holland, 1984; Holland and Tigges, 1981; Pizzi, 1983, 1986, 1990, 1993) advocate the use of open-systems approaches to create supportive environments.

OCCUPATIONAL THERAPY AS A COMPONENT OF THE HOSPICE TEAM

Clients usually enter the hospice system through physician referrals when it is believed that the client's status is terminal and the expertise of professionals dealing with end-of-life issues is required. Referrals may also be self-generated or made through family members or other knowledgeable sources, simply by contacting the local hospice agency. These authors have often recommended hospice to families while working in home health care because of the increased benefits provided by hospice. Home-based occupational therapy services still can be continued under the auspices of hospice.

Hospice team members usually include nurses, social workers, clergy, and physicians, and may include occupational, physical, speech, and respiratory therapists, counselors, pharmacists, dietitians, and volunteers. With medical care and pain control, the primary- or specialty-care physician solves problems daily and urgent concerns as needed and signs the plan of care. Clergy are available for spiritual needs and concerns and facilitate the completion of the person's life story in the context of their family situation. The social worker helps clients and families cope with grief and bereavement issues and assists with practical concerns such as burial and insurance matters. Volunteers who carry out daily tasks for client and family may develop activities at home (often in conjunction with occupational therapy practitioners) and can also offer respite to caregivers. A home health aide and/or caregiver also may be involved to provide support for activities of daily living and home management.

The nurse is the primary medical professional involved in the client and family's life, providing comfort care and advocating for medical and social support. Often, the nurse, who is aware of the power and efficacy of occupation in the client's life, is the person responsible for initiating appropriate referrals to occupational therapy and requesting a physician order for occupational therapy services. Any of the other disciplines involved in the client's care also can identify the client's occupational needs and initiate a referral. If needed, the occupational therapist may discuss the anticipated benefits of the referral with the referring professional, nurse, or physician.

In developing strategies to maintain and enhance occupational function, the occupational therapy practitioner collaborates with the various professionals and others who impact significantly on the dying person's life. Through a team approach, the priorities and needs of terminally ill persons and their families are met more effectively.

To increase an occupational therapy practitioner's visibility, number of referrals, and the potential for providing occupational therapy services in the hospice, specific strategies may be employed. These may include:

● Formal and informal in-service programs to hospice and home-care agency personnel
● Letters to the editor and articles for hospice and trade newsletters
● Written documentation about a special case for professional journals or the local newspaper

OCCUPATIONAL THERAPY INVOLVEMENT IN COMMUNITY-BASED HOSPICE

Hospice services are available to persons who can no longer benefit from curative treatment. The typical hospice client has a life expectancy of six months or less. However, many outlive their diagnosis, and some may be discharged from hospice care. Occupational therapists may be involved with hospice clients in the community through home-based care.

Hospice care is often associated with home-care models of service delivery. The basics of home-care consultation and practice apply to hospice when services are delivered in the home. Hospice care can also be provided in free-standing facilities that are growing in numbers throughout the United States. In 1998, approximately 28 percent of hospices were independent corporations. The remainder of hospice services were provided at hospitals, nursing homes, and through home health agencies (National Hospice Organization, 1999).

By far, the primary diagnosis of hospice clients is cancer. Other diagnoses include heart-related diseases, AIDS, Alzheimer's disease, and renal and pulmonary conditions. Related to environment of care, 77 percent of hospice clients died in their personal residence, 19 percent in an institutional setting, and 4 percent in other settings (National Hospice Organization, 1999). Community-based approaches to hospice care are much needed, given that the majority of hospice clients died at home. Direct care and the development of programs and consultation services are all appropriate roles for the occupational therapy practitioner in community-based care.

Jaffe and Epstein (1992, p. 678) discuss the role of the occupational therapist as a consultant and the development of an ecological/environmental perspective as a theoretical model for consultation:

> The total environment is an important concern for the clinician as well as the consultant/therapist. In both roles, he or she must recognize interactive environmental dynamics that influence the outcome of planned interventions.

They articulate future roles of therapists as consultants, such as environmental engineers to address architectural barriers or environmental managers to facilitate social and cultural change to support achievement of goals (Jaffe and Epstein, 1992, p. 678):

> Change can be facilitated through a collaborative and/or educational consultation approach. Thus, the therapist's role shifts to a consultative perspective within the larger treatment context, and consultation becomes part of the service delivery model.

Jaffe and Epstein (1992) delineate a synergism between consultation and treatment approaches. Using a combination of approaches is strongly recommended for the occupational therapist in community-based practice. Doing so affords numerous op-

   TABLE 13–1

TREATMENT APPROACH VS. CONSULTATION MODEL

Treatment Approach Steps	*Consultation Model Steps*
Referral	Entry
Screening	Needs assessment
Diagnostic evaluation	Diagnostic analysis
Needs identification	Goal setting and planning
Intervention plan	Intervention strategies
Intervention/adaptation	Intervention/adaptation and feedback
Ongoing reassessment	Evaluation
Termination	Termination
Follow-up	Renegotiation

Source: Jaffe, E.G., and Epstein, C.F. (1992). *Occupational therapy consultation: Theories, principles and practice* (p. 684). St. Louis: Mosby. With permission.

portunities for employment and services where none may exist. In both treatment and consultation, there are nine steps to the process, as identified in Table 13–1.

The most familiar treatment model is the direct-care approach. However, in the consultation model, the therapist may evaluate and analyze not just the client/caregiver (direct treatment) but also the system of hospice care or a part of the system. Thus, open-systems theory and use of models that support community-based care are essential. Because environment has a profound impact on the way care is delivered, many types of barriers to care, including architectural, financial/insurance, and social barriers such as stigma and discrimination, are important to identify.

RELEVANT OCCUPATIONAL THERAPY HOSPICE THEMES

Important themes relevant to the occupational therapist as a practitioner and consultant include meaningfulness and meaning of occupation; dignity in the dying process; the family as the unit of care; and loss, grief, and bereavement issues. Other themes, such as quality of life, temporal adaptation, locus of control, environment, pain and pain control, and adaptation, are covered in Pizzi (1993).

Meaning and Meaningfulness

One of the most important central themes of the hospice relevant to occupational therapy is meaning and the **meaningfulness** (significance, importance, or purposefulness) of occupation. Yerxa (1967, p. 170) states that "authentic occupational therapy is based upon a commitment to the client's realization of his own particular meaning." The meaningfulness of occupation is heightened at the end of life. New and different meanings are imparted to occupations such as crafts, cooking, and gift giving for family and friends. By engaging in one's chosen occupations, even the meaning of simple actions is enhanced. In light of the value, time, and effort for each task, the person can be spiritually enriched through the performance of, and the symbolism associated with, that activity. When the individual feels this spiritual nature of meaningful occupation, he or she also experiences a centered attention and enjoyment of participation. This may be in contrast to previous experiences when the action may have just been a task to complete. Meaning is influenced by, and must be viewed within, the context of the developmental, temporal, social, cultural, and environmental aspects of occupational behavior (Pizzi, 1993). Meaningful occupations to a person nearing the end of life may be participating in the preparation of the family's Thanksgiving meal, creating an autobiographical videotape for one's grandchildren, or making a baby blanket for a child yet unborn. These activities may enhance the individual's sense of connectedness and spirituality.

Meaning and the meaningfulness of occupation, particularly for those individuals with life-threatening illness, take on additional spiritual qualities. In March 1997, the *American Journal of Occupational Therapy* published a special issue on *Spirituality, Occupation and Life Meaning*. Peloquin and Christiansen's (1997) seminal work with this issue speaks directly to how meaning is derived by a person's life choices, experiences, and beliefs, and how meaningful activity (occupations) engaging mind, body, and spirit enhances a person's quality of life and spirituality. This is a vital component for the occupational therapist to incorporate into hospice practice. A transformation of illness to wellness, through engagement in meaningful occupation, is the essence of mind-body-spirit holistic practice.

Occupational therapy aims to provide an individual with meaning and purpose. Peloquin states (1997, p. 168):

> Occupation, the core of our therapy, animates and extends the human spirit; we participate in that animation. Gazing past the details of practice while led by their design to the point beyond, we discern a deeper aim. The discovery is awesome.

Community-based hospice practice in occupational therapy is best defined as the organization and implementation of a holistic program of care that facilitates living on all levels (including pain management) and thereby encourages active engagement in meaningful life occupations. This facilitates hope for the client and caregiver that each day will be a new beginning and that whenever closure to life occurs, more likely it will be a celebration of one's existence. As therapists begin to engage clients in meaningful occupation that is relevant to their choices and lifestyle, the other relevant themes emerge and blend.

Death with Dignity

Death with dignity, or allowing the dying person to have as much control over the dying process as possible, is a cornerstone of hospice care. Dignity can be maintained or restored when services to clients and caregivers are provided in the home and community. The environment is more natural, the care provided is more meaningful and relevant, and fewer barriers to caring exist. Providing choices and enabling control over one's physical and social environments to the degree desired enhance dignity during the dying process (Pizzi, 1984). Simple examples of adding dignity for the client is not being awakened for vital signs when asleep or during the middle of the night and allowing the client to determine how and when to complete his or her self-care activities such as grooming, dressing, and bathing.

Family as the Unit of Care

The family, or caregiver situation, is one of the crucial components of hospice care and like the client, necessitates intervention. The family provides the foundation and context for occupational development and adaptation. Performance of the members' roles is associated with optimal family functioning.

In recent years, the family is regarded as the unit facing the disease, where one member's terminal illness also disrupts the lives of the others. The integrity and functioning of the family system is threatened and role performances are impaired. Families vary in their adaptability to the impending death of their loved one based on the degree to which the illness disrupts the dying person's role performance, the ability of family members to compensate, and the burden imposed by added caregiving responsibilities.

Family members and significant others may perceive that performing tasks for their loved one is helpful. However, this may achieve a negative effect if more independence is desired and the help being provided is resented. Feeling uncomfortable and inadequate, family and friends may withdraw, leaving their dying loved one feeling more isolated and alone. According to Pizzi (1986, pp. 245–246),

> Appropriate recommendations to the family unit and significant others can alleviate stress and help individual members organize their routines and activities to better promote their own health and adaptive ways of living while caring for their dying loved one.

Grief and Bereavement

Grief, a universal phenomenon, is a normal reaction to loss. The loss is usually categorized as physical or symbolic. However, symbolic significance may be attached to physical losses (Rando, 1984). For example, breaking a piece of china is a physical loss, but it also may be a **symbolic loss** (a loss that represents something with emotional attachments or sentimental value) if the china was a family heirloom. Another type of symbolic loss might be decreased self-esteem due to a job layoff or from the limitations imposed by illness.

When dealing with loss and grief issues, four considerations that may be helpful to caregivers and practitioners are:

- An illness involves numerous losses that are both physical and symbolic in nature.
- Each of the specific losses must be identified.
- Each of these losses prompts and requires its own grief response.
- The importance of a loss will vary according to its meaning for the specific individual (Rando, 1984, p. 18).

Hospice practitioners must recognize the importance of grieving and its place in intervention and facilitate a client-centered grieving process.

Another essential component of hospice care is helping significant others and family members with the ongoing process of **bereavement** (suffering the loss of a loved one). Bereavement interventions can occur at any time during the hospice process. Occupational therapy's unique contribution is facilitating the role transitions and restructuring of daily living routines by family members. This may include a focus on meal preparation and money management for a person who has relied on the dying spouse for handling these responsibilities.

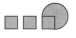 ## OCCUPATIONAL THERAPY'S ROLE IN HOSPICE

Bye (1998) analyzed data gathered by 10 occupational therapists working in hospice care. Nine conceptual categories were generated from the data, including making a difference, making a referral to occupational therapy, assessing the situation, setting goals building against loss, incorporating "normality within a changed reality," maintaining client control, providing supported and safe care, and facilitating closure. She concluded that the core principle of the analysis generated the theme "Affirming Life: Preparing for Death" and recognized that occupational therapists need to reframe their practice and thinking to effectively work in hospice care. According to Bye (p. 19),

> The outcome is not about independence or permanent rehabilitation to a normal life—hallmarks of traditional occupational therapy. It is about occupational therapists helping clients to realize their goals to connect with life, and people in their life, on a level beyond illness and receipt of care. The achievement of this outcome affirms clients' lives.

Hasselkus (1993) noted that caring for someone with a terminal illness presents a paradox between facilitating comfort and quality of life while simultaneously supporting approaching death. She states that "the ability to be comfortable with the latter role is most likely the distinguishing characteristic of the health professional who is fully competent to work with patients who are dying"(p. 722). This competence is both inherent and learned because one must have the passion and commitment to work with persons who are dying along with the technical occupational skills and clinical reasoning to competently implement occupational therapy services.

EVALUATION OF OCCUPATIONAL PERFORMANCE

Assessment of occupational performance areas and performance components includes neuromuscular, sensorimotor, and cognitive and psychosocial dimensions of daily living. The family context and the physical environment must also be assessed and incorporated into the plan of care.

Evaluation in hospice care relies on a variety of sources of data, including observations, interviews, information from charts and other team members, and occasionally, formal assessments. Active listening, skilled observations of the client, family, and environment, and therapeutic use of self are the essential components of the evaluation process in hospice practice.

A tool designed specifically for this setting, the **Hospice Assessment of Occupational Function (HAOF)** (Pizzi, 1993), integrates hospice and occupational therapy philosophy with principles of occupational science and occupational behavior. The instrument's holistic approach provides qualitative and quantitative data and can be used alone or as a supplement to traditional occupational therapy assessments.

HOSPICE INTERVENTION PLANNING

Adaptation and occupation are both the primary tools of occupational therapy and its desired outcome. Occupational needs, goals, and desires of clients and their families guide intervention planning. The following treatment principles are particularly cogent in hospice care. Well-designed occupation-based interventions

- Arouse interest, confidence, and courage
- Are applied systematically based on evaluation data
- Are graded according to client and family capabilities, which change over time
- Focus on the health of clients rather than on pathology
- Emphasize the expression of emotions
- Provide a total program of care (Pizzi, 1984)

Clinical reasoning in hospice care incorporates the philosophy and themes of hospice, knowledge of the dying process, and an understanding of loss, grief, and bereavement issues. An appreciation of the complex interplay of these elements and the integration of occupational behavior and occupational science principles provide the foundation for effective and meaningful interventions (Pizzi, 1992).

The strategy of grading occupations and environmental challenges through levels of increasing complexity to improve function is inappropriate when working with clients who have a terminal illness. Short-term, meaningful, and easily attainable goals are best. Acting as a facilitator, the occupational therapy practitioner engages the client in occupations that enhance the quality of life and provide emotional closure.

DOCUMENTATION AND REIMBURSEMENT

Congressional action in 1982 extended Medicare coverage to beneficiaries who qualified for hospice care. Eligibility criteria for Medicare hospice benefits include coverage with Medicare Part A and a terminal prognosis certified by a physician. Medicare hospice coverage may extend for two 90-day periods plus one 30-day period if necessary. If the lifetime limit of 210 days of hospice care is reached, or at any time elected by the client, coverage may revert back to regular Medicare. Eligibility requirements for hospice care may vary among other insurance providers.

Payment for hospice occupational therapy services under Medicare is covered by the hospice per diem rate. Although Medicare-certified hospices are required to contract with occupational, physical, and speech therapists, there is no stipulation that the services must be used. Some private insurance companies may cover occupational therapy hospice services. It is the responsibility of the hospice agency or the therapist to determine the client's insurance coverage prior to evaluation and intervention. When funding for therapy is inadequate, other sources for defraying the cost should be sought. These may include grants, private contributions, and fundraising.

Documentation requirements for routine Medicare reimbursement, such as demonstrating patient progress, do not apply for Medicare hospice coverage. For Medicare-certified hospice programs, the documentation must include a description of the treatment provided, the client's response, and changes noted since the prior visit. In contrast to routine Medicare coverage, functional improvement is not a prerequisite for reimbursement (Health Care Financing Administration, 1983).

 DEVELOPMENT OF A COMMUNITY-BASED HOSPICE PRACTICE

Creating hospice occupational therapy services in the community can be a rewarding challenge for the motivated and entrepreneurial occupational therapy practitioner. In developing any new niche, first a vision, then a commitment, and finally a plan of action and follow-up are needed. A clear definition of the role of occupational therapy and the ability to differentiate it from other professional services in hospice are essential. Most importantly, one must be able to effectively demonstrate that, although the field is perceived as a rehabilitation service, client care is approached from a holistic and wellness perspective, adapting tasks and environments regardless of the type or duration of the disease process. The basic principle of adaptation (a cornerstone for occupational therapy) is an essential ingredient when developing a proposal to create hospice occupational therapy services.

The proposal may be inadequate if the professional is not passionate about, and committed to, making it work for one's self, the consumer, and the organization. The professional's passion will be evident in the development of the proposal, its content, and the way it is marketed to potential employers. Several steps are necessary to properly develop a proposal.

STEP 1: NEEDS ASSESSMENT

Identifying the occupational problems and needs of people with life-threatening illness can be done via a literature review in the therapies and the fields of nursing, social work, and rehabilitation, via the Internet, or through development of a needs assessment. The needs assessment lists all the potential areas in which occupational therapy may serve clients. Hospice staff can identify clients who are having occupation-related problems (for example, dressing, mobility, cooking, and leisure participation), if any staff are providing assistance in those areas, and if the client may wish assistance in those areas. Pizzi developed a needs assessment survey for a hospice and included the question, "Does the client or caregiver wish to be more independent in any of these areas?" and then listed several occupational performance areas. All clients and caregivers stated they valued independence. This data helped to get the occupational therapist involved in both direct care and consultation.

STEP 2: FORMATION OF STRATEGIES

Once the data are collected in step 1, the practitioner needs to determine how to effectively propose occupational therapy services. Seeking answers to the following questions will assist the practitioner in effectively presenting the proposal:

- Who is the best person to meet with—the executive director, director of nursing, or business manager?
- What are the statistics on length of stay, services already provided, and where referrals come from?

- Can the occupational therapist help to generate referrals?
- Will occupational therapy services enhance the quality of life of clients?
- How will that happen? (Although therapists believe the answer to the preceding question is a resounding yes, what data are available to support this idea?)
- Will occupational therapy services decrease use of other services (e.g., nursing assistants) and be a cost savings service or expenditure?

STEP 3: PROPOSAL DEVELOPMENT

When the preceding information has been gathered, a proposal delineating answers from steps 1 and 2 can be developed. The proposal should include the following basic headings:

- Occupational needs of people with life-threatening illness
- What is occupational therapy/use of services for the hospice client?
- Occupational therapy evaluation and intervention issues
- Involvement of the caregiver in the occupational therapy process
- Costs and benefits of occupational therapy services
- Case studies
- References

STEP 4: MARKETING THE IDEA

The definition of **marketing** most acceptable for occupational therapy practitioners is that "marketing in the true sense means being sensitive to and responding to the needs of people as they perceive them" (Kotler and Andreasen, 1987, p. 7). People with life-threatening illnesses, as noted earlier, have many occupational needs that often go unmet.

The community-based occupational therapy practitioner committed to hospice care combines the particular needs of the hospice agency with knowledge of hospice principles to frame a proposal that will educate hospice personnel. The first step in marketing is identifying the need and the person(s)/organizations being served. Improving the awareness of hospice personnel to two types of needs can be helpful: (1) the lack of knowledge and visibility of occupational therapy services in hospice and (2) the limited identification of occupational dysfunction by hospice staff.

Marketing the proposal is probably the biggest challenge and, yet, the most rewarding. When the first author developed occupational therapy services in several already existing home-care-based hospices, the market was different. Monies were more available from a variety of sources to support services, thus simply setting up a meeting or in-service and demonstrating the benefits of occupational therapy as a powerful and unique service for the dying person was successful. The selling point emphasized continued independent functioning that translated into increased quality of life, happiness, and restoration of dignity for the client and caregiver. With the current trend in cost savings, a proposal must clearly outline how occupational therapy services will cut costs.

Social marketing theory is crucial to proposal development. MacStravic (1977) outlined five components of social marketing:

- Identification of constituencies
- Assessment of the marketing environment and its problems
- Selection and evaluation of marketing objectives
- Design of a marketing strategy

- Planning, implementation, control, and evaluation of marketing efforts (as discussed in Gilkerson, 1997)

Social marketing as a strategy is relevant to four focused areas of proposal development: (1) development of a clear plan with objectives and specific strategies, (2) market segmentation, (3) consumer benefits, and (4) identification of numerous benefits.

Development of a Clear Plan with Objectives and Specific Strategies

This should include a specific written plan for approaching hospice personnel, the contact person for a meeting, and the persons who are desired to be present at the meeting. Important to present is *what* are the benefits achievable through collaborative efforts explained as behavioral objectives for presenter and the involved hospice staff. If the presentation is clear in explaining the interface between occupational therapy and hospice and comes from a place of compassion and good business, the proposal will have a better chance at resulting in a partnership with the hospice community.

Market Segmentation

Market segmentation refers to *who* is being marketed to and *what* is being marketed. In this instance, the "product" is occupational therapy services. However, a meeting with ("marketing to") the social worker about easing the caregiving burden, and marketing to the executive director when discussing costs/benefits, might be most appropriate. Other considerations include geography of the hospice relative to services offered (rural vs. urban), demographics of the hospice clients (pediatrics vs. elderly), and attitudinal/perceptual factors ("How can a rehab professional help here when he or she works with disabled kids and stroke patients?").

Consumer Benefits

This is the area that will make or break a proposal. "Why should consumers (hospice clients and caregivers and/or the hospice organization) buy *this* product (occupational therapy services)?" In the proposal, this area must be so clearly explained that the consumers might wonder why they were unaware of the value of occupational therapy in hospice. The way to market the service is to demonstrate cost cutting, quality-of-life improvements, and continued functional independence in meaningful occupations via compassionate, occupation-centered practice.

Identification of Numerous Benefits ("Products")

The proposal should include a variety of interventions for the client and also how caregiver burden is eased, home environments are improved, tasks and environments are modified and adapted, and cost savings are added. All of these can be written up as hospice products delivered by the occupational therapy practitioner. Taking a businesslike approach to care, while maintaining compassion, forges new ground in the community-based practice arena.

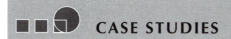 **CASE STUDIES**

SARA

Sara was a 78-year-old woman with metastatic liver cancer. The cancer had spread to her bones and likely to her brain, although this was unconfirmed. When Sara was first seen by occupational therapy, it was through a nursing referral in the nursing home.

(Note: Hospice care is "an environment of care" and referrals are not just in the home or a freestanding hospice.) The aides and the primary nurse "just knew" Sara could do more for herself than she said she could. However, she refused all care and was "angry with a fiery spirit." The OT referral was generated to increase Sara's self-care skills and possibly to ease the burden of the aides too. The first encounter with Sara ended with the therapist standing at the doorway and introducing himself from there, as Sara refused entrance to her room. Respecting her rights, the therapist from a distance discussed the benefits of occupational therapy and notified Sara that he planned to return the next day, a promise kept much to her dismay.

On the next visit, Sara allowed entrance to her room. The therapist sat at her bedside where an occupational history and a sense of her functional capacity were assessed. Sara was thought to be bedbound and unable to perform many tasks for herself. When this was mentioned, she shot straight up in bed and started swearing at the top of her lungs, at which time the therapist realized she certainly had more mobility than previously thought. The therapist told her that he'd return the following day, again keeping the promise.

By the third visit, Sara realized the therapist wasn't going to go away like many others had because of her language and behavior, so she finally began to cooperate. She sat up on the edge of the bed independently but was slow to come to a standing position or to transfer, primarily from fear combined with some weakness. Eventually, the OT sessions culminated in her being able to sit, stand, and transfer independently to a wheelchair. Sara also began to feed herself with adaptive equipment and began to wash and dress with minimal assistance. She soon won the hearts of all the nurses and aides and would tell wonderful stories of her life. Because of her increasing activity tolerance (strengthened by an increase in the attention and empowering support of others), the OT began to develop an out-of-room program of activity. During this time, the reason behind the fiery spirit and the often refusal of care from others began to be revealed and understood. Sara was raised as an only child and became an independent woman during the rise of feminism and equal rights. She married young, and her husband became blind soon after their marriage. They had no children. She helped him run his small business of selling fruits and vegetables and often struggled to make ends meet. Being in this very dependent environment and state of being, lacking attention from others, and having an unknown future had left her fearful, angry, and frustrated, and lacking spirit.

Sara wasn't very willing to leave the room. However, it was discovered that she loved to bake and often baked cakes and cookies to help support herself and her husband. A plan was developed for Sara to bake a cake in the kitchen upstairs for "all the wonderful girls who helped me." Sara recognized she was quite a challenge to them and wanted to do something special. By this time, the cancer had metastasized quicker than realized and she was rapidly weakening. The therapist adapted utensils and time frames for Sara to complete tasks, keeping her active enough to feel more independent and giving her the sense of control she needed. Sara used her favorite frosting recipe that she remembered from 50 years ago and frosted the cake. She got off the elevator with this huge cake and, as Sara was wheeled to the nursing station, all were moved to tears, acknowledging how wonderful this simple task of baking an "appreciation cake" (as Sara called it) was for all concerned. Sara received many hugs and kisses from everyone and some powerful moments of living with Sara were shared.

Soon thereafter, Sara began to lose her memory and judgment. The aides would get her up routinely, and she would sit with her friends at the nursing station. At this point, OT consisted of some gentle massage, music tapes Sara enjoyed, and engaging her in some light craft activities on which she formerly worked. One day, the therapist walked to the nursing station ready for Sara's session and was informed she had died the previous night. The therapist cried with the nurses because Sara was beloved by all and had taught much to her caregivers. Surface emotions and behaviors may not be what they seem to be. Often, there is a wonderful human being just waiting to be cared about and loved. From Sara, the therapist and others learned some important lessons about the power of occupation and how the mind and body, in concert with a loving environment, can work wonderful miracles, for both patient and professional.

BRYAN

Bryan was a 12-year-old living with a younger brother and sister and both parents in the home. He had hemophilia and had been infected with HIV at age 6. Bryan was referred to occupational therapy for developmental delay and for presenting as a cerebrovascular accident (CVA) affecting his dominant side as neurological sequelae secondary to HIV. He was an average student in the sixth grade, his family was very religious, and all were aware of his diagnosis. The OT program consisted of physical restoration activities, helping him adapt his life activities around one-handed performance and psychosocial interventions to help him and his family cope with current and future changes in living with HIV.

Bryan walked with a single crutch and would often get into fights at school because of being ridiculed for being "a gimp" (according to Bryan). According to his mother, he would often win his fights by using his crutch as his defense weapon. OT incorporated anger interventions and coping styles into the treatment program in conjunction with meaningful aspects of his life, such as his role as the eldest of three, his love of cooking with mom, and playing board games and sports. These motivated him to engage more actively in therapy and also helped him gain a sense of control with improved anger management. He liked being able to utilize his adaptive equipment to tie shoes, cut apples for making apple pie, and be more independent with all activities of daily living (ADLs). OT also used games and sports activities incorporating neurodevelopmental techniques to further increase function in his affected side.

The family was very supportive of Bryan. OT included his younger siblings into treatment as often as possible, especially in play activities and ADLs with which Bryan sometimes needed help. The therapist also had several conversations with family members about health-related activities, infection control and wellness/health promotion, and HIV. At times, his mother was concerned about Bryan's activity level and his risky play behaviors (he liked contact sports despite the risks for hemophiliacs). Discussions with his parents ensued about ways to set boundaries for their own emotional health and strategies to balance Bryan's need to play hard. The OT was also able to discuss more mind/body activities with them, including their religious beliefs, such as belief in their God and how that positively impacted on Bryan's health and his involvement in church activities. The research on social systems and the positive impacts of social support on general health and immune function were acknowledged. These activities and discussions further empowered them to see beyond a child with hemophilia and HIV to seeing a child adapting to changes in function but still engaging in life.

The OT worked with Bryan and his family off and on for about a year, until he became more drug-resistant. Eventually the viral load (increase in HIV) overwhelmed him. When he became more bedbound, he was still able to play board games and help mom with cooking activities. Adaptations in performing these cooking activities were made with him and his family so he could still be a major part of the family system. Bryan's death was mourned by many. Later, his mother sent the OT a letter from Bryan that he was glad the OT liked his apple pies and that he had "a lot of fun." The quality of life and the dignity that occupational therapy could preserve for Bryan and others like him is a great gift.

 CONCLUSION

This chapter provides information designed to enhance the reader's already rich knowledge of occupation and demonstrate its power when used in the context of the lives of people with terminal and life-threatening illness. Facilitating engagement of the mind, body, and spirit at the end of life is very rewarding when the practitioner realizes the quality added to a person's life. Health and healing are facilitated despite the lack of a cure.

Occupational therapy is an important component of hospice care as it provides the person with a terminal illness an opportunity for meaningful occupation. Meaningful occupation can facilitate a sense of continuity of life even in the dying process. Although physical restoration of function is not possible in the late stages of dying, important psychosocial needs of the client and family can be met through occupational therapy intervention.

According to Bolen (1996, p. 79),

> Work (as well as life) that calls upon us to use and develop our innate gifts is personally meaningful. Work that interests us, challenges us to grow, and provides opportunities for us to be creative engages us in life. We feel authentic and true to ourselves when we do such work. When what we do is what we love, work is an expression of our true nature.

It is the challenge of occupational therapy practitioners to create opportunities for clients to engage in the most meaningful work of their lives and, thereby, to be engaged in the work of their lives.

 ## STUDY QUESTIONS

1. Compare and contrast the philosophy of hospice with key concepts and principles of occupational therapy.

2. In today's health-care marketplace, is there a role for occupational therapy in grief and bereavement services? Why or why not?

3. Briefly describe appropriate assessment and treatment approaches for the following case: Bob, a 33-year-old male with end-stage AIDS, is a graduate student who is nearing completion of his degree. Recently, he has had a bout of pneumonia and has been discharged from the hospital to home with hospice services. He is cared for by his female roommate, who is a nurse. His significant other, Mark, has withdrawn from Bob and is unable to cope with the situation. Bob has many interests, including music, gardening, and reading. He has lived with AIDS for the past six years.

4. Identify a hospice provider in your local community, conduct a brief needs assessment, and write a short proposal to provide occupational therapy consultation services.

REFERENCES

Agich, G.J. (1978). The ethics of terminal care. *Death Education, 2*(1–2), 163–171.

American Occupational Therapy Association (1987). *Guidelines for occupational therapy services in hospice.* Rockville, MD: American Occupational Therapy Association.

Bolen, J.S. (1996). *Close to the bone: Life threatening illness and the search for meaning.* New York: Scribner.

Bye, R. (1998). When clients are dying: Occupational therapists' perspectives. *Occupational Therapy Journal of Research, 18*(1), 3–24.

Capra, F. (1982). *The turning point: Science, society and the rising culture.* New York: Bantam.

Corless, I.B. (1983). The hospice movement in North America. In C.A. Corr and D.M. Corr (Eds.), *Hospice care: Principles and practice* (pp. 335–351). New York: Springer.

Flanigan, K. (1982). The art of the possible . . . occupational therapy in terminal care. *British Journal of Occupational Therapy, 45*(8), 274–276.

Gammage, S.L., McMahon, P.S., and Shanahan, P.J. (1976). The occupational therapist and terminal illness: Learning to cope with death. *American Journal of Occupational Therapy, 30*, 294–299.

Gilkerson, G. (1997). *Occupational therapy leadership: Marketing yourself, your profession and your organization.* Philadelphia: F. A. Davis.

Hasselkus, B. (1993). Death in very old age: A personal journey of caregiving. *American Journal of Occupational Therapy, 47*(8), 717–723.

Health Care Financing Administration. (1983). Medicare program, hospice care: Final rule. *Federal Register, 56008–56036,* December 16.

Holland, A. (1984). Occupational therapy and day care for the terminally ill. *British Journal of Occupational Therapy, 47*(11), 345–348.

Holland, A., and Tigges, K.N. (1981). The hospice movement: A time for professional action and commitment. *British Journal of Occupational Therapy, 44*(12), 373–376.

Jaffe, E.G., and Epstein, C.F. (1992). *Occupational therapy consultation: Theory, principles and practice.* St. Louis: Mosby.

Koff, T. (Ed.). (1980). *Hospice: A caring community.* Cambridge, MA: Winthrop.

Kotler, P., and Andreasen, A. (1987*). Strategic marketing for non-profit organizations.* Englewood Cliffs, NJ: Prentice Hall.

Kubler-Ross, E. (1969). *On death and dying.* New York: MacMillan.

MacStravic, R.E. (1977). *Marketing health care.* Germantown, MD: Aspen.

National Hospice Organization. (1979). *Standards of hospice program of care.* Rosslyn, VA: National Hospice Organization.

National Hospice Organization. (1999). Web page. *http://www.nho.org/ques.html*

Peloquin, S. (1997). The spiritual depth of occupation: Making worlds and making lives. *American Journal of Occupational Therapy, 51*(3), 167–168.

Peloquin, S., and Christiansen, C. (1997). Special issue on occupation, spirituality and life meaning. *American Journal of Occupational Therapy, 51*(3). Rockville, MD: American Occupational Therapy Association.

Pizzi, M. (1983). Hospice and the terminally ill geriatric patient. *Physical and Occupational Therapy in Geriatrics, 3*(1), 45–54.

Pizzi, M. (1984). Occupational therapy in hospice care. *American Journal of Occupational Therapy, 38,* 252–257.

Pizzi, M. (1986). Care of the terminally ill, part 1: General principles. In *Role of occupational therapy with the elderly* (pp. 241–249). Rockville, MD: American Occupational Therapy Association.

Pizzi, M. (1990). The transformation of HIV infection and AIDS in occupational therapy: Beginning the conversation. *American Journal of Occupational Therapy, 44*(3), 199–203.

Pizzi, M. (1992). Hospice: The creation of meaning for people with life-threatening illness. *Occupational Therapy Practice, 4*(1), 1–8.

Pizzi, M. (1993). Environments of care: Hospice. In H. Hopkins and H. Smith (Eds.), *Willard and Spackman's occupational therapy* (8th ed., pp. 853–864). Philadelphia: Lippincott.

Rando, T.A. (1984). *Grief, dying and death: Clinical interventions for caregivers.* Champaign, IL: Research Press.

Saunders, C. (1965). The last stages of life. *American Journal of Nursing, 65*(3), 70–75.

Yerxa, E.J. (1967). 1966 Eleanor Clarke Slagle lecture: Authentic occupational therapy. In *A professional legacy: The Eleanor Clarke Slagle lectures in occupational therapy, 1955–1984* (pp. 155–173). Bethesda, MD: American Occupational Therapy Association.

ADDITIONAL READINGS

Benson, H., and Stark, M. (1997). *Timeless healing.* New York: Fireside.

Cousins, N. (1989). *Head first: Biology of hope.* New York: Dutton.

Dossey, L. (1996). *Alternative therapies: Special issue on love and human interconnectedness.* Thorofare, NJ: Slack.

Flowers, B.S., and Grubin, D. (Eds.). (1993). *Healing and the mind with Bill Moyers.* New York: Doubleday.

Moore, T. (1992). *Care of the soul.* New York: HarperCollins.

Moore, T. (1996). *The re-enchantment of everyday life.* New York: HarperCollins.

Pizzi, M. (1996). *HIV Infection and AIDS: A professional's guide.* Silver Spring, MD: Positive Images and Wellness.

Pizzi, M., and Burkhardt, A. (1998). Cancer and AIDS. In M. Neistadt and E.B. Crepeau (Eds.), *Willard and Spackman's occupational therapy* (9th ed., pp. 705–715). Philadelphia: Lippincott.

Pizzi, M., Mukand, J., and Freed, M. (1991). HIV infection and occupational therapy. In J. Mukand (Ed.), *Rehabilitation for patients with HIV disease* (pp. 283–326). New York: McGraw-Hill.

Pizzi, M., and Wilson, C.F. (Eds.). (1997). *Alternative and complementary care and the allied health professions.* Silver Spring, MD: National Center for Wellness and Health Promotion.

Siegel, B. (1986). *Love, medicine and miracles.* New York: Harper and Row.

Siegel, B. (1989). *Peace, love and healing.* New York: Harper and Row.

Tigges, K.N., and Marcil, W.M. (1996). Palliative medicine and rehabilitation: Assessment and treatment in hospice care. In *ROTE (role of occupational therapy with the elderly)* (2nd ed., pp. 743–763). Rockville, MD: American Occupational Therapy Association.

Weil, A. (1995). *Spontaneous healing.* New York: Ballantine.

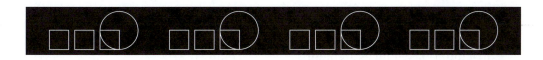

14 CHAPTER

Early Intervention Programs

Donna A. Wooster, MS, OTR, BCP

■ OUTLINE

Amplification

Curriculum-based measurement (CBM)

Early Intervention

Ecological evaluation

Eligibility

Family-centered philosophy

Free Appropriate Public Education (FAPE)

Individualized family service plan (IFSP)

Interdisciplinary teaming

Multidisciplinary team

Natural environments

Service coordinator

Solution-focused questions

Transdisciplinary teaming

LEARNING OBJECTIVES

This chapter is designed to enable the reader to:
- Describe legislation that has affected the development of early intervention programs.
- Explain the events demonstrating the need for early intervention services.
- Identify the components of early intervention programs.
- Discuss the role of the occupational therapist in early intervention programs.
- Identify and describe appropriate areas for evaluation and assessment instruments for early intervention occupational therapy services.
- Discuss the importance of family involvement in early intervention.
- Identify important aspects of quality occupational therapy services in early intervention programs.

 INTRODUCTION

Early Intervention is a federally mandated program implemented by states for children aged birth to 3 years. States are mandated to "develop and implement a statewide comprehensive, coordinated, multidisciplinary, interagency program of early intervention services for infants and toddlers with disabilities and their families, facilitate the coordination of payment for early intervention services from federal, state, local and private sources . . . " (34 CFR 303.1 [a][b]). The primary purpose is to identify children with delayed development who may be eligible for services and to provide necessary services to promote the family's ability to care for the child. The Individuals with Disabilities Education Act (IDEA) and now the Individuals with Disabilities Education Act Amendments of 1997 (H.R. 5) define the components of the programs. Part C covers centers and services to meet special needs of individuals with disabilities, while part H defines infants and toddlers with disabilities. The components requiring a **Free Appropriate Public Education (FAPE)** are in parts B, C, and H, which mandate the provision of education for all children with disabilities. States control the implementation and allocation of resources to the children. The 1997 amendments mandate a much more inclusive environment for these infants and toddlers, which includes providing services in **natural environments** such as day-care centers, day-care homes, and preschool programs. Children with disabilities should be in the community with non-disabled peers of the same age. The team's responsibility is to provide services to support these children's continued development in the community environments.

This chapter discusses the need for, and purpose of, early intervention and the legislatively mandated components of early intervention programs. Occupational therapy's participation in early intervention services is described, including evaluation, family involvement, parent instruction, and documentation. In addition, special considerations in early intervention are discussed and three case studies illustrate the major concepts.

 ## EARLY INTERVENTION PROGRAMS

The premise of early intervention service delivery is that the sooner the intervention begins, the better the outcomes for the family and child. Research has shown that an optimal environment is critical for the high-risk child to survive and thrive (Horowicz, 1982; Korner, 1987). The pioneer work done by Gordon (1969) taught parents to act as trainers for other parents. Gordon's research demonstrated that the children's development advanced significantly in this model program. The mothers showed improved teaching styles and became less directive and more supportive (Gray, 1976).

Current early intervention systems are intended to be "parent friendly," allow local communities to utilize and develop needed resources, facilitate a parent-professional collaboration, and attempt to minimize fragmentation and gaps in resources (Baldwin, Intriligator, Jeffries, Kaufmann, and Walsh, 1990). Research shows that families prefer informal methods to identify strengths and needs (Summers et al., 1990).

DEMONSTRATION OF NEED

In the past, parents were urged to place children with disabilities in institutions. Changes in society have contributed to the expectation that families will care for their child at home regardless of the child's disability. Some families need intense interventions and supports to competently handle this level of care. Research suggests that professionals can help families by providing information, emotional support, and continuous services (Featherstone, 1980).

Changes in the American family have resulted in many single parents raising children with disabilities. Job relocation is a factor that may result in having fewer extended family members locally as resources. This decreased child-care relief creates greater stress on the primary caretaker. Even in two-parent families, mothers, still the primary caretakers for these children (Crowe, 1993), are at risk for social isolation. They function better when provided with resources and consistent social supports (Anderson and Telleen, 1992).

Research shows that medically fragile children now have longer life expectancies than they did in the past (Fitzsimmons, 1993; Gortmaker and Sappenfield, 1984). Although the total size of the population of children with disabilities and chronic illness will probably remain stable, the longer life span will result in families with continued needs that will change over time as the child grows (Wallace, Biehl, MacQueen, and Blackman, 1997).

Additionally, many children with disabilities may live in poverty, dysfunctional families, and disadvantaged communities (Thompson, 1992). Poverty is associated with increased risk for disability and increased hospitalizations for problems related to chronic health conditions (Newacheck, 1989; Wissow, 1988), thus placing children with disabilities at greater accumulated risk.

The complex variety of health insurance providers adds to the confusion regarding meeting the needs of a child with a disability. Contracts that include copayments, preexisting conditions, deductibles, and primary care physicians as gatekeepers often confuse the family. State Medicaid systems establish variable eligibility criteria. Children who qualify for Medicaid in one state may not qualify in another state. Even children with private insurance coverage face capitation issues. Families need early intervention programs to fill the gaps and negotiate the system of service providers to ensure care for their child.

Each state has developed an early intervention system based on federal guidelines designed to address their specific needs and resources. The occupational therapist should seek information specific to the state(s) in which they practice. Most early intervention programs work in conjunction with the state department of education.

COMPONENTS OF EARLY INTERVENTION

Identification

Each state must establish a system to identify children who may be eligible for services and refer them to the early intervention system. Children with suspected developmental delays may be identified through a variety of sources, including occupational therapists, parents, physicians, other health providers, and community agencies. Professionals must seek verbal approval from the parents to make a referral. A central phone number (usually an 800 number) is typically available for referrals.

Eligibility Determination

One component of each statewide system is establishment of the "local lead agency." This appointed agency varies from state to state. Most often it is a part of the state department of education. The local lead agency schedules the evaluation with the parents to determine *eligibility*. **Eligibility** refers to whether or not the child qualifies, under the state's criteria, to receive early intervention services. Once written parental consent is obtained, the evaluation process is initiated. The evaluation can be done by a variety of trained professionals. The evaluation scores will be used to determine eligibility for services, which varies from state to state. A specific level of developmental delay (such as 25 percent) in one or more areas, or two standard deviations below the norm in any two areas, may constitute eligibility. In some states, an "at-risk" category based on professional opinions of high risk may qualify the child.

Evaluation and Assessment

The IDEA 1997 includes specific information about the evaluation process. Evaluations must be done within 45 days of referral and given in the native language or type of communication that suits the family. The assessment instruments must not be culturally or racially biased. Many states indicate a specific instrument as the assessment tool of choice and allow other informed clinical opinions to be expressed in writing to support the findings. Parents should be included in the evaluation process to provide information about the abilities of their child.

A variety of factors, such as the child's age, gender, ethnic background, native language, and culture, and information needs of the family and team, influence the selection of assessment tools. Assessments must be standardized test instruments that assess performance in five areas: (1) motor, (2) cognitive, (3) social-emotional, (4) communication, and (5) adaptive development.

Once the evaluation request is received, the child's chart is carefully reviewed. The chart may contain past medical history and previous testing, possibly indicating baseline skills and disabilities. If necessary, the therapist may request parental permission to obtain medical records and reports of previous tests.

Best practice research indicates that the evaluation of a child in multiple environments or contexts increases the reliability of the evaluation (Miller, 1994). If possible, occupational therapists should conduct observations of the child at home, in day care or nursery school, and in other natural environments. Factors that may be evaluated include response to different environments, effects of peer role models on performance, solitary versus group function, and social-emotional and communication skills with children and adults other than the parents. Gathering information across environments will help the therapist to use the person-activity-environment fit to match the child's abilities with the requirements of the activity and the features of the environment to enhance performance.

The early intervention program is primarily an educational model with teachers as the primary evaluators and providers. Early intervention teams must have many other professionals, including occupational therapists, physical therapists, speech language pathologists, audiologists, nurses, and others, available. One team member, usually a teacher, may perform the primary assessment. This person administers assessment tools and then, based on test findings across the five areas, calls in other services such as speech or occupational therapy. For example, occupational therapists may be involved in the evaluation process of infants and toddlers.

Another format is the arena-style evaluation. Multiple service providers gather to simultaneously observe the evaluation being conducted by one or two primary evaluators. Each team member records information and discusses the child's abilities. The team members discuss the observations and write a joint evaluation report. A child may be determined eligible for early intervention services based on the test scores. A report is written following the evaluation and an individualized family service plan (IFSP) is formulated, if warranted. The results and observations of the evaluation are used to make referrals to appropriate service providers, including occupational therapy. For example, if the child scored low on adaptive and fine-motor skills, then a referral is usually made for occupational therapy services.

The Individualized Family Service Plan (IFSP)

Once eligibility has been established, a written plan, called an **individualized family service plan (IFSP),** must be developed by the team (see Box 14–1). Only one IFSP is developed despite the involvement of a number of agencies. Family members are key participants in the development of the IFSP. All services required by the child must be documented in the plan, including which community agency will provide the service. The plan specifies the service providers, the frequency of treatment, the family goals, and the resources that will be involved. Expected outcomes are clearly stated. This process

---

BOX 14–1

The Individualized Family Service Plan (IFSP) Process

The IFSP process gathers information on the following:

- Child's current status
- Family resources, priorities, and concerns
- Major outcomes expected
- Specific services—frequency, duration, provider, and dates to initiate
- Need for other services, for example, medical
- Name of service coordinator
- Steps to support transition at age 3

will identify the child's needs, family resources, priorities, concerns, and supports. At the conclusion of the process, which also includes the appointment of a service coordinator and a family meeting, the nature and extent of services will be delineated.

Occupational therapy may be a primary service provider for the infant/toddler under the IFSP plan (Decker, 1992). Occupational therapy may be the only service provider or may be part of a team of providers. Each plan is customized to the needs of the child and the family. Any child with an identified need for occupational therapy must receive the service.

The **service coordinator** (see Box 14–2) functions as a consultant to the parents and providers. The service coordinator may be involved in training parents and other family members and professionals, coordinating appointments with medical personnel, participating in the team IFSP process, and establishing links with service providers. In addition, the service coordinator assists the family in planning for the transition to public school when the child is 3 years of age. The service coordinator has the most contact with the family and is able to view the needs of the family and child more holistically. This program model makes assumptions that the service coordinator is proactive, family centered, and enables and empowers families by promoting competencies (Bailey, Palsha, and Simeonsson, 1991; Dunst, Johanson, Trivette, and Hamby, 1991). An occupational therapist could also serve in the role of the service coordinator, which would decrease the number of professionals involved.

Parents have many rights associated with the IFSP process (see Box 14–3). The parents may review records at any time and can consent to share medical information with the IFSP team. A parent who is dissatisfied with the service provision or finds the documented IFSP services are not being provided has the right to due process. This is a legal proceeding that involves a hearing conducted by an impartial mediator to resolve disputes. This clearly illustrates the rights of the family in planning for the needs of their child who is receiving early intervention services.

The language in the law also states that services should be provided in *natural environments,* i.e., places children would normally find themselves, depending on age and activity. These include home, day-care provider's home, day-care center, nursery school, and playgrounds. Parents have input guiding the team in the choice of location(s) of service delivery. An occupational therapist may request to treat the child primarily in the home, with monthly visits to the nursery school, or vice versa. Decisions are made individually, based on the needs of the family and infant/toddler. The 1997 amendments strongly advocate for children to be placed in natural inclusive environments with peers. Service provision should be provided in these inclusive environments as well.

BOX 14-2

Role of the Service Coordinator

- Consulting with parents and providers
- Training parents and others
- Participating in team assessment and the IFSP process
- Coordinating early intervention and other health services
- Ensuring service access, contracts, and advocacy

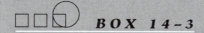

BOX 14-3

Summary of Parent Rights

- Consent necessary for evaluation of their child
- Review of their child's records
- Consent necessary to share medical information with team
- Written prior notice before services can be changed or refused
- Due process to resolve disputes
- Availability of impartial mediator

TEAM MEMBERS

Members of the early intervention team usually consist of the parents, teachers, therapists, and other individuals, including a variety of contracted service providers, working with the child. The occupational therapist can be one member of this team. The team's primary goal is to provide the needed services to the family as documented in the IFSP. Each team is formed based on the needs of the family. Some service providers will work together frequently and be familiar with each other. Often the team members are representative of a variety of agencies contracted for specific service provision. Teams that have a clear, focused statement of purpose, goals, and philosophies function more effectively.

Briggs (1993) describes 10 qualities as essential to a team's success. One of the most important qualities discussed is *communication.* Teams develop communication systems suitable to their situation. Today's technology allows more avenues for communication than ever before—fax, cellular phone, voice mail, pagers, and e-mail, which offer team members broader opportunities to seek guidance from others and share knowledge. Even when team members work in distant areas, they can develop creative means to communicate. A written set of rules that governs how members will communicate important information to each other is very advantageous in promoting good communications.

Problem solving is another key component of the early intervention team's work. Team meetings are essential and require a commitment of time and space from the agencies. Meetings should be decisive and productive. Briggs (1997) has pulled together information to assist teams to overcome obstacles in a positive and productive manner. A five-step decision-making model that can be used in problem-solving situations has been outlined in the literature (Briggs, 1991).

There are basically three different team models: (1) multidisciplinary, (2) interdisciplinary, and (3) transdisciplinary. The **multidisciplinary team** is an older model in which each professional conducts individual evaluations and writes his or her own goals. **Interdisciplinary teaming** involves individual evaluations with joint discussion for prioritization of goals, allowing for more coordinated services (Case-Smith and Wavrek, 1993). **Transdisciplinary teaming** involves overlapping roles, responsibilities, and functions among participating disciplines. It allows flexibility and relinquishes predetermined professional boundaries (Hutchison, 1978). All team members are involved in cross-training in preparation for this role. This cross-training is a process that takes time to develop and requires that team members have a solid foundation in child development and therapeutic intervention. Cross-training involves the team progressing through a series of developmental stages: role extension, role enrichment, role expansion, role exchange, role release, role support, and role transition (Briggs, 1993). The reader is referred to the reference cited for further information on these stages.

Obstacles or barriers to transdisciplinary teaming include philosophical and professional differences, legal liabilities, licensure limitations, variable education of service providers, inconsistent mastery of skills practiced in role release, and reimbursement policies (Orlove and Sobsey, 1991; Ottenbacher, 1983).

With a transdisciplinary team, generally one team member becomes the primary provider to the family. Team members are utilized for consultation as needed. This allows the team to develop a holistic program for the child and build stronger relationships with family members. In addition, the family has time to get comfortable with one primary service provider. This may be the best option for time efficiency and trust building with a family. Some programs that cover large rural geographical areas find this also helps to reduce traveling time and increases one-to-one time with families.

The certified occupational therapy assistant (COTA) can also be a vital member of an early intervention team. However, the demands of the transdisciplinary model may prohibit the use of the entry-level COTA. The OTR/ COTA will discuss the roles and responsibilities of the COTA, following the American Occupational Therapy Association (AOTA) Standards of Practice and Guidelines for Supervision as well as state laws pertaining to occupational therapy practice. Experienced COTAs can be primary service providers with supervision from the OTR as required. A COTA, in this role, must demonstrate excellence in clinical observation and reasoning, awareness of personal limitations, and good rapport building and communication skills. The OTR remains accountable for the quality of services and makes all final clinical decisions.

TRANSITION PLANNING

Transition planning must be part of any IFSP. Transitions are known to be a time of stress for the family. The early intervention team must make referral to the local education agency (LEA) at least six months or more before the child's third birthday. The LEA will determine preschool programs that are available to the child. The team works closely with the family to notify the school-based staff of any special equipment that will be required in the preschool environment. If possible, when given parental permission, the early intervention occupational therapist should contact the school occupational therapist personally to facilitate the transition. This may be helpful to provide pertinent information about techniques and procedures that have worked well as reinforcers, the amount and course of progress, and the treatment approach focus. If a mealtime protocol has been developed, providing it to the preschool program staff will improve continuity.

Transitioning into the preschool-based setting is stressful to families. The model changes from a family-friendly model to a special education school-based model. Early intervention teams should assist parents in developing assertiveness skills to request necessary services for their child. The early intervention team should encourage parents to speak up at meetings and ask for what their child needs. Informing them of their legal rights and educating them about the relevant components of the Individuals with Disabilities Education Act (IDEA) is also very helpful.

If the family is relocating, the therapist might offer to make a videotape of the current feeding/toileting/dressing programs with routines. This facilitates carryover of desired techniques. Notes about favorite toys and preferred activities can help new team members to plan successful transition sessions. If possible, adaptive equipment should be sent with the child and family. If that is not possible, team members can make a list of specific equipment and purchasing information for the parents and the new team. Including contact names and phone numbers will also be useful.

OCCUPATIONAL THERAPY SERVICES IN EARLY INTERVENTION

Occupational therapists may assume many roles in the early intervention process. They can be part of the evaluation team, provide direct services, provide consultation to other team members in a transdisciplinary model, or do any combination of these roles (Hanft, 1989). Occupational therapists can also be service coordinators.

OCCUPATIONAL THERAPY EVALUATION

Children, especially those at 7 or 8 months of age who may be experiencing stranger anxiety, may need time to adjust to the therapist before they will cooperate with an assessment. Allowing the parents to remain with the child initially is important. Also, during this time, the child should be approached slowly with time allowed for gradual interaction and play. Performance will be negatively affected when a child is crying or afraid.

Assessment instruments chosen should demonstrate high validity and reliability; accurately identify appropriate infants; include comprehensive health, social, behavioral, and environmental components; and involve the family as equal partners with the professionals (Hanson and Lynch, 1989).

Curriculum-based measurement (CBM) measures the academic skills that children are expected to acquire. This type of evaluation determines the child's level of competence in specific academic skills. The child's ability to match and name colors or shapes, or to place items in a shape sorter, may be evaluated (Deno, 1983).

Ecological evaluations determine the skills needed to be successful in various environments. For example, in preschool, the child's ability to generalize new skills to different environments is evaluated. This may include moving from his or her chair to a circle of chairs for an activity, removing outer clothing and placing on a hanger, requesting and going to the bathroom with prompts, and playing safely on the playground on various pieces of equipment. Ecological evaluation is very useful in allowing team members to assess practical functional changes in the child.

Play is assessed by occupational therapists because it is the primary occupation of children. A variety of assessments are available to assist the team in determining eligibility. Or they may provide more specific information about baseline performance of skills. This information can be incorporated into the decision-making process as well as treatment planning and scheduling of daily activities. Play offers opportunities to treat deficits in specific motor, cognitive, communication, and social-emotional skills.

The Transdisciplinary Play Based Assessment (TPBA) (Linder, 1990) is an observation-based, transdisciplinary assessment tool. It addresses normal developmental sequences of skill acquisition in the areas of cognition, social-emotional, communication, and sensorimotor skills and describes procedures for conducting a transdisciplinary arena-type assessment. The team evaluates the child in normal play in a natural environment.

The Revised Knox Preschool Play Scale is for children from birth to 6 years of age. It assesses four areas of play: (1) space management, (2) material management, (3) pretense/symbolic, and (4) participation. This requires play observation both indoors and outdoors in natural environments with peers over a minimum of two 30-minute observations. More detailed descriptions of the evaluation process and interpretation of play assessments can be found in *Play in Occupational Therapy for Children* by L. Parham and L. Fazzio (1997).

Sensory integration and sensorimotor functions are important components for the occupational therapist to evaluate. Understanding the body language of premature babies is especially important (Hussey, 1988). An examination of infant states is a way to evaluate sensory processing, and the Infant-Toddler Symptom Checklist by Degangi (1995) is available from Therapy Skill Builders. Other available tools for children under 3 years are listed in the Appendix.

Feeding is an especially important performance area to evaluate in infants and toddlers because good nutrition is essential for adequate growth and development, particularly of the nervous system. Infants who have motor delays, immature central nervous systems, or gastrointestinal abnormalities may experience significant difficulties with feeding. Morris and Klein (1987) suggest that sensory or medical problems that interfere with feeding develop into more complex emotional and behavioral issues. The occupational therapist must have a detailed understanding of normal feeding development. The normal feeding development sequence is the foundation for all feeding evaluations. Most children's hospitals have feeding teams available to conduct transdisciplinary feeding evaluations. This is the safest place to evaluate the medically complex and fragile child. Occupational therapists with less experience with feeding should develop a link with the team at the hospital for referrals. Establishing appropriate non-nutritive sucking and oral-motor stimulation programs for children is necessary for them to learn saliva control and become feeders.

Other assessment tools may be used to address specific skill areas such as fine-motor, visual-motor, and self-care skills. The types of assessments are numerous (see the Appendix). Some are specific to a diagnosis, while others are based on normal development. The recommendation is that at least one assessment tool be a developmental checklist that allows parents to report their observations as well. It also should cover all the areas designated by IDEA.

FAMILY INVOLVEMENT

A **family-centered philosophy** makes the assumption that the parents know best. The parents, viewed as partners with the service providers, are expected to be advocates for their child. The role of service providers is to meet the needs of the family by providing the information and instruction designated as important by the parents. To understand the family-centered philosophy, the provider must understand and have a family systems perspective (Bronfenner, 1976). For example, occupational therapists must learn to form partnerships with families. Accepting parental reports as reliable information, allowing parents to help define goals, letting parents lead the discussions, and allowing parents to have questions ready for the team to problem solve together are good starting places.

Family-centered philosophy differs from the medical model previously utilized by occupational therapists. The medical model often places the health-care providers in a superior role to advise the parents about what they should be doing for their child. The parents are the passive recipients of well-meaning advice, some of which may not fit the needs of their child. This deters the parents from being active or learning how to advocate for their child.

Occupational therapists must learn to communicate with the family in their native language or have a translator present to facilitate the process. Simeonsson and Bailey (1990) identified a hierarchy of parental involvement, representing a continuum from passive to active participation, for early intervention. Families will fluctuate in the levels, depending on the environmental demands and their coping abilities at the time. At the lowest level is *elective noninvolvement,* in which the family chooses not to be involved in the child's care. At the midlevel of the hierarchy is *family involvement,* which focuses on gathering information and developing skills. At the highest level, the family seeks *psychological change* in the family system. Identifying the level at which the family is functioning, at a given time, will assist the occupational therapist in determining appropriate caregiving roles within the family. Featherstone (1980) suggested that professionals could assist families by providing relevant and current information and providing emotional supports and needed services. Some families may need the help of the therapist to teach them how to be advocates for their own needs and empower them to make decisions for themselves and their child.

Observation of the child in the natural environment will provide valuable assessment information about family routines, roles, and communication styles. The concept of "amplification" may be a useful strategy for occupational therapists. **Amplification** is a process of "noticing, describing, and discussing an interactive event between family member and child that is likely to promote child change" (Andrews and Andrews, 1993, p. 42). This means that the occupational therapist discusses his or her observations with the family regarding any communication attempts the child makes and the responses of the parent that reinforce the child's behavior. This encourages the parents to notice and respond to nonverbal communication attempts. For example, during lunch, the occupational therapist might comment, "I just saw your child visually attend to you and move his head toward the spoon. Try placing the spoon just in front of his mouth again this time and see if he moves that way again." This encourages the parent to attend to this nonverbal communication and reinforces the child's efforts. This may be the first recognition of interaction, which can facilitate bonding between the child and parent. In some cases this interaction may be the beginning of some partial participation in the activity that can be recognized and built on. Occupational therapists take larger tasks, such as feeding, and analyze the many small steps it takes to complete the task. Partial participation is active involvement in any of the smaller component steps. This is especially important in many functional self-care tasks.

During the interview with the parent, the message that families are competent and in control of their child's life must be conveyed. One way to do this is to ask solution-focused questions (Andrews and Andrews, 1993). **Solution-focused questions** are worded such that they assume the family is already working toward improving the situation, giving the family credit for their efforts. For example, "I have noticed how carefully you position your child's head and arms when you place him in the infant seat. This is great. Do you do this in any other tasks or positions as well?" Another example, "Turning off the TV during feeding really seemed to help your daughter concentrate on feeding. Have you noticed other things you do that help her pay attention?" Important information, as well as trust building, can be gained from this approach.

Looking at the family's normal daily routine also is important. Families will be better able to carry over positioning and exercises if they are taught how to fit them into their established daily routine. Examples include performing range of motion exercises at times when the diaper needs changing or placing the child in an infant seat in a secure place with toys on the tray for play while the parent is cooking a meal or showering. The most effective suggestions are those that work within natural family routines.

The nature of the activity can also affect which family members are available to help. Every parent needs time for personal hygiene, meal preparation, and care of siblings. The therapist can demonstrate ways the child can be placed in a safe and independent play position when a parent is most likely to be busy. Siblings can be involved by showing them ways to play with and monitor the child. This, of course, depends on the age and abilities of the siblings. A therapist who arrives when the older siblings need to be leaving for school may be interfering with regular routines. Therefore, arriving 10 minutes earlier could be very helpful or very inconvenient. Therapists should allow the family to establish convenient times to visit.

Little information is available to measure the quality of the services provided to families. Safer and Hamilton (1993) have written suggestions on how to measure quality of services based on timeliness, effectiveness, individualization, transition, family-centered focus, and coordination (see Box 14-4).

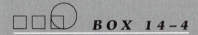

BOX 14-4

Best Practice Guidelines for Occupational Therapy in Early Intervention

- Regard parents as partners in decision making.
- Use clear, open, and collaborative communication style with all team members.
- Share responsibilities for service implementation with team members.
- Use knowledge to improve performance and functional outcomes.
- Deliver cost-effective quality treatment.
- View child's abilities in context of natural environments.
- Incorporate carryover into natural daily routines.
- Use amplification and solution-focused questions.

PARENT INSTRUCTION

Parent instruction is an ongoing process that includes modeling the practice of skills and specific behaviors. Research by Hinojosa (1990) demonstrated that mothers are unable to follow inflexible home programs and, instead, need programs that fit into the daily routine. Case-Smith and Nastro (1993) found that mothers preferred the use of written handouts with specific activities. Similarly, Rainforth and Salisbury (1988) have advocated programs that fit into the lifestyle of the parents. Multiple sets of instructions are confusing. Often, simple, clear diagrams, placed in strategic locations, can be great aids to reinforce positioning. Suggestions include placing pictures near the changing table (and just inside the diaper bag) demonstrating how to relax the child and change the diaper in a side-lying position, and placing a feeding positioning diagram on the refrigerator or near the table and a bathtub positioning diagram in the bathroom. Practicing techniques with parents and interested family members can provide reassurance.

EQUIPMENT AND SUPPLIES

The occupational therapist should have a variety of assessment tools, positioning equipment, feeding supplies, developmentally appropriate toys with switch access, and cleaning supplies for standard precautions readily available.

Positioning equipment, including a variety of supportive chairs and standers, is helpful if needed. Some vendors allow therapists to borrow equipment in preparation for purchase. Equipment should be selected to allow room for growth in both height and width, and should be durable, easy to clean, and adaptable. Corner chairs sometimes can be made by a carpenter or parent. Cardboard can be shaped to form positioning devices. Rolled towels, small beanbags, and filled sandwich bags can also be used as lateral supports. Other commercially available products can sometimes be used, such as child-sized lawn chairs for tub seats or infant/child car seats with a variety of positioning options.

Feeding kits are essential to the evaluation process. A budget for consumable supplies is also suggested because some items, such as toothbrush handles with a variety of textured ends and rubber tubes that slip on fingers with toothbrush-type bristles on the end, are often given to the families to use. Different nipples, cups, a scoop dish, utensils, and sensory items also are required.

Developmentally appropriate toys should be selected for durability and ability to be cleaned. Purchased materials are often adaptable for a variety of ages and purposes. These include bubbles, Play Doh, balloons with covers, balls, scooter boards, dress-up clothes, peg boards, blocks, dress-up dolls, fine-motor shape toys, and small toys to manipulate. Therapists can share creative ideas for making toys from a variety of recyclable or household items and in the process teach parents the properties of toys appropriate for their child.

Toys that require a variety of skills or offer alternative ways to play also are helpful. A toy-lending library is a great resource to early intervention teams, if available. Knowing how to make switch interceptors is helpful. Toys 'R' Us now carries a line of adaptable toys. Many companies make commercially available switch toys.

Cleaning supplies are essential. Items to have available include gloves for standard precautions and sanitary foam for handwashing. A mixture of bleach and water (at a mix of 1:10) can be used to clean toys after each use.

DOCUMENTATION

Documentation requirements may vary by agency, source of reimbursement, and type of treatment. Examples include daily progress notes, daily/monthly checklists, or quarterly reports. Usually, separate forms for travel time and expenses, meeting times, and direct and indirect service hours will be used.

Files, reports, original records, and the IFSP and parent instruction sheets should be stored in locked file cabinets at the early intervention center. These are confidential and should only be reviewed by essential team members. Originals of all notes and communication should be included in this file. Notes written by COTAs are to be reviewed by the OTR and countersigned before any copies are distributed. Therapists may keep copies of their notes in their personal files, including a summary of progress toward goals. These files are for personal use only and are not to be shared.

A progress note describing the child's progress includes the frequency and duration of treatment since the prior note; explanation of any changes in treatment approach or medical problems that interfered with therapy; and mention of transportation problems, missed visits, sickness, and other factors that enabled or impeded progress. Factors that altered parental stress are documented due to their effect on coping skills.

Concise, readable reports written in nonmedical language that parents understand is most helpful to the family. For example, instead of using the term "upper extremity," the term "arms" should be used. Similarly, instead of using "bilateral" or "ipsilateral," terms such as "on both sides" or "on the same side of the body" should be used.

All reports should explain and justify services, including their frequency and duration. IFSP forms have spaces for this information. Discharge notes summarize the child's abilities and progress and include the date and reason for discontinuation, type of program, the frequency and duration of treatment, and a summary of the interventions used and progress achieved. Information reported includes activities done during daily routines, effective reinforcers and treatment approaches for the child, and useful strategies that facilitated the parents' abilities.

 ## SPECIAL CONSIDERATIONS IN EARLY INTERVENTION

RURAL SERVICE DELIVERY

Providing skilled intervention services in rural areas requires much planning because distances between homes can be significant (see Box 14–5). Tips on auto and trip preparation may be found in Chapter 11 on home health care. As a safety precaution,

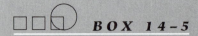

BOX 14–5

Rural Service Delivery

- Prepare the vehicle (cellular phone recommended).
- Plan schedule and check with families the day before.
- Plan visits with other team members.
- Check in with office—follow schedule.
- Be prepared for inclement weather.
- Know emergency procedures for natural disasters.

it is recommended that visits to secluded or less safe areas be scheduled during the morning or early in the day and that the therapist notify the agency on arrival and departure.

LARGE EXTENDED FAMILIES

Extended family members can be very helpful with treatment. However, excessive noise and movement may distract or overstimulate some children. If there are other children in the home, planning a group activity for them may be helpful so the parent can concentrate on working with the therapist. Siblings can volunteer or be selected on a rotating basis to engage with the team member and the child with special needs. This will enable siblings to learn appropriate interaction skills, possibly allowing them to help with some responsibilities involving their sibling.

Observing family meals provides information about the environment and the type of sensory stimulation provided. This allows for more appropriate suggestions to the family. A child's performance may be very different on a one-to-one basis than during a family meal. To give parents some relief, the therapist can encourage extended family members to learn the basic care routines of the child and to share chores.

When considering what toys to utilize for play, durability is a factor. It is inevitable that siblings will want to play with the new toy, and sharing can be encouraged. Using nonbreakable toys and materials can prevent many hurt feelings.

CULTURAL DIVERSITY

Practices regarding adaptive skills and social-emotional skills are very much dependent on the culture of the family. Views regarding child rearing vary greatly, including the involvement of other children in family decisions; the types of foods and the social climate of meals; hygiene; clothing habits and choices; behavioral expectations; and disciplinary actions and methods. The early intervention team must learn about the culture of the family and make the evaluation and treatment appropriate to this context. Children must learn to function first in their family and then in their community. The child's ability to participate in religious ceremonies, cultural activities, and school activities may be especially important for families.

Occupational therapists should seek information about the areas in which care will be delivered. Learning about community activities and discovering resources, including interpretive services, is very helpful.

PROFESSIONAL PREPARATION

Therapists who desire to work in early intervention should consider their abilities and seek additional continuing education. Experience in pediatrics, an understanding of medical testing, and knowledge of pediatric assessment tools are helpful. Knowledge of standardized and nonstandardized assessment tools and their use is essential. Familiarity with basal and ceiling age criteria, administering and scoring, and the interpretation of test scores is also important.

Awareness of the expertise that occupational therapy and other service providers bring to the early intervention team is important as well. Occupational therapy's expertise includes specialized knowledge in feeding, adaptive skills, task analysis skills, environmental modification, normal development, motor control, sensory processing, and the variety and progression of play skills.

Each state has created competencies that must be met by all early intervention team members. Specific continuing education and experiences are usually required but can vary by state.

Knowledge of community agencies, such as the local food bank, where to apply for Section 8 housing, the day-care center, secondhand clothing stores, and the types of department stores available is helpful. Toys, feeding utensils, and other products may be locally available.

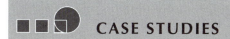 CASE STUDIES

MARLA

Marla, one of twins, was 3 months old when she came home from the hospital. Born at 32 weeks gestation and weighing 3 pounds 14 ounces at birth with APGAR scores of 4 and 6, respectively, she spent her first five weeks in the neonatal intensive care unit and then another five weeks in the nursery for premature infants. She displayed characteristic low tone and poor suck and was fed via nasogastric (NG) tube for the first four weeks. The occupational therapist worked on non-nutritive sucking, positioning, and sensory stimulation for arousal. While in the premature infant nursery, Marla was very slow to gain weight due to her weak sucking ability. She was transitioned to oral feeding with a squeeze bottle and longer nipple. During this time, she also had bradycardia and two febrile seizures secondary to an infection, which later cleared. Marla was discharged from the hospital to the family's mobile home in rural Alabama. Her twin sister, Mandy, was much larger and had been discharged at 2 weeks of age. There was some concern that Marla had cerebral palsy and left hemiplegia, the cause of which was uncertain at the time of discharge.

The early intervention team requested an occupational therapy evaluation and treatment. Marla was the fourth child in the family with siblings 4 and 2 years old. The mother was 20 years old and expressed fear about caring for her premature infant because this baby was so "different" and "tiny" compared to the others. The father worked full time at the local automobile repair shop and drove the family's only vehicle to work daily. Occasionally, arrangements could be made for him to get a ride to work if his wife needed the use of the car. The early intervention team collaborated with the family in the creation of a family service plan. Long-term goals for this infant and family included: (1) helping the family adjust to handling, feeding, changing, and playing with the twins; (2) being able to get out in the community and safely transport the children; (3) establishing feeding schedules for the twins that allowed for family mealtimes; and (4) providing play opportunities to facilitate development.

The occupational therapist helped the parents to schedule times for feeding the twins (both were on bottles), meal preparation, family meals, and necessary chores. In addition, the mother learned energy conservation techniques to pace herself throughout the day and to incorporate the other children into appropriate activities. The therapist suggested that the parents seek volunteers from community groups to provide child care. Three church members offered to assist with chores and activities with the children. This allowed the mother time to go grocery shopping and do other necessary errands.

Evening occupational therapy visits were scheduled in order to educate and involve the father and grandparents in child care. Each parent and grandparent learned how to feed, bathe, change diapers, and position the infants safely. Incorporated in this instruction were techniques to provide proprioceptive input and weight bearing on Marla's left side, to bring both hands to midline for play/exploration, to bring hands to mouth for feeding, and to position her in a variety of ways throughout the day to promote development. Positioning for Marla was based on the family routines and activities. Pictures of "good positioning" for the infant were placed in appropriate locations as reminders for the parents, grandparents, and volunteers.

Occupational therapy continued to address Marla's oral-motor skills and feeding abilities. She was able to suck more effectively and transitioned to a regular bottle with shorter nipple. A prefeeding program was implemented that included left-sided facilitation techniques and facial stroking toward midline. Gradually Marla was introduced to spoon-feeding.

Follow-up medical visits confirmed the diagnosis of cerebral palsy. The parents were assured that the early intervention team would continue its involvement with the family to meet their changing needs.

DANIEL

Daniel, an 8-month-old infant with Down's syndrome, has been receiving early intervention services for the last four months from a special education teacher and a physical therapist. The early intervention team is concerned about his sensory processing and self-help skills. The physical therapist has been addressing gross motor skills and positioning and will continue to treat him. Current testing reveals a gross motor age equivalent of 5 months and a cognitive age equivalent of 4 months. Parental concerns include his lack of grasping and interacting with toys, irritability, becoming easily afraid, crying when in different environments, and refusing to take infant food from a spoon.

Daniel lives in a small city with his parents and two siblings who are 10 and 12 years old. His parents are college educated. His father's job as an insurance adjuster requires frequent travel. His mother has just returned to work part time three nights per week as a nurse. No extended family members live in the area. A hired neighbor stays with the children when both parents are working. The siblings are old enough to offer some assistance.

Occupational therapy intervention addressed Daniel's sensory needs. The Infant/Toddler Symptom Checklist indicated some problems with self-regulation and bathing/dressing/touch. Through observation, the occupational therapist noted adverse responses to sensory stimulation to the face and palms of the hands, a dislike for vestibular changes associated with rapid movements, and a tendency toward overstimulation by visual and auditory information in the environment. Further assessment revealed low tone in the face and tongue and some fatigue with exertion.

Occupational therapy intervention addressed sensory and motor needs through parent education, environmental modifications, and a prefeeding program. The therapist provided parent education on sensory stimulation, identified the visual and auditory sources of distress, and suggested environmental modifications. These included turning off telephones and televisions during mealtimes, positioning the infant to minimize visual distractions, and simplifying verbal and nonverbal communication. Indicators of sensory overstimulation in Daniel included hiccuping, turning away, pushing into extension with his body, and crying. Calming activities, such as slow rocking, swaddling, holding securely, deep pressure input, low lighting, minimal talking, were taught and suggested for use before bedtimes, naps, and when the infant showed beginning signs of overstimulation. Due to Daniel's discomfort with rapid movement and the accompanying vestibular changes, the parents were taught to inform Daniel when they were going to move him and then move him slowly and securely.

Since Daniel was refusing to accept infant food from a spoon, a prefeeding program was implemented to improve his sensory tolerance in the oral-motor area. His mother selected calming music and, while it was playing, she provided slow-moving, constant pressure, stroking his face with her hands and then with a facecloth. Stroking was always done toward facial midline and lip closure. The mother used an infadent on her fingertip and slowly stroked the midline mouth area and then the gums. Next, the first in a series of mouth brushes (Nuk) was slowly introduced at midline and in front of the gums, gradually working back into the mouth. Over time, the brush was dipped in infant fruit to introduce flavors. As Daniel became more familiar with this touch, he gradually opened his mouth and became more accepting. Some facilitation techniques to the facial area and tongue were introduced to work on lip closure and tongue control. A spoon was gradually added, and his diet progressed to cereals and fruit.

TENISHA

Tenisha is a 1-year-old child recently placed in foster care by the court and child protection services due to a history of neglect and abuse. She has cerebral palsy with spastic quadriplegia and visual and hearing impairments. She is currently in the bottom 3 percent for weight and height for her age. She has had three hospitalizations for pneumonia and was hospitalized one month ago with a mild concussion. At that time, she was diagnosed as HIV positive. During that hospitalization, a video fluoroscopy was done, indicating severe aspiration. A gastrostomy tube (G-tube) was inserted for feeding, and she was discharged from the hospital to the foster home. The infant seems depressed and has organic failure to thrive. Some knee and elbow contractures are present. The early intervention team determined that the child needs nursing, occupational therapy, physical therapy, and a home trainer to assist her foster parents. A long-term placement in this home is desired. Occupational therapy, physical therapy, and nursing practitioners are visiting once a week, while the home trainer is visiting twice weekly. Physical therapy's focus is on contracture management, range of motion (ROM), inhibition of tone, and positioning. Occupational therapy's focus is on oral-motor stimulation, promoting play positions with multisensory toys, and parent education, including standard (universal) precautions.

An oral-motor program has been implemented to help Tenisha control saliva and improve oral muscle control, which may aid vocalization. The program focuses on inhibiting facial muscles and promoting lip closure and vocalizations. Multisensory cues and positioning are key elements in this process. The infant is placed supine on an elevated wedge or on the elevated thighs of the parents to promote face-to-face contact. Positioning and neurodevelopmental treatment techniques are used to promote lung expansion and exhalation. The foster parents are encouraged to complete the oral-motor program just before or during G-tube feeding to promote the connection of mouth stimulation and stomach satiation.

The occupational and physical therapists work together to develop a daily positioning program that fits in with the routines of the family. During the course of the day, the family is shown how to utilize positioning, ROM, and inhibition techniques while changing diapers, dressing, bathing, and playing with the child. Tenisha is placed prone on a blanket on the floor with a small half roll under her shoulders to facilitate knee extension. A head switch that activates a small vibrating toy is used to promote neck extension. In a side-lying position, bilateral hand skills are promoted to explore textured toys and materials and to promote reach and grasp. In a supine position, head control in flexion and pull-to-sit is encouraged, as well as reaching up for suspended toys. Sitting positioning is addressed in the infant seat, car seat, and carriage while providing opportunities for head control and hand skills.

The concept of partial participation in age-appropriate, self-care skills is utilized. Tenisha is provided hand-over-hand assist in order to remove hats and to place arms in/out of sleeves and legs in/out of shorts. The family is encouraged to develop a dressing routine, using consistent tactile cues to indicate desired behaviors. Over time, Tenisha has been improving her ability to initiate these movements.

Tenisha has been placed on a variety of medications at different times. This has required consistent communication between the early intervention team and the family to ensure awareness of possible side effects and to modify performance expectations of the infant as needed. With the assistance of the early intervention team, the foster family has been able to provide the level of care required for Tenisha. They work diligently to provide opportunities to promote her health and development and are rewarded by her loving and affectionate nature.

 CONCLUSION

Early intervention occupational therapy occurs in home and community environments. The skills required of an early intervention occupational therapist include evaluation and observation skills, flexibility with scheduling, good time management, knowledge of community agencies and resources, awareness of cultural and religious diversity, and excellent communication skills. Occupational therapists must learn to function on a variety of teams and with different team members. Respect for parents and the ability to establish rapport are necessary. Daily challenges and rewards abound. The diversity of the infants and toddlers and their families provide stimulation and excitement.

Community-based practice can be isolating at times and unique and challenging at other times. The use of computers for accessing information and resources can be a valuable tool to have available. Effective use of team members and other occupational therapists can be re-energizing to the therapist and provide needed professional support.

 STUDY QUESTIONS

1. Discuss how legislation has affected the development of early intervention programs.
2. What state licensure laws need to be considered for supervision and practice in early intervention?
3. Compare and contrast the characteristics of the three types of teams in early intervention programs.
4. List and describe the rights of parents in early intervention programs.
5. Describe strategies for facilitating family involvement in the therapy process.
6. Describe the variety of roles available to the occupational therapist in early intervention programs.
7. What are the key performance areas and performance components for the occupational therapist to evaluate and what tools are available to assess these?
8. List five characteristics of "best practice" for occupational therapy in early intervention programs.
9. If you needed to put together a "therapy kit" to keep in your car, what equipment, supplies, and forms would you need to include in the kit?

REFERENCES

American Occupational Therapy Association. (1989). *Guidelines for occupational therapy services in early intervention and preschool services.* Bethesda, MD: American Occupational Therapy Association.

Anderson, P., and Telleen, S. (1992). The relationship between social support and maternal behavior and attitudes: A meta-analytic review. *American Journal of Community Psychology, 20*(6), 753–774.

Andrews, M., and Andrews, J. (1993). Family centered techniques: Integrating enablement into the IFSP process. *Journal of Childhood Communication Disorders, 15,* 41–46.

Bailey, D.B., Palsha, S.A., and Simeonsson, R.J. (1991). Professional skills, concerns, and perceived importance of work with families in early intervention. *Exceptional Child, 58,* 156–163.

Baldwin, D., Intriligator, B., Jeffries, G., Kauffman, R., and Walsh, S. (1990). *Critical factors in the development of part H service systems.* Vienna, VA: The National Maternal and Child Health Resource Center.

Briggs, M. (1991). Team development: Decision making for early intervention. *Infant Toddler Intervention: The Transdisciplinary Journal, 1,* 1–9.

Briggs, M. (1993). Team talk: Communication skills for early intervention teams. *Journal of Childhood Communication Disorders, 15,* 33–40.

Briggs, M. (1997). *Building early intervention teams: Working together for children and families.* Gaithersburg, MD: Aspen.

Bronfenner, U. (1976). The experimental ecology of education. *Educational Research, 5*(9), 5–15.

Case-Smith, J., and Nastro, M. (1993). The effect of occupational therapy intervention on mothers of children with cerebral palsy. *American Journal of Occupational Therapy, 46,* 811–817.

Case-Smith, J., and Wavrek, B. (1993). Models of service delivery and team interaction. In J. Case-Smith (Ed.), *Pediatric occupational therapy and early intervention.* Boston: Andover.

Crowe, T. (1993). Time use of mothers with young children: The impact of a child's disability. *Developmental Medicine and Child Neurology, 35,* 612–630.

Decker, B. (1992). A comparison of the individualized education plan and the individualized family service plan. *American Journal of Occupational Therapy, 46*(3), 247–252.

Degangi, C. (1995). Infant toddler symptom checklist. San Antonio, TX: Therapy Skill Builders/Psychological Corporation.

Deno, S. (1983). Curriculum based measurements: The emerging alternative. *Exceptional Children, 52,* 219–232.

Dunst, C.J., Johanson, C., Trivette, C.M., and Hamby, D. (1991). Family-oriented early intervention policies and practices: Family centered or not? *Exceptional Children, 58,* 115–121.

Family Education Rights and Privacy Act of 1974. Public Law No. 93-380, 20 U.S.C. §1232, 34 C.F.R., Part 99.

Featherstone, H. (1980). *A difference in the family: Life with a disabled child.* New York: Basic Books.

Fitzsimmons, S. (1993). The changing epidemiology of cystic fibrosis. *Journal of Pediatrics, 122,* 1–9.

Gordon, I. (1969). Early childhood stimulation through parent education. Final report to the Children's Bureau, Social and Rehabilitation Services, Department of Health, Education and Welfare (HEW), ED 038–166.

Gortmaker, S.L., and Sappenfield, W. (1984). Chronic childhood disorders: Prevalence and impact. *Pediatric Clinics of North America, 31,* 3–18.

Gray, S. (1976). A report on the home-parent centered intervention programs: Home visiting with mothers of toddlers and their siblings. DARCEE, Peabody College, Massachusetts.

Hanft, B.E. (1989). Nationally speaking—early intervention issues in specialization. *American Journal of Occupational Therapy, 43,* 431–434.

Hanson, M., and Lynch, E. (1989). *Early Intervention: Implementing child and family services for infants and toddlers who are at risk or disabled.* Austin, TX: Pro Ed.

Hinojosa, J. (1990). How mothers of preschool children with cerebral palsy perceive occupational and physical therapists and their influence on family life. *Occupational Therapy Journal of Research, 10*(3), 144–162.

Horowicz, F.D. (1982). The first two years of life: Factors related to thriving. In S. Moore and C. Cooper (Eds.), *The young child: Review of research* (Vol. 3). Washington, DC: National Association for the Education of Young Children.

Hussey, B. (1988). *Understanding my signals.* Palo Alto, CA: VORT Corporation.

Hutchison, D. (1978). The transdisciplinary approach. In J. Curry and K. Peppe (Eds.), *Mental retardation: Nursing approaches to care*. St. Louis: Mosby.

Korner, A.E. (1987). Preventive intervention with high risk newborns: Theoretical, conceptual, and methodological perspectives. In J. Osofsky (Ed.), *Handbook of infant development*. New York: Wiley.

Linder, T. (1990). *Transdisciplinary play based assessment*. Baltimore: Paul H. Brookes.

Miller, L.J. (1994). Journey to a desirable future: A value-based model of infant and toddler assessment. *Zero to Three, 14*(6), 23–26.

Morris, S.E., and Klein, M.D. (1987). *Pre feeding skills*. San Antonio, TX: Therapy Skill Builders/ Psychological Corporation.

Newacheck, D.W. (1989). Adolescents with special health needs: Prevalence, severity, and access to health services. *Pediatrics, 84*, 872–881.

Orlove, F., and Sobsey, D. (1991). *Educating children with multiple disabilities: A transdisciplinary approach*. Baltimore: Paul H. Brookes.

Ottenbacher. K. (1983). Transdisciplinary service delivery in school environments: Some limitations. *Physical and Occupational Therapy in Pediatrics, 3*, 9.

Parham, L., and Fazzio, I. (1997). *Play in occupational therapy for children*. St. Louis: Mosby.

Rainforth, B., and Salisbury, C. (1988). Functional home programs: A model for therapists. *Topics in Early Childhood Special Education, 7*(4), 33–45.

Safer, N., and Hamilton, J. (1993). Legislative context for early intervention services. In W. Brown, S. Thurman, and L. Pearl (Eds.), *Family-centered early intervention with infants and toddlers: Innovative cross disciplinary approaches* (pp. 1–19). Baltimore: Paul H. Brookes.

Simeonsson, R.J., and Bailey, D.B. (1990). Family dimensions in early intervention. In S.J. Meisels and J.P. Shonkoff (Eds.), *Handbook of early childhood intervention*. Cambridge, MA: Cambridge University Press.

Summers, J., DeOliver, C., Turnbull, A., Benson, H., Santell, E., Campbell, M., and Siegel-Causey, E. (1990). Examining the individualized family service plan process: What are family and practitioner preferences? *Topics in Early Childhood Special Education, 10*, 78–99.

Thompson, T. (1992). For the sake of our children. In T. Thompson and S. Hupp (Eds.), *Saving our children at risk: Poverty and disabilities*. Newburg Park, CA: Sage.

Wallace, H., Biehl, R., MacQueen, J., and Blackman, J. (1997). *Mosby's resource guide to children with disabilities and chronic illness*. St. Louis: Mosby.

Wissow, L. (1988). Poverty, race, and hospitalization for childhood asthma. *American Journal of Public Health, 78*, 777–782.

ADDITIONAL READINGS

American Occupational Therapy Association. (1997). *Occupational therapy services for children and youth under the Individuals with Disabilities Education Act*. Bethesda, MD: American Occupational Therapy Association.

Bashaw, M. (1997). *Children with disabilities* (4th ed.). Baltimore: Paul H. Brookes.

Case-Smith, J., Allen, A., and Pratt, P. (1996). *Occupational therapy for children*. St. Louis: Mosby.

Ensher, G., and Clark, D. (1994). *Newborns at risk: Medical care and psychoeducational intervention*. Gaithersburg, MD: Aspen.

Hanft, B.E. (1989). *Family centered care: An early intervention resource manual*. Rockville, MD: American Occupational Therapy Association.

Krauss, M. (1990). New precedent in family policy: Individualized family service plans. *Exceptional Children, 56*, 388–395.

Parham, L., and Fazzio, I. (1997). *Play in occupational therapy for children*. St. Louis: Mosby.

Semmler, C., and Hunter, J. (1990). *Early occupational therapy intervention*. Gaithersburg, MD: Aspen.

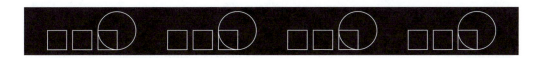

15 CHAPTER

Community-Based Mental Health Services

Marian K. Scheinholtz, MS, OT/L

■ OUTLINE

INTRODUCTION
MENTAL HEALTH DISORDERS
   Historical Aspects Associated with
     Occupational Therapy
   Etiology and Epidemiology
   Terminology
   Symptoms
INTERVENTION
  APPROACHES/MODELS
   Prevention
   Medical Treatment Approaches
   Rehabilitation Approaches

TREATMENT SETTINGS: A
  CONTINUUM OF SERVICES
   Ambulatory Behavioral Health Care
   Vocational Program Settings
   Home Health Services
FUNDING FOR COMMUNITY-BASED
  MENTAL HEALTH PROGRAMS
SPECIALIZED OCCUPATIONAL
  THERAPY ROLES
   Case/Care Management
   Consultation

Ambulatory behavioral health care

Americans with Disabilities Act (ADA)

Case management

Community mental health centers (CMHCs)

Community support program

Consultation

Diagnostic and Statistical Manual of Mental Disorders, Fourth Edition (DSM-IV)

Negative symptoms of schizophrenia

Partial hospitalization program

Positive symptoms of schizophrenia

Program for assertive community treatment (PACT)

Psychiatric rehabilitation

Psychoeducational approach

Psychopharmacology

Psychosocial rehabilitation

Psychotropic medications

Sheltered workshop

Stress-vulnerability model

Supported employment (SE)

Transitional employment (TE)

This chapter is designed to enable the reader to:
- Briefly describe the history of mental health practice as it relates to occupational therapy.
- Discuss the role of occupational therapy in community mental health settings.
- Explain the multidimensional etiology of mental disorders.
- Describe the relevance of the stress-vulnerability model to occupational therapy.
- Explain the principles of ambulatory behavioral health care.
- Describe the PACT approach to mental health rehabilitation.
- Identify opportunities and barriers to successful occupational therapy practice in community mental health settings.
- Discuss the specialized roles occupational therapy practitioners may assume in community mental health care.

 # INTRODUCTION

Occupational therapy had its genesis in the treatment of mental disorders. For patients who were hospitalized, occupational therapy provided activities to engage patients in habits of healthy living and meaningful and culturally relevant occupations, including handicrafts. Work also was used as an occupational therapy medium. With the shift in mental health care to outpatient settings, community-based services are on the rise. Accompanying this rise in services is an increase in the role of occupational therapy in community-based intervention.

This chapter describes the role of occupational therapy in community-based intervention for persons diagnosed with mental disorders, focusing on how occupational therapy practitioners can function within established or emerging service systems. Mental disorders addressed are those illnesses and disorders, other than substance misuse and addictive disorders, defined in the *Diagnostic and Statistical Manual of Mental Disorders, Fourth Edition* (American Psychiatric Association, 1994). The chapter describes program models, treatment approaches, and settings appropriate for occupational therapy practitioners. Embedded in the description of program models, approaches, treatment settings, and practitioner roles are values and beliefs essential to successful community practice in mental health. While many of the principles and mechanisms discussed can be applied to any population, the primary focus is on adults because of the special issues often encountered with children, adolescents, and the elderly. Indirect roles for occupational therapy practitioners and the transdisciplinary nature of community practice also are described.

 # MENTAL HEALTH DISORDERS

Mental health disorders also are called *brain disorders*. The term "brain disorders" has recently been introduced by the National Alliance for the Mentally Ill (NAMI) in an effort to dispel the stigma associated with the term "mental illness" (National Alliance for the Mentally Ill, 1996).

HISTORICAL ASPECTS ASSOCIATED WITH OCCUPATIONAL THERAPY

As part of the "moral treatment" movement, individuals with mental disorders were placed in curative institutions outside the large, crowded industrial areas. Here, occupational therapy consisted of engaging patients in activities that fostered healthy living and meaningful and relevant occupations, including handicrafts. Work, known as "industrial therapy," was also used as an occupational therapy modality. In military hospitals, soldiers were given "jobs" with lessened demands during their recovery. Since that time, most psychiatric occupational therapy services have continued to be delivered primarily in inpatient hospital settings. However, a clear role for occupational therapy exists in community-based services, which is consistent with the shift from a focus on minimizing symptoms to improving functional capability (Jeong, 1998).

Since the mid-1950s, several factors have contributed to the growth of services outside of inpatient settings for persons with psychiatric disorders. The introduction of neuroleptic or antipsychotic medications at that time significantly decreased psychotic symptoms, thus allowing many individuals to lead relatively normal lives outside institutional boundaries. Federal legislation had an even more significant impact on the mental health delivery system in the United States. The Community Mental Health Act and Title V training programs for mental health professionals (psychiatry, psychology, social work, and nursing) established a nationwide system intended to address the nation's mental health problems through a community-based network (Stein and Cutler, 1998). One of the primary purposes of these acts was to address the needs of the most severely ill individuals who were being discharged or diverted from institutional placement. As a result of the Community Mental Health Act of 1963, federally funded **community mental health centers (CMHCs)** were established to provide mental health services in the community as an alternative to state hospitals. However, it became apparent that the services of the CMHCs did not adequately meet the needs of those with serious mental illness (Ellek, 1991).

In the mid-1960s, the passage of the federal entitlement programs Medicare and Medicaid significantly impacted mental health care. These programs provided federal dollars to finance ongoing and fairly unlimited payment for professional services outside state hospitals. However, the state hospitals were primarily dependent on funding from state budgets. These state budgets provided money for payment of the total cost of caring for their institutionalized patients including housing, food, and medical/psychiatric services (L. Mosher, personal communication, 1987). Although both systems shared the burden of providing services to all who accessed them, the limited funding for state hospitals resulted in severe overcrowding and under-staffing. Additionally, the limited funding allowed for little or no follow-up on clients in community systems who were "noncompliant" with services. Community mental health centers were dependent on other agencies to provide aid to their clients who needed housing and social supports. Coordination of care and contact among agen-cies, hospitals, and the community mental health centers was fragmented, leaving many individuals to "fall through the cracks" (Ellek, 1991).

In the intervening years, numerous service models and intervention strategies were developed to address these problems. Many of these programs emerged because of the establishment in 1977 of the **community support program** by the National Institutes of Mental Health. States received funding to set up community-based programs to ad-dress the needs of persons with serious mental disorders who had been deinstitution-alized from state hospitals. Community support programs were designed to prevent rehospitalization by providing appropriate medical, rehabilitation, and support ser-vices in community settings (Stroul, 1984). Several of these community service mod-els, such as the program for assertive community treatment (PACT) in Madison, Wis-consin, and the Fountain House program in New York City, have consistently demonstrated positive outcomes, including decreased hospitalization and increased independence. However, a dearth of cost-effective interventions and support systems continues to exist for a large number of individuals diagnosed with mental health dis-orders in the United States. Many of these individuals are homeless or residents of shelters. As the state hospitals downsize even more, advocates note the sharp increase in the number of individuals in prisons and those who are homeless who have been diagnosed with a mental disorder (Frese, 1998).

While community treatment programs and funding for community treatment have grown during this time, occupational therapy has not necessarily been part of this growth. According to Nielson (1993), occupational therapy practitioners have continued to function primarily in inpatient settings, even while the occupational therapy litera-ture promoted practice in community mental health settings. She described three barri-ers to successful community practice for occupational therapists: (1) the need to assume alternative roles, i.e., from clinician to case manager, program director, or consultant; (2) the need to work in a transdisciplinary model, where professional boundaries and roles are flexible; and (3) the need to understand and influence the sources of power within the established systems. The sources of power exerting significant influence on systems of mental health care currently, and in the future, include the impetus to control costs through managed care, the Americans with Disabilities Act (ADA, 1991), the merging of public and private health-care systems, and the consumer/advocacy movement.

The major reorganization of mental health service systems resulted in interprofes-sional "turf" wars, another factor critically influencing the evolving system of care. An additional barrier to community practice is the reduced financial compensation of community practitioners relative to those in inpatient settings.

ETIOLOGY AND EPIDEMIOLOGY

Current understanding of mental health disorders points to multidimensional etiology (American Psychiatric Association, 1995). Biological factors, particularly genetic pre-disposition to illness and emotional state, have been strongly implicated in the gene-sis of mental disorders. Though no genomes have been identified specifically for psy-chiatric disorders, numerous structural and physiological anomalies have been linked to depression, bipolar disorder, and anxiety disorders. In addition, psychological and social influences, based in the individual's past and present environment, have an important role in producing conditions that precipitate the emergence and ongoing progression of the person's mental health disorder. Total symptom remission, periods of remission and exacerbation, and ongoing occurrence of symptoms varying in intensity may occur (see the stress-vulnerability model later in this chapter).

Epidemiological studies indicate that approximately one out of four persons in the United States experiences a mental health disorder in his or her lifetime. The occurrence of mental disorders in adults in any single year is estimated to be 22.1 percent. Severe mental illness is estimated to affect 2.8 percent of the adult U.S. population, or approximately 5 million adults (American Psychiatric Association, 1995). Approximately one out of 10 individuals experiences disability due to his or her mental disorder. In addition to the individual and family suffering caused by the disorder, the economic impact of both the cost of care and loss of productivity is significant. The cost of mental disorders is estimated to be $150 billion annually (National Institute of Mental Health, 1998). Advocates for parity in coverage of the treatment of mental disorders suggest that appropriately financed intervention and support services could decrease the economic and human costs. A recent study by the Substance Abuse and Mental Health Services Administration (Sing, Hill, Smolkin, and Heiser, 1998) indicated that the cost for parity for mental disorders would be no greater than an additional 3.6 percent of current insurance costs.

Mental health disorders also occur at a significant rate concomitantly with other conditions. Recent studies indicate a significant co-occurrence of substance misuse and mental health disorders, estimated at 50 percent or more. Developmental disabilities and physical disorders, such as traumatic brain injury, rheumatoid arthritis, and chronic pain, also co-occur with mental health disorders. Some therapists have noted the presence of sensory integrative disorders, such as tactile defensiveness or learning disability, in the histories of numerous individuals diagnosed as adults with paranoid schizophrenia and schizoaffective disorder, respectively (Learnard, 1998). In addition, individuals with mental health disorders have shorter life spans, possibly due to poor self-care, self-injury, lower socioeconomic status, and other reasons (Hyman, 2000; Hyman and Rudorfer, 2000). Some practitioners report that many individuals with a primary mental health disorder carry two or more additional diagnoses that may complicate their ongoing care and functional capacity.

TERMINOLOGY

Two major areas of terminology important to understand are the system of terms used to identify mental health disorders and the terminology related to medications. The *Diagnostic and Statistical Manual of Mental Disorders, Fourth Edition* (*DSM-IV*) (American Psychiatric Association, 1994) is the most widely used system for identifying psychiatric disorders in adults and children in the United States. The primary categories included are developmental, personality, psychotic, affective, addictive, anxiety, and organic brain disorders. A client is evaluated on five axes:

- Axis I is the primary psychiatric diagnosis (or diagnoses).
- Axis II identifies personality disorders and mental retardation (if applicable).
- Axis III includes physical and medical conditions.
- Axis IV is the level of environmental stressors experienced by the client.
- Axis V is the client's current level of functioning (American Psychiatric Association, 1994).

Axes IV and V are most relevant to occupational therapy treatment. Often the occupational therapist can be a key contributor in determining the rating of these axes.

Medications used to treat mental health disorders belong to the general drug class known as **psychotropic medications.** The science of their use is called **psychophar-**

macology. Numerous subclasses of psychotropic medications are available. For example, neuroleptic medications, typical or atypical (based on the characteristic response at dopamine receptors in the central nervous system), are usually used to treat psychotic disorders; mood stabilizers or antidepressants are used for treating affective disorders; and tranquilizers, antianxiety agents, and antidepressants are used for anxiety disorders. In many cases, individuals will take a combination of medications to treat their disorders or to control side effects of the primary psychotropic drug. In recent years, some medications not initially developed for treating mental health disorders are now regularly used for treatment. These include some epilepsy, cardiac, and thyroid medications.

SYMPTOMS

Although occupational therapists in community mental health settings may provide services to individuals with a variety of different mental health diagnoses, schizophrenia is probably the diagnosis seen most frequently and therefore deserves specific mention. Symptoms of a few of the other common mental disorders are listed in Table 15–1.

Individuals diagnosed with schizophrenia exhibit symptoms that have been identified as positive or negative (Andreasen and Olsen, 1992). **Positive symptoms of schizophrenia** are those that are present in a person with a mental disorder but are not present in persons who are mentally healthy. They are not part of normal life experiences. Positive symptoms in schizophrenia include delusions, hallucinations, and disorganized speech and/or thoughts. These symptoms have been fairly responsive to neuroleptic medications. However, standard drug treatment may not completely eliminate them and, in some individuals, may actually increase the negative symptoms of this disorder.

Negative symptoms of schizophrenia refer to those characteristics of mental health that are impaired in a person with a mental health disorder. In schizophrenia, negative symptoms may include:

● Affective flattening or blunting
● Alogia (poverty or latency of speech and/or thoughts)
● Avolition or apathy (including poor grooming and hygiene, lack of persistence in occupational roles, and infrequent spontaneous initiation of activities)
● Anhedonia (lack of pleasure)
● Asociality (withdrawal from others)
● Attentional impairment (Andreasen and Olsen, 1992)

These symptoms have been unresponsive to traditional drug therapy. However, new medications, such as clozapine (Clozaril), have been somewhat effective in controlling these symptoms. Occupational therapy intervention directly addresses the impact of negative symptoms on functioning.

While medications may relieve or diminish the symptoms of mental health disorders, many individuals continue to experience less severe residual symptoms, especially in certain environments or at times when they feel stressed. Numerous nonpharmacological interventions are used to address these symptoms and their impact on functioning. These include psychotherapy, counseling, cognitive-behavioral therapy, environmental modification, job coaching, and job accommodations.

Stress-Vulnerability Model

The **stress-vulnerability model** was originally proposed to explain the occurrence of the symptoms of schizophrenia through an understanding of the interaction of environmental "stressors" and personal "vulnerabilities" inherent in individuals diag-

TABLE 15-1

SYMPTOMS OF SELECTED MENTAL DISORDERS

Disorder	Symptoms
Major depressive episode	• Depressed mood • Diminished pleasure in almost all activities • Significant change in body weight • Insomnia or hypersomnia • Psychomotor agitation or retardation • Fatigue or loss of energy • Feelings of worthlessness or excessive guilt • Diminished ability to concentrate or make decisions • Recurrent thoughts of death or suicide
Bipolar disorder	• Chronic fluctuations between major depressive episodes and manic or hypomanic episodes • Manic episodes characterized by grandiosity, decreased need for sleep, talkativeness, flight of ideas, distractibility, psychomotor agitation, spending sprees, and increased sexual behavior • Significant impairment in social and occupational functioning
Obsessive-compulsive disorder	• Obsessions and/or compulsions • Recognition that the obsessions/compulsions are excessive • Obsessions/compulsions cause distress and interfere with normal functioning
Schizoaffective disorder	• Major depressive episode or manic episode concurrent with symptoms of schizophrenia • Delusions and/or hallucinations • Disturbance not due to the effects of a drug • Significant impairment in social and occupational functioning
Posttraumatic stress disorder	• Experience by the person of a traumatic event that threatened his or her physical integrity • Feelings of intense fear and helplessness • Recurrent and distressing thoughts and dreams of the event • Avoidance of stimuli associated with the trauma • Sleep disturbance • Exaggerated startle response • Difficulty concentrating • Irritability and emotional outbursts
Panic disorder	• Recurrent unexpected panic attacks • Persistent concern about having future panic attacks • Changes in behavior as a result of the panic attacks • Anxiety over the consequences of panic attacks • May include agoraphobia (fear of being in places where escape may be difficult or embarrassing)

Source: American Psychiatric Association. (1994). *Diagnostic and statistical manual of mental disorders, fourth edition.* Washington, DC: American Psychiatric Association Press.

nosed with this disorder (Neuchterlein, 1987; Birchwood, Hallet, and Preston, 1989). While originally conceptualized to explain schizophrenia, this model is particularly helpful in understanding the exacerbation and remission of symptoms in individuals with mental health disorders living in a community setting. Episodes of symptom exacerbation are usually accompanied by a decrease in the individual's ability to perform in functional tasks and occupational roles. According to this model, these episodes are prompted by "ordinary" environmental stress in vulnerable individuals (Neuchterlein, 1987). In a vulnerable individual this "ordinary" level of stress can also be responsible for a continuing period of significant symptoms and diminished functioning. An individual's personal vulnerabilities are believed to result from abnormal brain functioning. However, these vulnerabilities may also be linked to other physical illnesses or disorders such as addiction or developmental disability. The degree of intrinsic vulnerability is inversely related to the level of stress that provokes acute episodes of mental disorder (Birchwood et al., 1989).

As an individual becomes more handicapped by the disorder, the clinical condition is further impacted, resulting in deterioration of skills, narrowing of environmental parameters where the individual is able to function, and inability to perform responsibilities of occupational roles. Each relapse directly increases vulnerability and the likelihood of future relapse. Subsequent entry into institutions further isolates the individual and reinforces the life role of patient, increasing dependency, negativity, and hopelessness. Intervention in this cycle occurs through personal and environmental "protectors" that prevent or diminish the intensity of symptom recurrence (Birchwood et al., 1989).

 # INTERVENTION APPROACHES/MODELS

PREVENTION

With the rise in managed care and its focus on keeping consumers well to decrease costs and improve the quality of life, the concepts of prevention and health promotion have received increasing emphasis. While funding for these programs by health insurance companies is still tenuous, some health practices are becoming more a part of the national culture. Laws have established smoke-free environments at many workplaces, shopping areas, and dining establishments and have discouraged driving after consuming alcohol. The American Occupational Therapy Association's (1995) position paper on health promotion and prevention of disease and disability identifies the need to promote health and wellness as "the cornerstone of all therapeutic intervention." Occupational therapy programs addressing prevention have been established in workplace employee assistance programs (Maynard, 1986), in a senior center (Eilenberg, 1986), and within a health maintenance organization (HMO) (E. Cohen-Kaplan, personal communication, 1998). Topics addressed include social interaction, problem solving, physical activity, stress management, couples counseling, and role-strain issues. Prevention programs offer another potential area for occupational therapy involvement in the community.

MEDICAL TREATMENT APPROACHES

The primary medical treatment approach for individuals with mental health disorders is pharmacological intervention. Daily oral medications may be prescribed or the client may require periodic injections of a long-acting formula. Additionally, new medications have been recently introduced and found to be more effective in the treatment of severe types of mental illness, such as schizophrenia and bipolar disorder. These medications have been associated with fewer side effects and have been found to be more effective in controlling symptoms. For example, the atypical antipsychotic medication, clozapine (Clozaril), has had a remarkable effect on individuals with schizophrenia. Although the drug requires monitoring for a rare but potentially fatal side effect, agranulocytosis (low white-blood-cell count that can lead to serious infection), clozapine has enabled many people to live more functional lives, return to school, hold a job, and have satisfying social relationships.

Another important medical approach that takes many different forms in the current treatment environment is psychotherapy. Traditional insight-oriented therapy may be used, but its application is limited due to the duration of treatment needed and the capacity for insight required. With this approach, the person develops insight into his or her current behavior by understanding how past events shaped the behavior and then makes changes based on that insight. Supportive and brief psychotherapy focuses more on current behavior and ways to cope with problems encountered without relying on the development of insight over time. Some techniques in this type of therapy may be more directive, based on the professional's understanding of clients' needs and desires.

Cognitive-behavioral therapy is a special type of psychotherapeutic intervention based on the theory that an individual's feelings, actions, and reactions are based on one's thoughts and perceptions of the world. If these thoughts or perceptions can be challenged or changed, then negative feelings of hopelessness, despair, and poor self-esteem may also be modified.

In the current managed care environment, limits on the number of treatment sessions and demands for functional outcomes are common. The combination of less time for psychotherapy, a greater reliance on medication compliance, and brief crisis intervention responses to mental health disorders has led to a "revolving door" phenomenon where clients are treated, discharged, and often return to treatment after a short time with increased symptoms and decreased functional capacity.

REHABILITATION APPROACHES

Rehabilitation is part of a triad of services that includes *treatment* to lessen the symptoms and impairments of the illness, and emotional *support* and practical *assistance* to sustain a better quality of life, including negotiating complex social and health-care systems. Rehabilitation services are delivered continuously to clients to promote functioning in adult life roles of employment, activities of daily living, and social performance.

Program for Assertive Community Treatment (PACT)

The **program for assertive community treatment (PACT),** also known as the assertive community treatment (ACT) model, is a comprehensive community-based treatment model for persons with severe mental illness. This program began in 1972 in Madison, Wisconsin, during the closing of some state hospital units. One hospital ward's treatment staff moved into the community with their patients, providing intensive treatment, rehabilitation, and support services to clients in their homes, at their jobs, and in social settings (Allness and Knoedler, 1998).

In this approach, a multidisciplinary mental health staff is organized as a type of mobile mental health agency. The members function as a transdisciplinary team, fulfilling their own unique role (e.g., physician, psychiatric nurse, psychologist, occupational therapist, social worker, counselor, and vocational specialist) and taking on other roles to provide seamless, uninterrupted services that are available when and where clients need them. The team is the primary provider of services and the "fixed point of responsibility" for the client.

Based on a comprehensive evaluation, services are highly individualized in intensity. The manner of delivery is based on the individual client's current needs and preferences. PACT services are delivered continuously and over a long term. The occupational therapist contributes to the initial comprehensive evaluation in the areas of occupational and social functioning and to the ongoing assessment of effectiveness of interventions on impaired areas of functioning. As members of the team, occupational therapy practitioners provide rehabilitation services to clients and rehabilitative expertise to the team.

The PACT team assists clients in structuring their time on a day-to-day basis in normal daily activities, rather than referring them to other day-treatment programs or sheltered workshops. Clients are helped to establish a daily plan of what needs to be accomplished and how it is to be done. The PACT team provides support to varying degrees and at varying levels, based on the client's needs and goals. Clients may be seen up to five to seven times per day for a combination of rehabilitation and other services. This includes assistance with employment, personal and instrumental daily living activities, social relationships, and use of leisure time.

Helping clients find and keep a job is central to the PACT model. All clients are involved in the vocational rehabilitation process. Employment-related services are delivered in a community-based setting, emphasizing real jobs. Once employment is attained, the team provides support and assistance to clients and their employers. Rather than disincentives, entitlements are viewed as financial support while the client is preparing for competitive employment.

The methods used by the PACT team in providing rehabilitation services are congruent with occupational therapy theory and values and have been proven to be effective in accomplishing client goals. These methods can be applied in many of the community settings and programs where occupational therapy practitioners work (Box 15–1).

Research on the effect of the PACT program and replication programs have demonstrated effectiveness in producing successful outcomes (Santos, Henggeler, Burns, Arana, and Meisler, 1995). These positive outcomes include significantly fewer hospitalizations and significantly shorter stays for those who are hospitalized, more time employed and more earnings from competitive employment, overall greater time in independent living situations, fewer symptoms and greater satisfaction with life, and modestly increased social functioning. However, studies indicate that when clients are discharged from the program, their gains are not sustained. This seems to indicate a need for ongoing services for persons whose mental impairment is likely to be long term (Allness and Knoedler, 1998).

Psychoeducational Approach

In the **psychoeducational approach,** information about the illness and its management is provided to consumers and families to foster active engagement in the treatment and recovery process, giving them a sense of control over the illness. Bloomer (1978) noted that in addition to a right to information about their illness and a choice of services, consumers have a right to safety and a right to be heard. These rights are consistent with occupational therapy philosophy and facilitate the process of consumer self-determination, resulting in increased self-efficacy and self-esteem (Bloomer, 1978). When used by professionals, psychoeducation is more than merely imparting information. Information that is carefully selected and provided in a manner helpful to the consumer and his or her family is crucial to the success of this approach.

The psychoeducational model for families, developed by Anderson, Hogarty, and Reiss (1980), involves four phases: (1) connection with the family, (2) survival skills workshop, (3) repetition of opportunities to apply and practice these new skills, and (4) continuing family therapy or disengagement. Occupational therapists have uti-

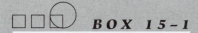 **BOX 15-1**

Occupational Therapy Use of PACT Methods

● *Helping clients establish and maintain normal daily routines.* Clients are assisted in scheduling activities of daily living, employment, and social leisure time activities. The team schedules are developed after the client's schedule is established, based on client's need for assistance to engage in the activities. Clients are then informed as to when to expect to see team members.

● *Lending side-by-side assistance to establish or re-establish adult role activities.* Team members actively participate with the client in planning and carrying out living, working, and social activities. The team member may initially do the bulk of the activity, but service intensity decreases when routines are established and client stamina and ability to concentrate are increased. This is especially important with home maintenance, money management, dealing with social service providers such as public welfare or social security, and structuring leisure time.

● *Modeling (demonstration), rehearsal (practice), coaching (prompts), and feedback.* Strategies are provided individually or in groups with clients and in real-life situations in the community. Feedback from families, roommates, employers, landlords, and others are regularly scheduled with team members to provide valuable information to both the client and the team.

● *Environmental adaptations to meet client needs.* Environmental adaptations are based on assessment of clients and their surroundings to determine when the environment is creating an obstacle to clients' successful performance of life activities. These adaptations may include limiting the length of holiday visits with family when a full-day visit is too long, scheduling frequent breaks during work hours for a client with a short attention span, and helping a client who is experiencing paranoia while riding a bus to work to find housing within walking distance.

lized the psychoeducational model to develop life skills programs. In partial hospitalization (McFadden, 1992) and day treatment (Tomlinson, 1994) programs, consumers receive individual and group instruction on goal setting, stress management, social skills, leisure planning, time management, budgeting, and other instrumental activities of daily living. In some programs, an educational milieu is established. Consumers take the student role in place of the "patient" role and attend classes, do homework, and use educational media. Consumers practice skills learned in classes as homework and report back on successes and failures (Lillie and Armstrong, 1982).

Psychiatric or Psychosocial Rehabilitation

Psychosocial rehabilitation represented an attempt "to apply the principles of physical rehabilitation to mental illness in order to achieve independent functioning in the community" (Cara and MacRae, 1998, p. 556). It was originally a separate approach from psychiatric rehabilitation because it excluded medication management (Cook and Hoffschmidt, 1993). On the other hand, **psychiatric rehabilitation,** based on the medical model, focused on symptom reduction and pathology, offering little hope for improved function. These models merged, integrating a rehabilitation approach with medication management. Currently, the terms psychosocial and psychiatric rehabilitation are used interchangeably (Cara and MacRae, 1998). In this approach, services focus on an extensive evaluation of individual strengths and weaknesses determined from detailed history taking and personal review. Then the individual is assisted in setting personal goals for optimal community function. Community supports are identified and the need for environmental modification is determined. Restoration of skills is desired and can be set as goals. If skills cannot be improved, goals are modified and/or environmental supports are utilized. Practical techniques are used to directly address vocational, social, housing, and recreational areas. Every individual is perceived as having the ability and need to be productive through paid or unpaid employment or another productive social role such as homemaker or volunteer (Anthony and Blanch, 1987).

This model has much in common with the occupational therapy principles that contributed to its development (Munich and Lang, 1993). The similarities include a focus on function rather than intrapsychic processes, the belief that health is achieved through meaningful occupation, and the understanding that change can be effected through "client choice and engaging in activities that promote skill building, exploration, education and community role development" (Jeong, 1998).

Fountain House Model

The Fountain House model is an example of a structured psychosocial rehabilitation approach. Fountain House was founded by a group of patients who had been discharged from a state mental facility during the deinstitutionalization movement. In addition to difficulties with meeting their basic needs for food and shelter, they felt socially isolated and disconnected from the community and meaningful daily activities. Fountain House was founded to try to meet these needs (Beard, Propst, and Malamud, 1975). The philosophy of Fountain House is that all former patients who participate in the program are considered members of the club. They are referred to as "members," which affords rights and privileges as well as expectations. Members are needed and wanted by the club. They are expected to come to the club on a daily basis and to participate in the club's work units at whatever level they are capable. All members are considered capable of being productive and are guaranteed a right to work in paid employment through the club's transitional work program. In this model, being productive and needed is considered extremely important for its regenerative and generative properties. The opportunity to socialize with others and the need to have decent living arrangements are also primary to the philosophy of this model.

Fountain House structures daily occupation into a work unit structure in order to perform necessary club functions, including meal preparation, clerical work, and maintenance of the clubhouse. The Fountain House, or clubhouse, model has been replicated or its concepts incorporated into programs throughout the United States, Canada, and the world. Occupational therapists have been involved in some clubhouse programs (Kavanagh, 1990; Urbaniak, 1995), often focusing on the vocational and prevocational aspects of the program.

In this model, occupational therapy practitioner roles range from clinical to administrative. Clinical roles include member evaluation, usually done in vivo and using naturalistic observation and interview techniques; direct interaction (modeling and coaching) with members in work units or social programs; clinical case management; and development, monitoring, and revision of members' individual service plans with other members of the intervention team. Administrative roles include managing the clubhouse program, supervising staff in the implementation of the service plan, and managing and developing the vocational programs. Work support groups (Kavanagh, 1990), work adjustment training units (W. Starnes, personal communication, 1998), and transitional employment placement management (Urbaniak, 1995) are examples of the vocational programs. The transitional employment concept originated with Fountain House and continues to be used in many clubhouses. Job coaching and other types of supported employment models are also used to expand the range of employment opportunities in clubhouse programs.

 # TREATMENT SETTINGS: A CONTINUUM OF SERVICES

Mental health services have traditionally been provided in a variety of inpatient treatment settings, including the state hospital, acute psychiatric units in general hospitals, and freestanding psychiatric hospitals. More recently, an array of community-based programs has emerged, including ambulatory behavioral health programs, vocational programs, and home health services for persons with mental disorders.

AMBULATORY BEHAVIORAL HEALTH CARE

Ambulatory behavioral health-care services have been described (Kiser, Lefkovitz, Kennedy, and Knight, 1996) as a continuum supported by several underlying principles. These principles include the following:

1. Ambulatory services are designed for people of all ages who do not require 24-hour care but do need psychiatric care that is more intense than can be provided by outpatient visits.
2. A comprehensive evaluation of client needs is performed and a coordinated array of active treatment components are implemented to address them.
3. Services are delivered in a manner that is least disruptive to and/or simulates daily functioning.
4. Community and family are involved in the treatment process.
5. The nature of these services makes them cost effective because they are delivered in the least restrictive environment, with reliance on client strengths, and using existing resources and family/community support systems.

Three levels of ambulatory behavioral health-care services are proposed in this continuum (Kiser et al., 1996).

Level 1

Level 1 is defined as **partial hospitalization programs** and other intensive services, such as home-based crisis intervention or stabilization, which divert the person from hospitalization. As an alternative to the hospital, the goal is to reduce acute symptomatology and provide crisis intervention. Persons at this level exhibit severe symptoms that cause significant functional disability, possibly resulting from an acute illness/episode or the exacerbation of a chronic illness. Services are usually provided on a full-time basis with attendance in a daylong program at least four days per week (National Model Medicare Local Medical Review Policy Committee, 1998) or at least daily contact in the clients' home or community environment. Partial hospitalization programs, which may be attached to a hospital program or a community mental health center, may differ somewhat in the medical staff that is present. However, program intensity, types of clients seen, and staff composition are similar.

Occupational therapy practitioners are often involved in the treatment of clients at this level. Therapy services include evaluation of functioning, especially safety issues, and individually planned therapeutic intervention delivered in both group and individual modes. Intervention is focused on easing symptoms and promoting function in occupational performance. Occupational therapy is specifically listed as a covered service by Medicare in partial hospitalization programs in the *Medicare Intermediary Manual.* Some concerns have been raised about occupational therapy services in this setting (Allen, 1998). However, these concerns seem to be related to the particular clients admitted to the program. That is, in some areas of the country, individuals who are more suited to a long-term, rehabilitative focused program (more like ambulatory level 2 services) have been inappropriately admitted to partial hospitalization programs.

Occupational therapy practitioners play a significant role in partial hospitalization programs due to the extremely short length of stay following client admission and the need for intense aftercare services upon discharge. Occupational therapy practitioners have a long history of treating patients in hospital settings when longer lengths of stay allowed for the stabilization of symptoms and improvement of functioning. Now stabilization and improvement frequently occur while clients are receiving partial hospitalization services.

Level 2

Ambulatory level 2 services are those that have a structured staff-supported milieu and involve active treatment with a rehabilitation or transitional focus. The program extends into the community and client attendance is flexible, based on need. Milieu-based intensive outpatient programs and psychosocial rehabilitation programs are examples of this level. Persons at this level may be functioning adequately in one of their occupational roles, needing moderate to maximum level of support by service providers or family.

Ambulatory level 2 programs include day-treatment or day-care programs, possibly involving clients for extended periods and various types of psychosocial rehabilitation programs. Tomlinson (1994) described a variety of therapeutic interventions used by occupational therapy in a day program. These include extensive assessment to determine functional abilities and needs; setting of realistic expectations based on the assessment; a gradual return to work program; and a milieu providing social interaction and a variety of occupational opportunities. Group programs include those focusing on exercise, social skills development, art, crafts, prevocational counseling, and psychoeducational seminars for clients and families. Informal activities are typically recreational, such as playing ping-pong, using a personal computer, and growing plants in a greenhouse. The focus of the day program is "to frame . . . occupational opportunities as an exploration for the client to rediscover the skills and interests they still have, in spite of the illness process" (Tomlinson, p. 6).

While they do not necessarily have a treatment focus, shelters and programs for homeless persons sometimes provide rehabilitation services. In New York City (Barth, 1994), occupational therapists are involved in a day program that provides treatment and rehabilitation services for homeless persons who have a mental illness. Many of these persons also have an addiction and/or are HIV positive. Client goals focus on developing self-trust and self-responsibility in this program. An assessment by the occupational therapist focuses on the clients' real world and their perception of it. Therapy attempts to help the client achieve mastery in everyday activities by building coping skills and functional capabilities.

An occupational therapist in the state of Washington treats homeless teens and young adults at a program known as "The Working Zone" (Joe, 1998). Funded by the U.S. Department of Housing and Urban Development (HUD), the program's goal is to promote housing stability by improving the client's employability. Many of the youths have learning disabilities, attention deficit disorder, addictions, and other mental health disorders plus a background of trauma or neglect. Although clients receive services by a number of professionals, the occupational therapist works exclusively on employability.

A special program for homeless women was started by the District of Columbia Occupational Therapy Association as part of an effort to address the general public's recognition of the value of occupational therapy. An occupational therapy activity group was started at an existing program that served dinner to the women, many of whom had a history of mental illness and/or substance abuse. The group's purpose was to increase a sense of trust, decrease isolation, increase positive social interaction, practice task and prevocational skills, and have the women transfer the skills learned in the community. Activities chosen had the following characteristics: (1) the activity would take no longer than one or two sessions; (2) performing the activity would provide a success experience; (3) the client would make a usable finished product; and (4) the activity would encourage interaction and appropriate emotional expression. Two occupational therapy practitioners and students from a local occupational therapy school staffed the program.

Other occupational therapy educational programs have used this same concept. Students are placed in environments where an occupational therapy program or an existing mechanism for funding occupational therapy services is not present. Supervision is usually provided by a faculty member. Though the purpose of these endeavors is to provide training for students, in some cases occupational therapy becomes a funded part of the program (M. Scaffa, personal communication, 1997; C. Helfrich, personal communication, 1998).

Level 3

Ambulatory level 3 services are delivered as part of a coordinated treatment plan, but do not necessarily involve structured program activities. These services are less extensive than ambulatory level 2 services but more extensive than outpatient care, involving more hours of intervention, a variety of treatment modalities, and the availability of 24-hour crisis intervention. Clients at this level usually function adequately in at least one occupational role and have family or other community support. Examples include outpatient occupational therapy individually or in groups, outpatient medication management group, and/or case management services in addition to doctor visits and therapy sessions.

VOCATIONAL PROGRAM SETTINGS

Consumers have identified that work is extremely important in the process of recovering from a mental illness and developing the ability to live a normal, satisfying life (Leete, 1989; Deegan, 1988). Work is seen to have a stabilizing effect, reducing the chance of relapse and promoting improved health and well-being.

While occupational therapy practitioners once were actively involved in work adjustment and other prevocational programming, involvement diminished in the 1950s with the adoption of the medical model of diagnosis and treatment (Jeong, 1998). In the past three decades, community treatment and rehabilitation programming for persons with mental disorders have undergone significant development by those outside the field of occupational therapy. Psychiatric or psychosocial rehabilitation, previously described, has been the pioneer in promoting employment and independent living of persons with mental illness (Jeong, 1998).

Place and Train Model

To achieve positive outcomes in vocational programming, a partnership among consumers, families, employers, and vocational and social service providers is necessary (Tryssenar, 1998). Currently, this appears to be best accomplished through a "place and train" model rather than the hierarchical "train and place" model.

The train and place model has been popular for decades in vocational rehabilitation, notably in state-run residential facilities where they may be most familiar to occupational therapy practitioners. In this model, consumers are evaluated, receive rehabilitation services, and then begin vocational training. Following this, the individual is assisted with placement and services end when a job is obtained.

The place and train model, or the "choose, get, and keep" model as it is known in psychiatric rehabilitation, is reversed. The consumer is assessed, focusing on work history, skills and interests, and daily living skills. From this, the consumer selects an area of employment with the assistance of the vocational specialist. Sometimes an on-the-job observational assessment is conducted on a job site in the area of employment chosen by the consumer, often to validate his or her choice and comfort with the job. Skills and skill deficits relative to the job or supporting living skills are noted. Skill deficits are addressed via direct training and/or modifying the physical or social environment. The consumer is then trained on the job directly by the employer with the support of his or her job coach, as appropriate.

A variation of this model has been used by occupational therapists in a community support program. In this program the "train, place, train" model is used. Consumers are involved in a clubhouse day program and a supervised living program. They join the work adjustment training unit if they are interested in employment. In this unit, they undergo an evaluation process during individual and group sessions where they identify goals related to becoming employed. The initial "train" phase includes these sessions where work habits are being developed (W. Starnes, personal communication, 1998).

Volunteer Work

Volunteer work can be used for work adjustment or as a final outcome by establishing a productive life role for a person living with a mental illness. Some clubhouses have group volunteer programs. A successful group volunteer project in one clubhouse where the author was employed involved having members take animals to a local nursing home for regular visits and pet therapy. Members did other activities with the elders including helping with simple craft activities and holiday visits.

Tryssenar (1998) notes the value of the volunteer opportunity as a way for consumers to be "altruistic and contribute to society." Further, consumers can choose their own hours and type of activity. Volunteer job matching, education of the volunteer agency/workplace, and volunteer job accommodations improve the effectiveness of placement. Volunteer work placements throughout the Clinical Center at the National Institutes of Health have been utilized by occupational therapists for many years as "work therapy" for persons with affective disorders, schizophrenia, and Alzheimer's disease.

Sheltered Workshops

Sheltered workshops are protected environments where persons with disabilities are paid for low-skilled, factory-type assembly work. These programs have been criticized for creating dependency and not preparing workers for real-life employment (Stein and Cutler, 1998). Sheltered workshops continue to be part of the spectrum of vocational programs for people with mental illnesses and developmental disabilities. However, many of the remaining programs are in institutional facilities. Those in the community are mostly used for vocational evaluation and as work adjustment training followed by job placement and support.

Consumer-Operated Businesses

Consumer-run businesses are part of many clubhouse programs and allow members to earn salaries of varying amounts. Clubhouse staff facilitate the business by assisting members with community contacts, preparing for work assignments, and performing the actual work as needed. Examples of these types of businesses include hot dog vendor carts, lawn maintenance services, weekly newspaper delivery service, thrift shops, and courier services. Some businesses are run solely by consumers, possibly subsidized by grants and sometimes by contracts with state departments of vocational rehabilitation. In addition, some of these businesses are partnerships with private individuals or corporations. Examples of these include a coffee shop/bakery and a computer-repair business. The role for an occupational therapy practitioner in consumer-run businesses is to develop and monitor work evaluation and work adjustment programs. In addition, the therapist could recommend programmatic or individual job site accommodations.

Transitional Employment (TE)

Transitional employment (TE), developed as part of the Fountain House/clubhouse model, involves the procurement of a job in a normal place of business that pays the prevailing wage and will allow job coaching on the job site. The TE job is shared by several members of the club for a predetermined time period, usually three months. The purpose of TE is to give members an opportunity to practice both their work and social interaction skills on a part-time basis. Because of time limitations, the member does not need to feel "stuck" in an entry-level job. The job belongs to the club, and a member must be willing to give it over to another member when his or her time is completed. Many members complete several TE experiences before going on to their own job.

The club guarantees that someone will do the job even if the member is unable. This is advantageous to the employer, especially if the work is less than desirable. This is one of the ways the clubhouse negotiates jobs with employers. Club members participate in the club's work units to demonstrate that they are ready and able to perform TE. In this way, TE serves as a motivation for club members to participate in the club work units. Occupational therapy practitioners serve as managers of TE and, in this role, learn the job, train members, and provide job coaching, utilizing the skills of task analysis and task and environmental modification (Urbaniak, 1995).

Supported Employment (SE)

Supported employment (SE) began in the field of developmental disabilities. Supportive strategies were developed to assist persons with developmental disabilities to work in places of competitive employment instead of sheltered workshops. Currently, SE is used extensively in the field of psychosocial rehabilitation in clubhouse programs or those providing primarily vocational services.

Following an assessment, the person is matched to a job as described previously. The job coach works with the employer to train the individual to perform the job and makes recommendations for appropriate accommodations. The job coach or agency provides education to employers about mental illness, focusing on the abilities and reliability of workers. The job coach is available to help the employee with difficulties encountered on the job or by supporting daily living functions. The job coach works in conjunction with a case manager or other mental health professional to assist the consumer with recurring symptoms, medication changes, or other issues that might interfere with successful job performance.

Occupational therapy practitioners can play a role in supported employment during the initial evaluation of the consumer, during the job matching process, and in the development of necessary accommodations. While salaries for job coaches are generally modest, this might be an appropriate role for an occupational therapy assistant who would be supervised by an occupational therapist.

Work Support Groups

Work support groups are run in many clubhouses for members on TE or in competitive employment. Similar groups have been held for outpatients after hospital discharge as they are returning to work. These types of groups usually involve discussing the work week, including specific work difficulties and successes. Some clubhouse groups prepare a meal and socialize prior to the discussion of work.

Assessments for Vocational Programming

For any of the vocational program settings described, assessment is important. Occupational therapy assessments suggested by Jeong (1998) for use in this setting include the following:

● Allen's Cognitive Level test to determine cognitive level of functioning, need for supervision and assistance in problem solving, and type of instruction needed
● Jacob's prevocational skills assessment to evaluate basic problem solving, categorizing, and sequencing
● Bay Area Functional Performance Evaluation (BAFPE) social interaction scale to determine difficulties and strengths in interpersonal interaction
● Cognitive Assessment of Minnesota to assess complex problem solving and memory retention

Additional assessments that have proven helpful in vocational treatment include:

● Assessment of Motor and Process Skills (AMPS) to determine status of motor and information-processing skills that underlie the ability to perform activities of daily living and work tasks
● Self-Assessment of Occupational Function
● Occupational history to determine past work and school performance and factors related to success in those endeavors

All of these assessments are cited and described by Asher (1997).

Naturalistic observation of the consumer performing a work task is often the best type of assessment because it can personify the type of demands and stressors of a real job. In a clubhouse program, this can be done in one of the work units. Simulated work tasks have also been used for this purpose. The observation techniques and rating system used in the AMPS are very helpful when observing naturalistic task activity to determine areas of need.

Reasonable Accommodations/Working with Employers

The **Americans with Disabilities Act (ADA)** (1991) guarantees workers the right to reasonable accommodations on the job, provided they can perform its essential functions. The business community is required to comply with the ADA for workers with physical and psychiatric impairments. While the interpretation of the law for persons with psychiatric impairments is extensive, employers still need assistance to understand the appropriate types of accommodations and the limits around which they must comply. Occupational therapy practitioners have worked with employers prior to, and since, the passage of the ADA to address accommodations for persons with physical disabilities. The same opportunity exists for those with psychiatric disabilities.

Advocacy is an integral part of this work, initially to educate employers about the causes and treatment of mental illness, then to dispel the stigma, and finally to help employees succeed. Some specific accommodations include structuring the work environment to eliminate distraction; providing frequent supervision, flexible work hours and breaks, job coaching, and time off for doctor or therapy appointments. Assessing the work environment prior to the client beginning work may be helpful to determine if the job is a good match and if accommodations can be made. For accommodations to occur, the employee must disclose that he or she has a psychiatric disability sometime after being hired. In the past, occupational therapists often assisted consumers to determine how best to answer questions so as not to reveal their illness. Now it is necessary to assist consumers to determine the positive and negative side of disclosure and to know their rights according to the ADA.

HOME HEALTH SERVICES

Occupational therapy practitioners provide home health services to persons with psychiatric disorders following the same general guidelines for services provided to persons with a physical illness. However, psychiatric home health services are less common, especially those utilizing occupational therapy services. Psychiatric home health services are provided to individuals with acute symptomatology, who are unable to leave their homes except for short periods and/or accompanied by a caregiver. Diagnoses include, but are not limited to, major depressive episode, agoraphobia, obsessive-compulsive disorder, schizophrenia, and dementia.

Psychiatric nurses are most commonly the first professionals involved with home-bound clients diagnosed with mental illnesses. The nurses' role is to assess mental status and home safety and to administer and monitor medications. Social workers providing home health care address legal and financial issues, family dynamics, and use of community resources (Earle-Grimes, 1996). The occupational therapy practitioner's primary focus is rehabilitative, a fundamental difference from that of the nurse or social worker. The occupational therapist evaluates the impact of "severe anxiety, immobilizing depression, memory impairments, agoraphobia, impaired judgment, impaired safety awareness and paranoid delusions" on function (Azok and Tomlinson, 1994, p. 1). Occupational therapy intervention focuses on how clients manage daily activities, meet social needs, cope with stress, and resolve problems in daily living (Earle-Grimes, 1996). "The occupational therapy practitioner identifies meaningful and purposeful activities, assesses cognitive functioning, instructs family and caregivers about cognitive deficits, and teaches adaptive techniques for enhancing self-care and home-care management" (Earle-Grimes, 1996). Time management, compensatory strategies for sensory-motor deficits, and community re-entry skills are other areas of therapeutic intervention.

Home treatment allows the professional to observe the actual environment in which consumers perform their daily living activities and make suggestions to improve safety and effective performance. For example, living space may be extremely chaotic and disorganized, leading to frustration and lack of motivation. In addition, home treatment provides direct access to family and caregivers who can significantly impact consumers' ability to function. Therapeutic collaboration with families can result in problem solving and adaptation to make the consumer more independent. Also, the occupational therapy practitioner can model more effective responses and interventions for the family (Azok and Tomlinson, 1994).

Due to the unfamiliarity with psychiatric home care and occupational therapy's role in this area, education of consumers, professionals, and home health agencies may be necessary. Home health care has been a covered benefit for both physical and mental health disorders by Medicare and may be covered by third-party payers and managed-care companies. In addition to education about the service, marketing the viability of such services to third-party payers and managed-care companies may be necessary. Since these payers are focused on cost and quality, demonstration of ways that home health care could decrease costs, such as by returning consumers to work more quickly and possibly avoiding further hospitalization, may be needed.

 ## FUNDING FOR COMMUNITY-BASED MENTAL HEALTH PROGRAMS

Several sources of funding for community mental health programs involving occupational therapy services are available. These include the federal entitlements, Medicare and Medicaid (state directed), private insurance, grant funding, and state block grants.

Partial hospitalization programs (PHPs) are based in hospitals as outpatient services or in community mental health programs. This appears to be the community setting where the largest numbers of occupational therapy practitioners in mental health are employed. Medicare and private insurers pay for these programs. Occupational therapy is specified as an included, but not mandated, service in the Medicare partial hospitalization benefit.

In 2000, PHPs came under a prospective payment system. Unlike the prospective payment system for skilled nursing facilities, there are no categories that account for patient severity. The daily rate is an average of all patients. Occupational therapy is "bundled" into the day rate, which is $208 (Health Care Financing Administration, 1999). The American Occupational Therapy Association, in meetings with the Health Care Financing Administration, has made it clear that this system makes it difficult for occupational therapy to continue as a viable service in PHPs and has suggested potential alternatives.

Community rehabilitation programs usually receive funds from a variety of sources. These include Medicaid, state block grants, and other grant funding. In addition, some receive funds from departments of vocational rehabilitation if they have an approved work adjustment and placement program.

Medicaid funding as to what constitutes required and optional benefits varies from state to state. Many states are now contracting with managed-care companies to manage the Medicaid benefit program. Mental health benefits may be "carved out" and managed by behavioral health-care companies.

Each state receives about 10 percent of its state mental health budget from the federal government through the Substance Abuse and Mental Health Services Agency (SAMHSA). A requirement of this funding is that each state have a mental health advisory planning council which provides input on how the money is spent. The membership of these councils must be comprised of at least 50 percent consumers and their families, with the rest made up of other stakeholders. This is an opportunity for occupational therapy practitioners to be involved at the planning stage and possibly influence the inclusion of occupational therapy in more community programs.

 # SPECIALIZED OCCUPATIONAL THERAPY ROLES

A variety of community practice occupational therapy roles, both direct and indirect, have been described in previous sections. The therapist may provide evaluation and treatment services directly to consumers, serve as a program or project manager, or be a member of a transdisciplinary community treatment team. Training and supervision of paraprofessional and professional staff are other roles. As a team member, the occupational therapy practitioner may have a traditional role as primarily a rehabilitation service provider or possibly serve in a variety of specialized roles (Table 15–2).

In the following section, some special roles for occupational therapy practitioners are described. These roles are found in the growing practice of case management and the role of the independent practitioner providing community consultation.

CASE/CARE MANAGEMENT

Several different models of **case management** currently are being used in mental health. One involves primarily an administrative role in which the case manager serves as a broker responsible for coordinating all aspects of a client's care. This type of case management is common in managed-care systems where the purpose is to contain costs and assure delivery of appropriate services while maintaining quality care (Cottrell, 1998).

TABLE 15-2

OCCUPATIONAL THERAPY ROLES IN COMMUNITY MENTAL HEALTH

Roles	Functions
Direct service provider	Evaluate the client. Analyze job site and residence. Intervene with client, employer, and housing staff.
Consultant	Assess problem situations. Develop plan of correction (with staff input). Train staff. Design environments/programs.
Supervisor	Train and oversee staff. Develop and review treatment plans and progress updates. Guide staff problem solving and "troubleshoot." Train students. Evaluate staff. Contribute to budget and program development.
Program manager	Provide day-to-day program direction. Assume overall budget responsibility. Supervise midlevel staff. Participate in grant development. Participate in program development. Perform public relations.
Case manager	Coordinate client's service delivery. Collaborate with other community providers. Manage entitlements. Interact with families and significant others regarding client's services.

Another model is clinical case management. In this model, the case manager addresses the overall maintenance of each individual's physical survival and personal growth. This encompasses both his or her recovery and adaptation to the mental illness and participation in community life (Kanter, 1989). While the primary role of the case manager is to ensure access to community services and resources, he or she also assists in the development of independent living skills such as money management, social interaction, and cognitive skills (e.g., decision making and problem solving) to varying degrees.

Cooper (1998, p. 580) notes the following characteristics common to clinical case management in mental health:

1. Services are provided in vivo.
2. Goals are to reduce hospitalization, maintain the client in the least restrictive community setting possible, and maintain quality of life.
3. A team or an individual . . . serves as a fixed point of responsibility.
4. Service is of unlimited duration.
5. Service will provide continuity of care over time and across referral agencies.

While not a distinct case management service, advocacy is frequently part of accessing services and resources.

Much of the training and skills of occupational therapy practitioners are applicable to case management. A holistic approach to healthy living, the ability to assess underlying components of skills and performance contexts, an emphasis on daily living, and a focus on functional outcomes are skills and perspectives of occupational therapy consistent with community case management. Occupational therapy practitioners can be especially effective in this role through their understanding of the impact of clients' functional deficits on their ability to use community services. Based on the findings of a functional assessment, the practitioner can modify the service and assist the client in using it. In addition, the occupational therapist may make recommendations to existing programs or services to modify their structures in order to better accommodate the clients who use them (Moeller, 1991). Unlike the hospital or even community rehabilitation setting, case management focuses on assisting the client in gaining the basic life necessities, managing their mental illness, and participating in community life. The generalist approach helps the client solve practical day-to-day problems.

CONSULTATION

Consultation involves providing information and expert advice regarding program development and evaluation, supervisory models, organizational issues, and/or clinical concerns. A model of a successful consultative occupational therapy community practice exists in Maine, where the focus is on evaluation and direct service to clients referred by various local and state agencies (Learnard, 1998). This practice will be described to illustrate the occupational therapy role of consultant.

Persons with mental health disorders are referred by agencies such as adult protective services, state departments of mental health and public welfare, and local school systems. They are sometimes referred for a specific reason, such as community placement from state facilities, but often they are seen by the occupational therapist because they are "somebody's problem" (Learnard, 1998). Services are financed by the referring agency and are provided upon request, although several of the agencies purchase a day of services weekly or monthly. In addition to individual service, consultation has also included designing a community residence for a group of individuals who had been hospitalized in a state facility for many years.

The philosophy of this consultative service is crucial to its success in the community. The practice combines the art and science of occupational therapy to achieve effectiveness (Robnett, 1998). This includes the science of function that is unique to occupational therapy, the understanding of environmental context and its impact on functional performance, and the ability to analyze tasks and activities.

The art of practice starts with offering the client a sense of positive hopefulness built on a relationship of mutual respect and trust. Hopefulness is fostered when the professional accepts the person exactly as he or she is; listens to his or her story, dreams, and needs; and finds in the person something he or she does or did well. The client's future is built on these current and past abilities. While the person may have been referred by an agency that has its own priorities, the occupational therapy practitioner must attend to the needs and desires of the person and envision possibilities of a future based on those desires. This involves truly accepting the person for what he or she is, not for what the practitioner wishes the person to be. The professional must visualize hope, not barriers, and anticipate future function and possibilities. He or she also must envision an environment that would support and enable that functioning (Robnett, 1998).

In this practice, each person served is seen as a citizen of the community and as an individual. Services are arranged or designed specifically for that individual. According to Robnett (1998, p. 33), the occupational therapy practitioner's job is "to create circles of support that will facilitate a functional environment for that person . . .

(the circles) can and should include a vast array of people and resources . . . friends, family, neighbors, religious leaders, and the shopkeeper down the street, as well as . . . traditional team members."

Community rehabilitation is more than simply "treating a client." It involves:

● Understanding the person's current ability to perform necessary tasks
● Analyzing the skills needed to perform those tasks
● Adapting the environment to promote the highest level of function
● Identifying supports to provide assistance that they cannot or do not wish to provide for themselves and if desired by the person
● Developing strategies and methods to build skills

These core beliefs, values, and technical skills have contributed to the success of this occupational therapy consultation practice.

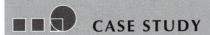 **CASE STUDY**

JAMES

James is a 26-year-old male diagnosed with schizoaffective disorder. He first experienced symptoms at age 13 and dropped out of school in the 10th grade. He was admitted to the Walnut Creek Community Rehabilitation Program one month after discharge from an eight-day inpatient hospitalization at the Walnut Creek Memorial Hospital for exacerbation of symptoms and suicidality. James has been hospitalized six times since he was first diagnosed. He lives in a group home and receives SSI and Medicaid. James' family, his mother and two brothers, live in the same community. His mother is unemployed. His older brother is a postal worker and his younger brother attends community college. James has used marijuana, alcohol, and crack cocaine in the past but has been sober since his discharge.

James is currently seen by a psychiatrist at the Walnut Creek Community Mental Health Center and was prescribed olanzapine (Zyprexa) and paroxetine (Paxil). He experiences mild side effects from these medications. James has had difficulty in the past remaining on his medication, but he does not want to receive injectable medication due to the side effects.

The Walnut Creek Program. The Walnut Creek Community Rehabilitation Program operates under the clubhouse model, consisting of a supervised apartment program, a day program, and an employment program. It also has an assertive community treatment team. An occupational therapist provides consultation to all the programs. She supervises three certified occupational therapy assistants (COTAs) who work in the employment program, the day program, and the apartment program, respectively. The COTAs are responsible for case management, program development, and program implementation. They assist in assessment of clients through naturalistic observation and completion of paper and pencil assessments such as the role checklist, activities configuration, and self-assessment of living skills (developed by Walnut Creek clients). The occupational therapist develops treatment plans cooperatively with the client and other members of the treatment team, including direct service workers, psychiatric nurse, social worker, and psychiatrist.

The day program follows the clubhouse model, with a food unit, clerical unit, maintenance unit, and outreach unit. Peer counselors run an evening and weekend social program, consisting of a drop-in center and scheduled small-group activities in the community. The program also has an arrangement for its members to join the local YMCA at a significantly reduced cost.

Evaluation. James states that his goals are to find a job and live in his own apartment. He has worked sporadically as a dishwasher but has lost employment due to absences and an inability to complete his shifts. He last worked 18 months ago. James reports he did not like dishwashing due to the long hours standing, bending, and lifting. Also, he sometimes heard voices that disturbed him while he was working. His reading and math skills, at a third-grade level, have limited his past employment. James briefly received vocational rehabilitation services, but these were discontinued shortly after starting because he did not keep appointments.

James' grandmother lived with his family while he was growing up, and she taught him basic cooking and baking skills. He retains these skills but cannot follow written recipes or directions due to his limited reading skills.

James likes to play basketball and shoot pool, and he enjoys socializing with others when his symptoms are "not bothering" him. James has no gross- or fine-motor or perceptual problems that impair his functioning. He can attend to moderately complex tasks for 15 minutes. He has difficulty resolving novel problems and sometimes asks for help from a supervisor. He can follow one- to two-step directions.

James is independent in his self-care, is neatly groomed, and dresses appropriately. He reports that his grooming deteriorates when his symptoms increase. He can do his own laundry and perform simple home maintenance tasks (e.g., dishwashing, vacuuming, dusting, changing light bulbs, etc.). James can make change and use money for commerce. He has no budgeting skills and has never had a checking or savings account. The group home operator gives James $25 per week from which he buys cigarettes, toiletries, and clothing. He often runs out of money before the end of the week.

Prior to starting at Walnut Creek, James was sleeping 12 hours per day. He spent most of his remaining time watching television with short trips into the community to buy coffee and cigarettes. His mother has been to visit him twice since his discharge, and he reports she is supportive and helpful to him.

Intervention. After one week of orientation in the clubhouse, James met with the occupational therapist to develop his plan. He indicated that he would like to become involved in the vocational program that meets half days, twice weekly for discussions, goal setting and review, and role plays of work situations. To develop tolerance for work, he decided to participate in the clubhouse food unit on the alternating three days. Though he would like to join the YMCA to improve his stamina and lose weight, James feels anxious about going there alone. He decided to participate in the clubhouse leisure program first.

The therapist believes that James has potential for working if a good job match can be made, his work tolerance improves, and he can remain sober and take his medication regularly. She suggests that he use a pillbox and have the boarding home operator supervise him filling it each week. She will further assess his reading and math skills and will set up a program for him to improve these skills. An occupational therapy student intern will carry out this program individually with James under the supervision of the therapist. The program will also address budgeting his spending money.

The therapist will also advocate for James with the vocational rehabilitation department to reopen his case. They have additional services to improve literacy, and the occupational therapist believes James may benefit from further training in food services as a potential for employment in the future.

 ## CONCLUSION

Future roles for occupational therapy practitioners in community mental health may be rooted in current trends. The development of new roles for occupational therapy will be dependent on the demand of the marketplace, consumer advocacy, and the marketing of the profession to the public. Two initiatives undertaken by the American Occupational Therapy Association in 1997 to 1998, the National Awareness Campaign and the Mental Health Partnership Project (Joe, 1998), may have an impact. The National Awareness Campaign is a public relations campaign designed to increase public awareness of occupational therapy with the message "occupational therapy: skills for the job of living." In its first year, the campaign significantly increased the number of consumer calls received by the association. The Mental Health Partnership Project is a grassroots effort to encourage occupational therapy practitioners to collaborate with consumer, advocacy, and other mental health associations and organizations to address issues of mutual interest. In some states, this may involve becoming allies in the effort to pass mental health parity legislation. In other states, occupational therapy may have the opportunity to have a voice in the redesign of state-supported mental health services as the Medicaid program comes under managed care. These efforts are crucial, as are the efforts of university faculty who are introducing occupational therapy to the community via student fieldwork placements.

As these activities progress, occupational therapy may find an expanded role in community mental health, where the skills, values, and purpose of the profession can be used. Through this process, mental health consumers can be assisted in their recovery process to have more satisfying and productive lives (Frese, 1998).

 ## STUDY QUESTIONS

1. Describe three strategies to increase the participation of occupational therapy practitioners in community mental health settings.
2. Discuss how legislation has impacted community mental health services.
3. Explain how vulnerability to stress impacts functional performance and the development and progression of mental illness.
4. Explain the four methods of rehabilitation used in the PACT model.
5. Identify the levels of ambulatory behavioral health care, describing the role of occupational therapy practitioners at each level.
6. Describe the four phases of the psychoeducational approach to rehabilitation.
7. Identify mental health programs in your community that do not currently employ occupational therapy practitioners and investigate the reasons why occupational therapy is not utilized in these settings.

REFERENCES

Allen, C.K. (1998, April). *Teaching the Allen cognitive levels and diagnostic module.* Institute presented at the American Occupational Therapy Association Annual Conference, Baltimore, MD.

Allness, D.J., and Knoedler, W.H. (1998). *The PACT model of community-based treatment for persons with severe and persistent mental illnesses: A manual for PACT start-up.* Arlington, VA: National Alliance for the Mentally Ill.

American Occupational Therapy Association. Commission on Practice. (1995). *Occupational therapy in the promotion of health and the prevention of disease and disability (position paper).* Rockville, MD: American Occupational Therapy Association.

American Psychiatric Association. (1994). *Diagnostic and statistical manual of mental disorders, fourth edition.* Washington, DC: American Psychiatric Association Press.

American Psychiatric Association. (1995). *Mental illness awareness guide for decision makers.* Washington, DC: American Psychiatric Association Press.

Americans with Disabilities Act (ADA) of 1990, P.L. 101-336, §2,104 Stat. 328 (1991).

Anderson, C.M., Hogarty, G.E., and Reiss, D.J. (1980). *Schizophrenia and the family.* New York: Guilford.

Andreasen, N.C., and Olsen, S. (1992). Negative versus positive schizophrenia: Definition and validation. *Archives of General Psychiatry, 39,* 789–794.

Anthony, W.A., and Blanch, A. (1987). Supported employment for persons who are psychiatrically disabled: A historical and conceptual perspective. *Psychosocial Rehabilitation Journal, 11*(2), 5–23.

Asher, I.E. (1997). *Occupational therapy assessment tools: An annotated index* (2nd ed.). Bethesda, MD: American Occupational Therapy Association.

Azok, S.D., and Tomlinson, J. (1994). Occupational therapy in a multidisciplinary psychiatric home health care service. *Mental Health Special Interest Newsletter, 17*(2), 1–3.

Barth, T. (1994). Occupational therapy interventions at a shelter for homeless, addicted adults with mental illness. *Mental Health Special Interest Newsletter, 17*(1), 7–8.

Beard, J.H., Propst, R.N., and Malamud, T.J. (1975). The Fountain House model of psychosocial rehabilitation. *Schizophrenia Bulletin, 13,* 131–147.

Birchwood, M.J., Hallet, S.E., and Preston, M.C. (1989). *Schizophrenia: An integrated approach to research and treatment.* New York: New York University Press.

Bloomer, J.S. (1978). The consumer of therapy in mental health. *American Journal of Occupational Therapy, 32,* 621–627.

Cara, E., and MacRae, A. (1998). *Psychosocial occupational therapy: A clinical practice.* Albany, NY: Delmar.

Cook, J.A., and Hoffschmidt, S.J. (1993). Comprehensive models of psychosocial rehabilitation. In R.W. Flexor and P.L. Solomon (Eds.), *Psychiatric rehabilitation in practice.* Boston: Andover.

Cooper, N. (1998). Case management. In E. Cara and A. MacRae (Eds.), *Psychosocial occupational therapy: A clinical practice.* Albany, NY: Delmar.

Cottrell, R. (1998). *Mental health case management: Developing OT's competency for expanding clinical roles.* Unpublished paper.

Deegan, P. (1988). Recovery: The lived experience of rehabilitation. *Psychosocial Rehabilitation Journal, 11,* 11–19.

Earle-Grimes, G. (1996). Psychiatric home health care: New horizons for occupational therapy. *Mental Health Special Interest Newsletter, 17*(2), 3–4.

Eilenberg, A.O. (1986). An expanded community role for occupational therapy: Preventing depression. *Physical and Occupational Therapy in Geriatrics, 5,* 47–57.

Ellek, D. (1991). The evolution of fairness in mental health policy. *American Journal of Occupational Therapy, 45,* 947–951.

Frese, F.J. (1998). Occupational therapy and mental illness—a personal view. *Mental Health Special Interest Section Quarterly,* September.

Health Care Financing Administration. (December, 1999). *HCFA Medicare hospital manual. Transmittal 747.* Washington, DC: U.S. Government Printing Office.

Hyman, S.E. (2000). Schizophrenia. In D.C. Dale and D.D. Federman (Eds.), *Scientific American medicine* (Section VII, pp. 1–5). New York: Healtheon.

Hyman, S.E., and Rudorfer, M.V. (2000). Depressive and bipolar mood disorders. In D.C. Dale and D.D. Federman (Eds.), *Scientific American medicine* (Section II, pp. 1–19). New York: Healtheon.

Jeong, G. (1998). Vocational programming. In E. Cara and A. MacRae (Eds.), *Psychosocial occupational therapy: A clinical practice.* Albany, NY: Delmar.

Joe, B.E. (1998). Joining hands on mental health. *OT Week, 12*(23), 12–13, June 4.

Kanter, J. (1989). Clinical case management: Definition, principles, components. *Hospital and Community Psychiatry, 40,* 361–368.

Kavanagh, M.R. (1990). Way station: A model community support program for persons with serious mental illness. *Mental Health Special Interest Newsletter, 13*(1), 6–8.

Kiser, L.J., Lefkovitz, P.M., Kennedy, L.L., and Knight, M. (1996). *The continuum of ambulatory behavioral healthcare services.* Alexandria, VA: Association for Ambulatory Behavioral Healthcare.

Learnard, L. (1998, April). *Payment and programming in behavioral health care.* Short course presented at the American Occupational Therapy Association Annual Conference, Baltimore, MD.

Leete, E. (1989). How I perceive and manage my illness. *Schizophrenia Bulletin, 15,* 197–200.

Lillie, M.D., and Armstrong, H.E. (1982). Contributions to the development of psychoeducational approaches to mental health service. *American Journal of Occupational Therapy, 36,* 438–443.

Maynard, M. (1986). Health promotion through employee assistance programs: A role for occupational therapists. *American Journal of Occupational Therapy, 40,* 771–776.

McFadden, R.S. (1992). *Learning for life: A guide to the design and delivery of psychoeducational groups.* Unpublished manuscript.

Moeller, P. (1991). The occupational therapist as case manager in community mental health. *Mental Health Special Interest Newsletter, 14*(2), 4–5.

Munich, R., and Lang, E. (1993). The boundaries of psychiatric rehabilitation. *Hospital and Community Psychiatry, 44,* 661–665.

National Alliance for the Mentally Ill. (1996). *Mental illnesses are brain disorders: What everybody needs to know.* (Pamphlet). Arlington, VA: National Alliance for the Mentally Ill.

National Institute of Mental Health. (1998). *Mental illness in America: The NIMH Agenda.* National Institute of Mental Health Online at *www.nimh.gov*

Neuchterlein, K.H. (1987). Vulnerability models for schizophrenia: State of the art. In J. Haffner, W.F. Gattaz, and W. Janzarik (Eds.), *Search for the causes of schizophrenia.* Heidelberg: Springer-Verlag.

Nielson, C. (1993). Occupational therapy and community mental health: A new and unprecedented turn. *Mental Health Special Interest Newsletter, 16*(3), 1–2.

Robnett, R. (1998). Paradigms of community practice. *OT Practice, 2*(5), 30–35.

Santos, A.B., Henggeler, S.W., Burns, B.J., Arana, G.W., and Meisler, N. (1995). Research on field based services: Models for reform in the delivery of mental health care to populations with complex clinical problems. *American Journal of Psychiatry, 152,* 1111–1123.

Sing, M., Hill, S., Smolkin, S., and Heiser, N. (1998). *The costs and effects of parity for mental health and substance abuse insurance benefits.* Rockville, MD: Substance Abuse and Mental Health Services Administration, U.S. Department of Health and Human Services.

Stein, F., and Cutler, S.K. (1998). *Psychosocial occupational therapy: A holistic approach.* San Diego: Singular Publishing Group.

Stroul, B. (1984). *Toward community support systems for the mentally disabled.* Rockville, MD: National Institute of Mental Health.

Tomlinson, J. (1994). The dimensions of occupational therapy in day programs. *Mental Health Special Interest Newsletter, 17*(1), 5–6.

Tryssenar, J. (1998). Vocational exploration and employment and psychosocial disabilities. In F. Stein and S.K. Cutler (Eds.), *Psychosocial occupational therapy: A holistic approach.* San Diego: Singular Publishing Group.

Urbaniak, M.A. (1995). Yahara House: A community-based program using the Fountain House model. *Mental Health Special Interest Newsletter, 18*(1), 1–3.

ADDITIONAL READINGS

Adams, R. (1990). The role of occupational therapists in community mental health. *Mental Health Special Interest Newsletter, 13*(1), 1–2.

Adams, R. (1992). GROW: An occupational therapist's experience with a peer support program. *Mental Health Special Interest Newsletter, 15*(2), 3–4.

Baxley, S. (1994). Options for community practice: The Springfield Hospital model. *Mental Health Special Interest Newsletter, 17*(1), 3–5.

Del Vecchio, A.L., and Kearney, P.C. (1990). Homeless women's dinner program: Adapting traditional interventions to a nontraditional environment. *Mental Health Special Interest Newsletter, 13*(1), 2–4.

Equal Employment Opportunities Commission. (1997, March 25). *EEOC enforcement guidance on the Americans with Disabilities Act and psychiatric disabilities.* 915.002.

Farabaugh, S. (1994). Occupational therapy opportunities at a community mental health center. *Mental Health Special Interest Newsletter, 17*(4), 3–4.

Jaffe, E. (1981). The role of the occupational therapist as a community consultant: Primary prevention in mental health programming. *Occupational Therapy in Mental Health, 1*(2), 47–62.

Klugheit, M. (1994). An appreciation for the role of occupational therapy in community mental health treatment. *Mental Health Special Interest Newsletter, 17*(1), 1–3.

Merryman, M.B., and Kannenberg, K. (1994). Occupational therapy for individuals with serious mental illness. *Continuum, 1*(3), 153–162.

Tomlinson, J.L. (1992). Joining consumerism through a psychoeducational approach. *Mental Health Special Interest Newsletter, 15*(2), 1–3.

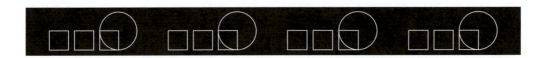

16
CHAPTER

Community-Based Approaches for Substance Use Disorders

Penelope A. Moyers, EdD, OTR, FAOTA
Virginia C. Stoffel, MS, OTR, FAOTA

■ OUTLINE

Brief interventions
Compulsive drug-taking behavior
Crisis intervention
Formal intervention programs
Occupational alienation
Occupational deprivation
Prevention

Problem drinking
Self-help programs
Stages of change
Substance abuse
Substance dependence
Tolerance
Withdrawal

LEARNING OBJECTIVES

This chapter is designed to enable the reader to:
- Define basic concepts of addiction.
- Describe the impact of substance use disorders on the community.
- Discuss the effects of substance use disorders on occupational behavior.
- Describe the stages of change, including precontemplation, contemplation, determination, action, maintenance, and relapse.
- Describe a variety of types of community-based interventions for substance use disorders.
- Identify the role of occupational therapy in community-based programs for substance use disorders.

 ## INTRODUCTION

With the advent of managed care, most intervention for substance use disorders occurs in outpatient settings (Pollack, 1996) and is typically short in duration. Strong financial pressures are being exerted to determine the most economical and most efficacious ways of delivering intervention for clients with substance use disorders (Finney and Monahan, 1996). To examine the issue of providing economical and efficacious intervention, characteristics of intervention other than just duration must be considered. Duration of intervention, or the total length of treatment, receives much attention from third-party payers due to its apparent relationship to cost. However, this relationship certainly is not as simple as it seems. Instead, the relationship between cost and duration is complicated by the factors of:

- Intervention modality (e.g., cognitive-behavioral or 12-step program)
- Intensity (e.g., frequency of intervention)
- Format (e.g., group vs. individual)
- Setting (e.g., outpatient office vs. outpatient treatment center)
- Therapist qualifications (e.g., alcohol and drug counselor or occupational therapy practitioner)
- Intervention goals (e.g., abstinence vs. moderation) (Miller and Cooney, 1994)

This chapter supplies the reader with a foundation for providing economical and effective community-based intervention unique to occupational therapy, but one that effectively complements the work of psychology, social work, nursing, medicine, and counseling. This chapter reviews the idea of problem drinking and the concepts of addictive behavior by defining diagnostic terminology. The extent of substance use in communities is examined, noting the drug use trends that have recently developed. The impact of substance use disorders on the community are

319

discussed in terms of violence, crime, unemployment, health-care costs, and family abuse and neglect.

This chapter also examines the influence of substance use disorders on occupational performance, specifically focusing on occupational alienation, occupational deprivation, and habit dysfunction. **Occupational alienation** is the sense of isolation or estrangement a person experiences as a result of engagement in occupations that are not personally meaningful and fulfilling (Wilcock, 1998). **Occupational deprivation** refers to circumstances beyond the person's control that result in limited occupational choices (Wilcock, 1998). The client can be taught to abandon the negative cycle of occupational alienation and deprivation, replacing it by entering the stages of positive change and recovery. Community intervention programs are described, highlighting the relationship between the outcomes of these programs with the progression through the stages of change. The potential contributions of occupational therapy to these community programs through lifestyle redesign and environmental modification to better support recovery behaviors are reviewed.

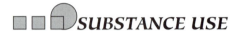 *SUBSTANCE USE*

The *Diagnostic and Statistical Manual of Mental Disorders, Fourth Edition* (*DSM IV*) (American Psychiatric Association, 1994) defines various substance-related disorders according to groups of substances or 11 classes of drugs. These include: (1) alcohol, (2) amphetamines, (3) caffeine, (4) cannabis, (5) cocaine, (6) hallucinogens, (7) inhalants, (8) nicotine, (9) opioids, (10) phencyclidine (PCP), and (11) sedatives.

DISORDERS

The substance use disorders include substance dependence and substance abuse. Substance dependence and abuse can be applied to every class of substance, with some exceptions. Therefore, the characteristics of these two diagnoses are similar across the various drug classes. However, saliency of a symptom may vary, and some symptoms are not present in a given drug class. Some symptoms are more or less pronounced, depending on the drug involved. For example, withdrawal symptoms are not typically present for hallucinogen dependence.

Substance Dependence

The chief feature of **substance dependence** is that "despite significant substance-related problems, the individual continues use of the substance . . . with a pattern of repeated self-administration that usually results in tolerance, withdrawal, and compulsive drug-taking behavior" (American Psychiatric Association, 1994, p. 176). **Tolerance** can be observed when increasing amounts of the substance are ingested to achieve the desired effect or when, with the same amount, less or little effect on the individual occurs. Tolerance does not necessarily develop across all classes of substances; however, it is fairly common in alcohol, narcotic, and tobacco use. **Withdrawal** is "a maladaptive behavioral change, with physiological and cognitive concomitants, that occurs when blood or tissue concentrations of a substance decline in an individual who had maintained prolonged heavy use of the substance" (American Psychiatric Association, p. 178). To avoid withdrawal, the person with substance dependence might ingest more of the substance. **Compulsive drug-taking behavior** typically includes the following:

1. Drinking or using the substance for a longer time period or in greater quantity than originally planned

2. Having difficulty cutting down on use of the substance
3. Organizing one's life around seeking the drug
4. Obtaining and being under the influence of the substance
5. Giving up or reducing important social and recreational activities

Additionally, the individual continues to use the substance despite having recurrent physical or psychological problems caused or exacerbated by the substance. Should an individual have three or more of these symptoms within a period of one month, substance dependence would be diagnosed. It is possible to have this diagnosis without the presence of withdrawal and tolerance. If these two particular symptoms are present, the diagnosis of dependence is modified to include a physiological dependence specifier.

Substance Abuse

Substance abuse is identified as "a maladaptive pattern of substance use manifested by recurrent and significant adverse consequences related to the repeated use of substances, such as failure to fulfill major role obligations at work, school or home" (American Psychiatric Association, 1994, p. 182). Occupational therapists are in an excellent position to evaluate occupational roles and to detect the impact that substances may have on an individual's performance. In addition to role performance problems, taking physical risks, such as driving a car while under the influence of a substance, incurring repeated legal problems related to substance use, or displaying social and interpersonal problems as the result of intoxication, are behaviors that contribute to the diagnosis of substance abuse. Only one of these symptoms need be present in the last year to meet this diagnostic category. The person, though, must never have been diagnosed in the past with substance dependence.

Problem Drinking

Epidemiological data suggest that within the general population, many more problem drinkers exist than those classified as having a substance use disorder (Hester, 1995). In the past, this population of problem drinkers was largely ignored. Only recently have professionals made an effort to provide these individuals with help in modifying their problem drinking. **Problem drinking** is the use of alcohol that is clearly above the norm (Doweiko, 1993). At this level of use, friends and relatives may express concerns about the person's drinking, and the drinking may begin to interfere with social relationships, financial affairs, and job performance. Problem drinking is differentiated from substance abuse by the significance of adverse consequences sustained while drinking. For instance, problem drinkers experience less severe role disruptions, take only minimal physical risks, and have fewer legal and social problems. However, close friends or family may notice beginning problems in controlling the use of alcohol, and the individual may be concerned about the effect of using alcohol on his or her behavior.

Intervention targeted toward the problem drinker often focuses on drinking in moderation instead of on abstinence. Drinking in moderation may be an intervention goal important for attracting a broader range of drinkers with alcohol problems. People who are successful in moderating their drinking eventually shift their behavior to abstinence (Hester, 1995). Inability to achieve this goal, however, may mean that the person is really misdiagnosed as a problem drinker and would benefit from intervention targeted to his or her substance use disorder. Even though unsuccessful in moderating drinking, the therapist has most likely established a relationship with the person and may influence the individual to take the next step in treatment. To offer only one treatment alternative in the form of abstinence may inadvertently turn away a large population in need of services.

EXTENT OF USE

Alcohol

In 1992, more than 7 percent, or nearly 13.8 million people, in the United States aged 18 years and older had problems with drinking. Of that number, 8.1 million people were considered alcohol dependent. Almost three times as many men (9.8 million) as women (3.9 million) had problems with alcohol. Prevalence of problems with alcohol was highest for both sexes in the 18-to-29-year-old age group (National Institute on Alcohol Abuse and Alcoholism, 1994, pp. 243, 245). About 64 percent of high school seniors report that they have been drunk on several occasions, and more than 31 percent of these students say that they have had five or more drinks in a row during a two-week period (Johnston, O'Malley, and Bachman, 1997). Approximately 43 percent, or 76 million people, in the United States have been exposed to alcohol in the family. This exposure occurs by growing up in an alcoholic home, by marrying a person with alcohol problems, or by having a blood relative with alcohol problems (National Center For Health Statistics, 1991, p. 1).

Drugs

According to the preliminary results of the 1999 National Household Survey on Drug Abuse (U.S. Department of Health and Human Services [USDHHS]), the number of current illicit drug users in 1999 was 14.8 million or 6.7 percent of the population 12 years of age and older.

In 1999, more than half of youth aged 12 to 17 reported that marijuana was easy to obtain. About one-quarter reported that heroin was easy to obtain. Fifteen percent of youths reported being approached by someone selling drugs in the month prior to being surveyed. In addition to the survey demonstrating the accessibility of illicit drugs, the results showed youths as perceiving a decrease in the risk for using illicit drugs. For example, the percentage of youths who perceived great risk in using cocaine once a month decreased from 63 percent in 1994 to 49.8 percent in 1999. The percentage of youths aged 12 to 17 who perceived great risk in using marijuana once a month decreased from 40 percent in 1990 to 33 percent in 1994, to 29 percent in 1999 (USDHHS, 1999).

MARIJUANA. An estimated 2.3 million people started using marijuana in 1998. This translates into approximately 6,400 new users each day (USDHHS, 1999). The resurgence in marijuana use continues, especially among adolescents. Along with this resurgence of marijuana use there seems to be a concomitant rise in the treatment and arrest of adolescents using this drug. Two factors may be contributing to the dramatic leap in adverse consequences: (1) higher potency and (2) the use of marijuana in combination with other dangerous drugs. Marijuana cigarettes often include crack, may be dipped in PCP, or sometimes are dipped in embalming fluid.

COCAINE. Crack cocaine continues to dominate the illicit drug problem in the United States, involving about 1.8 million people in 1998. Most cocaine users are older, living in urban inner-city areas that are often dominated by crime and prostitution. Even though this number represents a reduction in use from a peak of 5.7 million in 1985, supplies of cocaine remain abundant in nearly every city. An estimated 730,000 Americans used cocaine for the first time in 1997 (USDHHS, 1998). These new users of cocaine include teenagers who smoke crack cocaine with marijuana, middle-class suburban dwellers who use cocaine hydrochloride in powder form, and females in their thirties who start using crack with no prior drug history.

HEROIN. An increasing trend in new heroin use has occurred since 1992, with the estimated number of heroin users in one month increasing from 68,000 in 1993 to 149,000 in 1998. Many of these new users are young people under age 26 who try a variety of methods for ingesting heroin, including smoking, snorting, or sniffing (USDHHS, 1999). One concern is that young heroin snorters may shift to needle injecting because of increased tolerance, nasal soreness, or declining purity of the drug. Injection use, through the sharing of needles, increases risk for AIDS (Pinger, Payne, Hahn, and Hahn, 1998).

STIMULANTS. Methamphetamine availability and use are sporadic in diverse areas of the country, but use seems to have increased in rural areas. Availability in rural areas prompts some concern because it indicates spread outside of the areas of endemic use (i.e., the West Coast) (Pinger et al., 1998). Methylphenidate (Ritalin) abuse continues among heroin users. Adolescents are buying ephedrine-based products at convenience stores, truck stops, and health food stores. In fact, many states have banned the sale of such products in an attempt to curb this escalating abuse among adolescents.

DEPRESSANTS. Persons frequenting nightclubs in several cities are using gamma hydroxybutrate (GHB) and ketamine ("Special K"), often mixing these two drugs with alcohol to form a special mixture called "Special K-lude." This mixture is popular because its effects are similar to those produced by methaqualone (Quaalude). Flunitrazepam (Rohypnol) use continues in many areas of the country; however, its widespread availability has declined since the federal government placed a ban on its importation. Clonazepam (another pharmaceutical benzodiazepine) or "roofies" are used to enhance the effects of methadone and other opiates (Pinger et al., 1998).

HALLUCINOGENS AND PCP. Phencyclidine (PCP) is often used in combination with other drugs, such as marijuana mixed with or dipped into PCP. Also, PCP may be combined with crack to create "spaceballs." Lysergic acid diethylamide (LSD) remains widely available in most cities and in suburban and rural areas as well (Pinger et al., 1998). An estimated 1.1 million Americans used hallucinogens for the first time in 1997 (USDHHS, 1998).

COMMUNITY IMPACT OF SUBSTANCE USE DISORDERS

In addition to being a mental health problem, substance use disorders are a major factor in many medical, public health, social, and safety issues within a community. As a medical problem, substance use, including alcohol use, contributes to diseases of the liver, pancreas, and digestive tract. Depending on the drug of choice, the respiratory, nervous, and cardiovascular systems also may be affected. High rates of comorbidity with other psychiatric diagnoses complicate and increase the cost of treating schizophrenia and bipolar disorders (Dickey and Azeni, 1996; Kwapil, 1996). Persons with schizophrenia are six times more likely to develop a drug use disorder and three times more likely to develop an alcohol problem when compared to the general population. Persons with a bipolar disorder are 7.9 times more likely to develop problems with substances (Kwapil, 1996).

As a community public health problem, substance use disorders have been linked to AIDS, tuberculosis, and neonatal defects (Weisner, 1995). Community social problems, such as unemployment and homelessness, are also strongly associated with substance use disorders (Weisner, 1995). Persons with drug and alcohol dependence obviously have the more serious medical problems and contribute the most to public health concerns. In contrast, the large numbers of problem drinkers in a community actually produce most of the drug-related costs sustained by a given community, (e.g., drunk driving, days of missed work, and domestic violence) (Sobell, Cunningham, and Sobell, 1996).

In terms of other safety issues within a community, the relationships of substance use with crime, industrial accidents, drownings, and cold temperature-related injuries are well established. Possibly as many as 79 percent of head and spinal cord injuries are related to drug and alcohol use (Hubbard, Everett, and Khan, 1996). In fact, preinjury prevalence of alcohol dependence has been found to be as high as 68 percent of persons with head injuries. Additionally, persons with spinal cord injuries who have heavy alcohol use participate less in rehabilitation as well as in vocational and educational activities and thus are more likely to require financial support from community resources.

The impact of substance use on the family cannot be underestimated. Persons with substance abuse or dependence typically have extensive marital and family problems (Rotunda, Scherer, and Imm, 1995). Research indicates that genetic and environmental exposure of children to alcohol dependence may lead to a predisposition to alcohol and drug abuse or dependence (Grinspoon and Bakalar, 1990; Tarter and Vanykov, 1994). In addition to developing dependence themselves, these children are considered to be at high risk for experiencing other difficulties, including cognitive, emotional, social, and academic problems (Moyers, Jones, Mirchadani, and Sherwood, 1993). The home environments for the children are characterized by more marital conflict, parent-child conflict, and child abuse when compared to the environments of children with parents who do not use substances (Rotunda et al., 1995). In addition, negative consequences, such as separation and divorce, are much more common in marriages containing an addicted partner in comparison with couples in the general population.

SUBSTANCE USE DISORDERS AND OCCUPATION

Thus far, the impact of substance use on the community as a whole has been examined. A successful and thriving community depends on the performance of multiple occupations by many individuals. "Just as particular occupations may promote health and well-being in individuals, so may the patterns of occupation that characterize particular cultures affect the health of towns, nations, cities, neighborhoods, and communities" (Clark, Wood, and Larson, 1998, p. 18). Therefore, attention is now placed on the relationship between the substance use of an individual and that person's subsequent engagement in occupations.

Occupations are the day-to-day activities or goal-directed pursuits that typically extend over time, have meaning to the performer, and involve multiple tasks (Christiansen, Clark, Kielhofner, and Rogers, 1995). Normally, when an occupational therapy practitioner thinks of an occupation, only those occupations that are health enhancing, positively valued by the culture, or necessary for daily survival come to mind. However, it is equally important for occupational therapy practitioners to understand those occupations that lead to negative consequences or that are considered to be deviant from socially acceptable norms. "Whereas some occupations and patterns of occupation are health promoting, others may be health compromising" (Clark et al., 1998, p. 18).

Using substances can be thought of as an occupation because of its many associated tasks and activities, which may include:

● Raising money for the drugs
● Purchasing or making the deal to obtain the drug supply
● Protecting the supply from others
● Removing barriers to using, such as ignoring family members who object to the person's behavior

● Creating situations for using
● Seeking persons with whom to use
● Spending time using
● Recovering from the effects of using
● Resuming the drug using process all over again (Moyers, 1997).

These "using" tasks and activities are directed toward the goal of achieving the desired drug-induced state. As the substance use progresses, these using-related activities extend over more time, often to the point of being all inclusive of one's day, evening, or night. It is not uncommon for clients to report a drug- and alcohol-using history that spans multiple years, even decades.

These drug-using tasks and activities have meaning to the user. This meaning often is incomprehensible to others who do not use drugs and alcohol (Moyers, 1997). The person using alcohol and drugs may report that the chemicals fulfill the need to escape, have fun, relax and sleep, avoid physical and emotional pain, gain confidence, increase sexuality, feel less inhibited and more creative, or increase energy and activity levels (Moyers, 1992a).

In addition to these meanings, alcohol and drugs are the objects to which the person gives over control of his or her life. Eventually, freedom to live differently or to engage in occupations other than drinking or using drugs becomes severely restricted. According to Mattingly and Fleming (1994), the person has lost intentionality, the creation of reasons for doing. Reasons for doing are the basis of volition or making choices for occupational behavior. The seductive ability of alcohol and drugs to create positive effect and euphoria during times of emotional stress is a powerful motivator for engagement in drug-using types of occupational behavior. When the individual is intoxicated or stoned, the person fails to enact intentions for doing other important tasks and activities. Instead the person becomes focused on maintaining the euphoria associated with using substances. This single intention of drinking or using is magnified to the detriment of all other intentions, however noble or important.

Reasons for doing are also symbolically expressed and structured by the daily habits and routines that characterize one's daily life (Mattingly and Fleming, 1994). Consider the daily routines of someone dependent on alcohol and drugs. Gradually, the day becomes organized by habits associated with drinking and drug use, such as stopping at the same liquor store or the drug dealer's house on the way home from work. Thus, drinking and using drugs leads to a habit dysfunction perpetuating the addiction. Because one's occupational behavior represents "the meaning that we make of ourselves acting in the world" (Kielhofner, 1995, p. 59), persons addicted to substances have gradually assumed a negative self-image. The "Big Book" (the nickname given by Alcoholics Anonymous (AA) members to the main text titled *Alcoholics Anonymous* [Alcoholics Anonymous World Services, 1976]) is replete with many stories that describe this distorted view of the self and this loss of freedom to select how one acts in the world. For example (Alcoholics Anonymous World Services, p. 199):

> Long since I had come to believe I was insane because I did so many things I didn't want to do. I didn't want to neglect my children. I loved them, I think, as much as any parent. But I did neglect them. I didn't want to get into fights, but I did get into fights. I didn't want to get arrested, but I did get arrested. I didn't want to jeopardize the lives of innocent people by driving an automobile while intoxicated, but I did. I quite naturally came to the conclusion that I must be insane.

As performance in occupations other than drinking or using substances progressively deteriorates, the individual becomes more and more alienated from normal occupations and becomes deprived of his or her healthy effects. Further engagement in nonusing occupations becomes devoid of usual meanings, only meaningful to the extent that these occupations serve as barriers or facilitators to drinking or using drugs.

Thus occupational alienation is complete. Further engagement in nonusing occupations is typically avoided as a method of protecting the ego from future failures, thus perpetuating the negative cycle of occupational alienation and deprivation. Unfortunately, occupational alienation and deprivation interfere with the person's biological need for occupations. Wilcock (1993, p. 20) stated that "occupations help individuals meet their bodily needs of sustenance, self-care, shelter, and safety"; that "occupations develop skills, social structures and technology aimed at superiority over predators and the environment"; and that occupations "exercise and develop personal capacities enabling the organism to be maintained and to flourish."

Occupational therapy practitioners use *Uniform Terminology* (American Occupational Therapy Association, 1994) to assist in analyzing the influence of substance use on occupational performance and the ability of the individual to satisfy the biological need for occupations. The occupational therapy evaluation addresses whether the person's activities of daily living have been affected by substance use, whether work and productive activities have been impacted, and whether engagement in leisure has been influenced (see Fig. 16–1).

The occupational therapist hypothesizes about the underlying causes of the occupational performance problems by evaluating the impact of substance use on performance component functioning. More specifically, are there any sensorimotor, cognitive, or psychosocial/psychological impairments that might be attributed to a substance use disorder? If so, are these impaired performance components expected to recover over time during abstinence? Will these impairments be slow in recovering? Will there be residual deficits in the performance components?

Questions regarding the context of performance are also raised. When, where, and with whom is the client more or less likely to engage in substance-using behaviors? What are the physical environmental cues that facilitate or inhibit substance use? What are the features of the social or cultural environment that support or interfere with substance use? Is the client's stage of development or life cycle important in understanding the client's potential for recovery?

STAGES OF CHANGE

Given the negative, self-perpetuating cycle of occupational alienation and deprivation inherent in substance use, is there a positive cycle that once entered can lead to recovery and long-term sobriety? Kielhofner (1995, p. 251) suggested that "therapeutically supported change" occurs when the individual, through his or her own efforts, accomplishes the primary change process. Therapy simply supplies the support for the client in assuming responsibility for his or her own health and the lifestyle choices made in relationship to the use of drugs and alcohol.

Not all people who experience problems with their use of substances are ready to change. The substance use literature has historically framed this response as *denial.* The concept of denial is now being challenged and perhaps deters professionals from providing help. Instead of breaking through this denial and forcing change, the focus in treatment is now on helping people prepare themselves for the next stage of change. It is not necessarily the goal to help the client go through all the stages of change. Because the substance use disorder often took years to develop, it is recognized that change may take years to fully occur. Therefore, each professional, through a consistent effort to bring the addiction to the client's level of awareness, can impact the client's change process but may not actually be the professional who finally supports the client's efforts to implement or sustain the change.

Prochaska and DiClemente (1982, 1986) have studied the change process and have identified these **stages of change** as follows: (1) precontemplation, (2) contemplation, (3) determination, (4) action, (5) maintenance, and (6) relapse. These six stages of

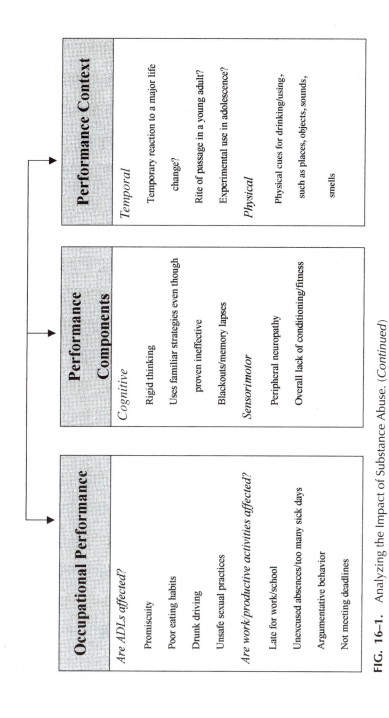

FIG. 16–1. Analyzing the Impact of Substance Abuse. (*Continued*)

change are arranged in a continuous cycle in which the person may enter or exit at any point, may progress or regress, or may remain in a given stage for an undetermined length of time. Furthermore, a person may skip stages in the change process while progressing or regressing.

A client seen in occupational therapy at the *precontemplation* stage would express surprise if the practitioner identified the client as having a drinking or drug problem.

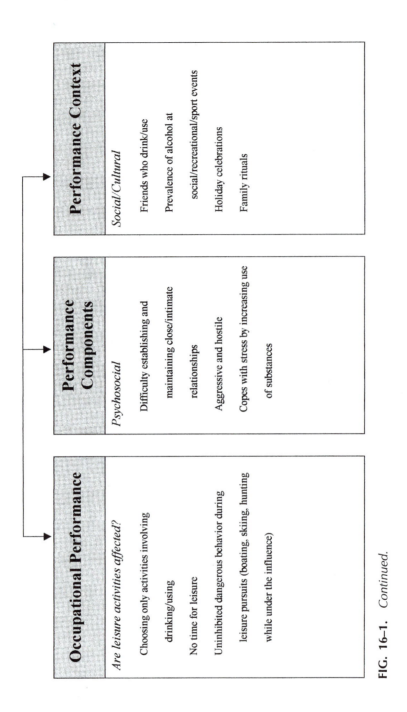

FIG. 16–1. *Continued.*

Typically, a lack of awareness of the relationship between the problems the client is experiencing and the use of chemicals is present. As the individual becomes more self-aware over time, he or she may find that there are, in fact, good reasons to change and may move into the next stage, or *contemplation*. At this stage, the client may be ambivalent about changing, as demonstrated by fluctuations in wanting to change and finding reasons not to change. Consequently, the client is not sure of the right direction in which to move toward recovery. When this back and forth process occurs and the balance tips toward change, the next stage of *determination* emerges. The client begins the preparation process for change, such as brainstorming about all of the possible change strategies, considering the pros and cons for each, and making decisions about the steps to take. *Action* is what comes next as the individual tries the strategies selected. As the actions become more a natural part of the person's day-to-day coping, the *maintenance* phase is entered.

For many clients, changing from a drinking or drug-using lifestyle to one of finding balance, abstinence, and maintenance of health habits can be most challenging. Persons in recovery from substance use disorders commonly experience the final stage of change or *relapse*. It has been reported that over 90 percent of clients will drink or use drugs again after completion of their substance abuse intervention program (Ouimette, Moos, and Finney, 1998). Therefore, learning how to prevent "a slip," which may involve having one drink or using limited amounts of the drug of choice, from turning into a full-blown return of the substance use disorder is the focus of this final stage of change. Seeing relapse as "just another step in the process of change that leads to stable recovery" (Miller, 1995, p. 92) allows the client and therapist to develop additional change strategies that must be implemented before the maintenance stage becomes fully operational.

COMMUNITY INTERVENTIONS

Substance use and addiction intervention can occur in a variety of medical and community settings (see Box 16–1). The stages of change provide a framework for analyzing each intervention program in terms of the contribution to recovery and the types of clients best suited for the program.

Prevention

Prevention of substance abuse, dependence, and problem drinking is accomplished through health education offered by schools, colleges and universities, employee assistance programs, and public health departments. Successful prevention programming helps individuals to identify risky behaviors for substance use disorders or for problem drinking and then helps the individual enter the cycle of change in order to modify these risk factors. The goals of prevention as related to the stages of change involve:

- Bringing the risky behaviors to the person's attention
- Helping the person to determine the need to change these risky behaviors
- Facilitating the decision to change and selecting strategies for change
- Implementing the change strategies
- Maintaining the new healthy behaviors
- Reinstituting the healthy behaviors when lapsing into old habit patterns and behaviors

As an aspect of helping the person move from precontemplation to contemplation in the change cycle for prevention purposes, occupational therapy practitioners educate individuals about the effects of substance use on the performance areas of activities of daily living, work and productive activities, and play and leisure. The goal of occupational therapy prevention programming is to improve such general life skills as healthy coping abilities, interpersonal communication, and successful occupational performance.

Targeting this prevention education to parents is also an important prevention strategy. Research indicates that parents teach norms to their children regarding the use of alcohol and other drugs (Rotunda et al., 1995). Occupational therapy practitioners can

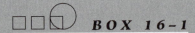

BOX 16-1

Sites of Specialized Addiction Service Delivery

Institutions
- Addictions and dual-diagnoses inpatient units
- Detoxification units
- Partial hospitalization programs
- Prisons

Outpatient
- Intensive outpatient programs
- Aftercare programs
- Outpatient office visits

Community
- Community mental health centers
- Schools, colleges, universities
- Halfway houses
- Employee assistance programs
- Wellness centers and programs
- Homeless shelters
- Community centers
- Sheltered workshops
- Battered women shelters
- Mobile crisis units/crisis intervention programs
- Public health departments
- Church ministry programs

work with parents to evaluate their current value system and to incorporate the following beliefs (Stoffel and Moyers, 1997):

- Using substances is not essential for occupational performance unless prescribed for specific medical reasons.
- Using substances uncontrollably is a health problem and interferes with occupational performance.
- Using substances to solve emotional problems is dangerous and may lead to permanent impairments in performance components, skill erosion, and habit dysfunction.
- Achieving an artificially altered emotional and cognitive state is not acceptable and disrupts occupational performance.
- Learning coping strategies is important for managing life problems and facilitating occupational performance.

Crisis Intervention

Crisis intervention refers to the management of alcohol or other drug emergencies. These crisis situations may be due to overdose, adverse drug reactions, or catastrophic psychological responses. Similar to those services provided to persons with other mental health diagnoses, such as depression, crisis intervention often occurs as the result of suicide gestures made either during intoxication or when the individual is experiencing a rather severe withdrawal syndrome. In a way, persons in crises are really acting out, although negatively, their desire to change. Thus, family members, community officials, and professionals must take advantage of this momentary opportunity for change by offering specific and structured forms of help. In fact, sometimes a crisis situation is helpful in moving the client swiftly from precontemplation to contemplation, determination, and action. However, a crisis or "hitting bottom" is not necessary for motivating change as was once believed by health professionals. Through the use of the stages of change model, "motivation is now understood to be the result of an interaction between the drinker [or drug user] and those around him or her. This means that there are things a therapist can do to increase motivation for change" (Miller, 1995, p. 91). In crisis intervention, the goal is to address the immediate psychological, criminal, or medical dangers. Once out of danger, the goal changes to implementing consequences for the behavior, such as implementing treatment for the substance use disorder.

Intervention by the police may be necessary when substance use produces violent and unpredictable behavior, particularly when overly high doses of the drug are ingested or when the content of the drug is laced with some other unknown mixture. For instance, amphetamine abuse and dependence may lead to a psychosis with a close resemblance to paranoid schizophrenia (Kaplan and Sadock, 1996). Marijuana dependence may lead to delirium or to a psychotic or anxiety disorder.

Medical crises may result when lethal mixtures of alcohol and barbiturates are taken or when the person with alcohol dependence suffers from delirium tremens as the result of an unsupervised withdrawal (Kaplan and Sadock, 1996). The specific life-threatening conditions associated with the abuse of amphetamines, including cocaine and crack, include myocardial infarction, severe hypertension, cerebrovascular disease, and ischemic colitis. Inhalant use can lead to respiratory depression, cardiac arrhythmias, irreversible hepatic or renal damage, epilepsy, and a decreased intelligence quotient along with other neurological signs and symptoms.

Crisis intervention thus involves evaluation of the lethality of suicidal or homicidal gestures; the potential for violence or other negative and unpredictable behaviors; the danger of medical symptoms related to overdose, withdrawal, or combinations of multiple drugs and alcohol; and the extent of injuries related to trauma sustained as the result of intoxication. This evaluation may initially occur over the telephone, with instructions to proceed to the nearest emergency room, mental health hospital or unit of a hospital, or to an alcohol and drug rehabilitation hospital or unit. Paramedics and police may also provide the initial evaluation and thus may arrest the individual as being dangerous to self or others. Emergency room personnel now routinely evaluate persons with traumatic injuries for alcohol and drug problems, once medical stability has been achieved (Rumpf, Hapke, Erfurth, and John, 1998). Being drunk and disorderly, committing public intoxication, or driving while under the influence, although crises, may only trigger involvement of the legal system. However, many courts mandate intervention in place of, or in conjunction with, incarceration.

Brief Interventions

The stages of change theory has led to creative thinking about ways that professionals can change the environment and change interactions with the client so that the client must eventually face the need to change the substance-using behaviors. **Brief interventions** involve offering clients well-written educational materials, conducting health screenings, discussing information about substance use, or providing information about resources (Heather, 1995). Brief intervention strategies have been found to be effective in motivating change (Miller, Zweben, DiClemente, and Rychtarik, 1992) and to be feasible, practical, and cost effective for implementation by a wide range of professionals. Occupational therapy practitioners are able to integrate these strategies into the intervention plans of their clients in multiple settings, even though the client may be initially referred for other reasons such as a hand injury (Moyers and Stoffel, 1999).

One type of brief intervention is information provided in a written format, such as self-help manuals, educational materials, pamphlets, and brief self-scoring questionnaires. These materials can be supplied in the waiting rooms of any occupational therapy clinic and thus do not need to be formally discussed with the client unless the client asks specific questions. The idea is to promote client responsibility while still providing information that moves the client into the next stage of change, such as from precontemplation to contemplation or from determination to action.

Miller and Munoz (1982) developed a self-help manual to supplement treatment. This manual has been shown to successfully enhance intervention outcomes. Thus, occupational therapy practitioners might do well to review their client education materials for content related to prevention and treatment of substance use disorders and problem drinking. This educational focus on substance use can be incorporated into other wellness information about health and the importance of occupational performance. Populations for which occupational therapy practitioners provide services could each have specifically designed materials addressing the problems related to substance use, prevention strategies, and resources for intervention. When this information is presented in the context of the health condition that is of most concern to the client, it may have a greater likelihood of being used by the client.

Motivational enhancement therapy (MET), developed by Miller et al. (1992), involves four highly structured sessions. The sessions include a drinker's check-up (DCU) and the FRAMES approach to interviewing for change (Miller and Sanchez, 1994). The DCU is a comprehensive assessment offered as a health check-up for persons with problem drinking. In addition to asking the individual quantity and frequency-of-use questions, other screening tools measuring the impact of problem drinking are administered, the most common tool being the CAGE (Ewing, 1984).

CAGE stands for the four questions that are asked about: (1) the need for *cutting* down on drinking, (2) feeling *annoyed* by others criticizing one's drinking, (3) feeling *guilty* about drinking, or (4) needing an *eye opener* (a drink the first thing in the morning or whenever the person wakes up). Positive results on the quantity and frequency questions is indicated by the person drinking 12 or more drinks (each drink equals 12 ounces of beer, 5 ounces of wine, or 1 ounce of distilled spirits) per week if a woman or 15 or more drinks per week if a man (Cooney, Zweben, and Fleming, 1995). Two positive answers on the CAGE would indicate a need to address the drinking problem.

The DCU would then proceed by using more specific questionnaires, such as the Michigan Alcohol Screening Test (MAST), which analyzes the social, medical, legal, and psychosocial consequences associated with problematic drinking, such as blackouts, loss of employment, and drunk driving arrests (Selzer, 1971). An occupational therapy practitioner would add an occupational history, highlighting the impact of the substance use on occupational performance to the DCU (Moyers and Stoffel, 1999). Blood testing for alcohol and urine testing for drugs may be conducted, along with medical laboratory screens that assess the functioning of liver and other systems impacted by long-term use of chemicals.

Results from the DCU are used to provide feedback so that the individual can successfully move through the successive stages of change. Miller and Sanchez (1994) developed the FRAMES model of interviewing for carefully imparting the information obtained from the DCU. FRAMES is a mnemonic device that stands for feedback, responsibility, advice, menu, empathy, and self-efficacy. Throughout the interview, the professional gives clear and specific *feedback* from the assessment that supports the need for change. The information is not accusatory and the focus is not on diagnostic labeling. Instead, the emphasis is on the person's *responsibility* to interpret and act on the information. The interviewer does give *advice* in relationship to the medical consequences for continued use. The professional supplies a *menu* of change options, ranging from self-help programs or manuals to hospitalization. Throughout the interview, the professional is *empathetic* and avoids hostile confrontations, power struggles, and judgmental and paternalistic attitudes. Additionally, the professional's attitude promotes the *self-efficacy* of the client or a belief in the individual's ability to make decisions about when and how to change.

The key to effective brief intervention strategies is to establish rapport and to use appropriate open-ended questions based on a topic that is of concern to the individual (Rollnick and Bell, 1991). Depending on the clinical circumstances, the occupational therapy practitioner may find that the FRAMES process rarely occurs in one session. Rather, it occurs over time. The individual may be able to absorb only some feedback, with emphasis on the client's own responsibility during a single interview. If a client, after a series of brief interventions, indicates a willingness to plan and take action about the substance use, the occupational therapy practitioner readily helps the client make specific and realistic plans. The occupational therapy practitioner should offer to initiate a referral and to provide support for implementing other change strategies on the menu of options.

Formal Intervention Programs

Miller (1995) indicated that treatment typically occurs when individuals are at the action stage of the change process. **Formal intervention programs** include inpatient medical detoxification, outpatient and partial hospitalization programs, dual-diagnoses programs, and aftercare programs. All these programs equip the person with the skills and strategies to stop drinking and using and develop the behavioral flexibility necessary for maintaining abstinence. People who seek out formal addictions intervention programs have often tried other methods (personal contracting to cut down or stop their alcohol/drug use or seeking support through church or self-help groups) but have found their efforts to be unsuccessful. Occupational therapists, after using brief intervention techniques to facilitate change, may find that referral to specialized addictions services is indicated to better meet their client's needs. Awareness and knowledge of available alcohol and drug programs in the community is important for making this referral. Communication with the staff of the alcohol and drug program about the initial referral, as well as follow-up, is important. A number of studies have shown that 70 percent to 90 percent of persons referred to alcohol treatment programs for alcohol abuse fail to enter or remain in treatment (Babor, Ritson, and Hodgson, 1986; Soderstrom and Cowley, 1987).

Miller (1995) has suggested that, despite formal intervention programs focusing on the action stage, for treatment to be effective, all stages of change need to be recognized and addressed. Therefore, addiction intervention must include the full continuum of services, which typically includes group, individual, and family programming; employee assistance programs; and support and self-help programs. In addition, addictions intervention programs should provide the appropriate level of intensity and ensure integration with other services to fully address the life issues impacted by the substance use disorder. Formal addictions programs are broadening the scope of services to include serving those whose alcohol and drug use problems are not at the severe level where dependence occurs. Consequently, Zweben and Rose (1999) advocate the integration of brief interventions into all medical and social service programs, including those programs staffed by occupational therapy practitioners.

Self-Help

Involvement of clients in **self-help programs** (those programs that do not rely on professional intervention but on the support of group members) is particularly important given the push by managed-care programs to drastically reduce both inpatient and outpatient treatment days. The occupational therapy practitioner encourages and recommends participation in a variety of 12-step-type self-help programs, such as Alcoholics Anonymous (AA), Cocaine Anonymous, and Narcotics Anonymous.

The most influential self-help program is Alcoholics Anonymous, with 2 million members worldwide and 95,166 groups in 150 countries (Alcoholics Anonymous World Services, 1996). Research has indicated the effectiveness of AA when combined with more formal intervention (Emrick, Tonigan, Montgomery, and Little, 1993; Humphreys and Moos, 1996; McCrady and Miller, 1993; Ouimette, Moos, and Finney, 1998). Miller (1998) stated that spirituality based programs, such as AA, are more likely to help people remain abstinent when compared to psychological therapy devoid of spirituality. In general, AA sees the most pervasive problem of alcoholism as the spiritual decay that results from the distorted perception that the self, rather than a higher power, is at the center of life. (Alcoholics Anonymous World Services, 1976). Committing to abstinence, decreasing preoccupation with the self, and living a lifelong program of spirituality are the essential elements of sobriety according to AA (Alcoholics Anonymous World Services, 1970). Achievement of these goals occurs by "working the 12 steps of recovery" and is facilitated by group participation and the support of a sponsor.

Rational Recovery (RR) (Trimpey, 1992) and Secular Organizations for Sobriety-Save Our Selves (SOS) (Christopher, 1989) were developed for those who are not comfortable with a spiritual emphasis. Rational Recovery, although peer led like the other programs, has a professional advisor. Abstinence is considered important by Rational Recovery, but the group also recognizes that some persons may be able to return to drinking in moderation. The Women for Sobriety (WFS) program was developed on the premise that women experience drinking in a different way and therefore require an alternate approach. WFS emphasizes the idea that because women are competent, they do not need alcohol and drugs to cope (Women for Sobriety, 1976).

Computer technology has made it possible to access self-help resources through e-mail and the Web. The home pages of many of these self-help groups provide information about the organization, about group locations and meeting times, and about ordering literature; some may actually conduct meetings on line. With technology, support for staying sober is immediately available at any time right in the home.

OCCUPATIONAL THERAPY AND COMMUNITY PROGRAMS

Research has examined the short-term effectiveness of intervention for persons with alcohol and drug substance use disorders (Finney and Monahan, 1996). The concern is that these studies may "overstate long-term remission and recovery rates because a significant proportion of alcoholic patients do not maintain gains achieved in the year following discharge" (Humphreys, Moos, and Cohen, 1997, p. 231). In fact, most long-term studies do not support the view that intervention has a lasting impact on the course of substance use disorders (Finney and Moos, 1992). This is not surprising given that intervention typically has emphasized short-term intervention for acute problems such as medical, personal, and legal crises. Because substance use disorders are chronic and often involve multiple remissions and exacerbations, short-term intervention focused on the immediate crisis consequently may not make a lasting impact. Additionally, the negative life context experienced by clients after discharge may counteract any effects of intervention and may actually create a sense of hopelessness or a belief in the impossibility of remaining drug-free (Moos, Finney, and Cronkite, 1990).

In answering the question of what predicts the long-term course of recovery, several factors have been delineated (Humphreys et al., 1997). Individuals who are unmarried, lack stable family situations and employment, and live in low-income communities tend to experience poor long-term intervention outcomes (Humphreys et al., 1997). Financial stress and problems related to continued substance use after intervention intertwine to create more complicated situations, making the solution of either problem increasingly difficult (Humphreys, Moos, and Finney, 1996). Substance use disorders are thus inextricably linked to the individual's social environment. Research has shown, for instance, that recovery is positively influenced by involvement in religious organizations, self-help programs, and strong relationships with extended family, friends, and a spouse/partner (Humphreys et al., 1996).

These findings support the involvement of occupational therapy practitioners in designing community intervention programs that focus on lifestyle issues and the modification of the context from one supporting engagement in "using" occupations to one supporting engagement in healthy occupations leading to successful occupational performance. Jackson, Carlson, Mandel, Zemke, and Clark (1998) originally described the concept of lifestyle redesign for occupational therapy in relationship to programs promoting healthy occupations for older persons in assisted living settings. Marlatt (1985) has described similar principles for persons using substances and has named this approach "lifestyle modification." However, Marlatt's approach focuses exclusively on developing coping strategies such as relaxation, exercise, and rest, and interpersonal communication skills. Adding techniques for environmental modification to support change and adding methods of re-establishing successful occupational performance enhances the work of Marlatt.

Lifestyle redesign is a client-focused approach in which the occupational therapist asks the client to determine the occupational performances that require intervention in order to achieve a greater life satisfaction. To identify these occupational performances, the occupational therapist may use an occupational interview or history to highlight for the client the loss of intentionality and the progressive abdication of control over one's life to alcohol and drugs. Reasonable goals are then collaboratively developed to help the client change the deficient occupational performance. For instance, it is important that the client receive help in finding a job and in locating suitable living arrangements. These are two of the critical factors that support the person in recovery. Additionally, the client may need social and leisure counseling and opportunities to attend drug-free social clubs.

In addition to helping the client improve occupational performance, the therapist also incorporates into the intervention plan the idea that occupations are opportunities "to progressively reinvent the way in which the self is understood" (Moyers, 1997, p. 211). Therapeutic occupations are used to reinvent the self as abstinent by creating rationales for being sober, developing habits of sobriety, and producing peak experiences when sober. Daily occupations are organized into basic habits such as getting rest, eating balanced meals, keeping the body neat and clean, and following the therapy regimen necessary for maintaining abstinence. Occupations also help to define abstinence as a meaningful and enjoyable experience, important given that ordinary daily activities may not compete with the seductive memories of a positive affect associated with drug use. Miller (1998) has noted through a review of 12 different studies that addiction is associated with a lack of meaning and purpose in life. Finding meaning is a spiritual process because the person attempts to discover his or her purpose or reasons for being in the world and clarifies within that scheme the importance of interpersonal relationships, daily events, and goals. Thus, rationales for staying sober are firmly established through meaningful occupations that promote spirituality and one's connectedness to the world.

Occupational therapy practitioners help the person newly recovering from substance use disorders to discover that particular occupations are symbolic of this self-reinvention process. The occupation serves as a metaphor for healing or for the positive changes associated with recovery. For example, engaging in daily exercise may be symbolic of the need to care for the self after years of neglect, thus reinventing a physical body that is more consistent with meanings ascribed to abstinence (being healthy). Occupations help re-establish intentionality as the individual deliberately selects occupations according to a variety of goals, values, or interests. In fact, occupations may serve as a transition to a valued future goal and thus provide the context for learning and applying new skills needed for personal growth. For instance, occupational therapy intervention might help the client redefine his or her qualifications, select and begin a program of intensive retraining, and eventually obtain a more satisfying and interesting job.

Underlying factors or performance components that contribute to declines in occupational performance are also key recovery factors identified and targeted for intervention. Cognitive integration and cognitive components are two of the most important aspects of functioning requiring evaluation and intervention. Recovery for some sensorimotor and cognitive components can be quite slow, or in some instances nonexistent, depending on the drug abused (Roehrich and Goldman, 1993). Independent occupational performance is highly dependent on the person's ability to analyze and solve novel problems. Occupations are designed to stimulate cognitive recovery (Moyers and Barrett, 1992), or task and environmental modifications are made to reduce the cognitive complexity of occupations when cognitive recovery is slow or nonexistent due to damage from long-term use of the substance.

To illustrate the influence of components of functioning on occupational performance, consider the individual who states that drug and alcohol use negatively affects school performance and interferes with the goal of graduating from college with a degree in accounting. In analyzing the underlying factors or performance components, the client and the occupational therapist determine that managing time, coping with stress and financial worries, developing study habits, and socializing with classmates who are truly supportive of the client's objectives are all important for achieving the goal of obtaining a degree.

The intervention plan outlines strategies to improve skills in time management, coping, academics, and socialization. Coping skills training is important for the client to learn how to cope with frustration when engaging in routine occupations. Coping skill training usually involves learning relaxation techniques, meditation strategies, alternate coping behaviors, specific control skills (limit setting, planning ahead for potential difficulties), drug refusal skills, and self-monitoring of emotional extremes and negative thinking. However, this training may be ineffective due to the disruption of these skills by the presence of drug-using cues in the environment. Contextual factors, including the physical, social, and cultural environments that facilitate or inhibit recovery, are also identified as a part of the intervention plan.

Exposure to drug cues in the environment is a significant relapse variable (Moyers, 1992a). *Drug cues* are those objects, persons, and places that trigger memories of alcohol and other drugs being able to produce positive effect or to remove negative affect (Moyers, 1992a, p. 105). A drug cue could be the presence of beer or wine in the refrigerator or the playing of music to which one traditionally listened when using the substance. These cues evoke compelling memories of drug use. These memories, if strong, also invoke a physiological response experienced as "craving." *Craving* involves a strong urge to consume the drug, positive outcome expectations for drug use (e.g., expecting the drug to help the individual relax and feel better), and physiological activation (i.e., strong anticipation of pleasure or reward).

Occupational therapists enable the person using substances to evaluate the environment and examine situational circumstances surrounding the typical episode of substance using. The individual is helped to explore the typical thoughts, feelings, and behaviors that precede the drug-using routines. Therefore, intervention must incorporate methods to remove the cues from the environment as well as to decrease the strength of cue reactivity. For removing cues, the client may choose to avoid typical drinking environments, such as the local bar, and avoid those friends who encourage drinking. However, situations will arise when the client is unable to avoid cues. Instead, the client will need to decrease the reactivity to the cue and manage the craving experience through coping techniques.

To decrease the cue reactivity, the occupational therapy practitioner coaches the individual to produce an adaptive response in place of the drug-using behavior. It is impossible to emit maladaptive behavior simultaneously with adaptive behavior. For example, when seeing an advertisement on television for beer, the client is aware of an urge to drink but "follows the addiction through" by quickly remembering a negative instance when beer drinking led to an arrest for driving under the influence. Because the craving lasts only a short time, the client also "out waits" the craving by redirecting attention to enjoyable activities such as roller-blading or going to a movie or by contacting persons supportive of the client's efforts to remain sober (Stoffel, 1992). These persons may be members of self-help groups that the client has chosen to attend.

Environmental modification also involves working with the family to help the person create a supportive atmosphere for change. Family behavior has been established as playing a role in the development and maintenance of alcohol and drug use. Typical family behaviors, such as reinforcing drug use through attention and care-taking, protecting the individual from the consequences of substance use, and punishing for infractions related to drug use, have been noted to increase the likelihood of continued substance abuse. Excessive ongoing family conflicts may contribute to relapse when the individual is attempting to recover. However, the family not only affects the person using substances, but also the individual's substance-related behaviors affect family members.

Occupational therapy practitioners work with members of the family to improve their function in performance areas and in components of function (Moyers, 1991, 1992b; Stoffel, 1994). The goals are to help family members learn to cope with their emotional distress and to concentrate on their own motivations for change in performance areas, regardless of whether the individual decides to change his or her substance use.

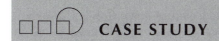

CASE STUDY

MARTIN

Martin is a 17-year-old who is a junior in high school. He lives with his mother and father, both natives of Mexico, who moved to the United States 20 years ago. Martin has an older sister, Anna, aged 18 and a senior in high school, and younger twin brothers, Michael and Peter, aged 10. Martin's high school has an occupational therapist in the counseling department who has been contracted through the local hospital to help troubled teens, after they are discharged from the hospital's behavioral health program, get back to school. The occupational therapist splits her time between the high school and the hospital, where she provides primarily outpatient services.

Martin has never been hospitalized before, but he is friends with several of the boys his age who work with the occupational therapist. These friends had expressed their concern about Martin to her and were worried that Martin was suicidal, especially when he became drunk. The occupational therapist stopped Martin in the hall and told him his friends were concerned and that she was available to talk to him if he would like to do so. She handed him several pamphlets with questions to help him determine whether he had a drinking problem. Martin appeared angry and walked away, causing her to believe he might be in the precontemplation stage of change. Several hours later, Martin came to the office of the occupational therapist and told her he thought he needed help. Apparently, the brief intervention with the pamphlets was helpful. She could see that he was contemplating change and was starting to move into the determination stage. The occupational therapist screened him for suicidal thoughts and their lethality. The results were positive, indicating Martin was planning to shoot himself with his father's shotgun.

The occupational therapist immediately reported the problem to the principal, who contacted the parents. The parents came to the school and talked to the principal and the occupational therapist, who planned to implement a modified version of the FRAMES approach to motivational interviewing. It was important to motivate the parents to take action; however, the parents were not convinced that Martin had a problem. During the meeting, Martin persuaded his parents that he was only having a "bad day." Martin was still in the contemplation stage where he was obviously ambivalent about what he should do. His parents believed he was just "going through a phase." At this point, the occupational therapist provided Martin's parents with information about the signs and symptoms of suicide and the importance of taking such threats seriously. At the minimum, removal of potential weapons and protection of the individual was absolutely essential. Martin's father said he would remove the shotgun from the house and both parents would watch Martin carefully. The principal gave Martin's parents a statement to sign, indicating they had been informed of the screening results, given information about suicide, and that further evaluation to determine intervention needs had been recommended by the school personnel. Additionally, the parents acknowledged receipt of information regarding community resources for evaluation and intervention.

Martin's parents did take him to the emergency room three days later because he had three successive nights of drinking binges, which affected his ability to attend school. During these binges, he was becoming increasingly threatening and aggressive toward his parents and siblings. In this way, Martin demonstrated movement into the determination and action stages of change. His behavior forced change to occur.

Martin was hospitalized a total of three days for the purpose of detoxification and assessment of his potential depression. During the first 24 hours of hospitalization, Martin spent most of the time in bed. He was somnolent and complained of severe stomach cramping, dry mouth, and headache. During the second day, Martin participated in an evaluation with the occupational therapist he had met at the high school. Martin seemed genuinely glad to see her. He admitted that her caring and insistence that he needed help impressed him. He was angry with his parents for not believing that anything was wrong. Martin indicated that he hated school and found it boring. He admitted that his academic performance had declined since entering high school to a grade point average of 1.2 out of a possible 4.0. He had received As and Bs in middle school. He reported meeting with one of the guidance counselors and stated that they had set academic goals for improvement. Martin stated he had made little effort to meet these goals. Martin had spent a month in an alternative school during his sophomore year due to excessive tardiness and absences. He reported his freshman year went much better as he had enjoyed track and field and had participated in the photography club. When asked what changed from his freshman to his sophomore year, Martin admitted that he had started drinking heavily in the summer between these two years and that, once school started, he could not stop.

The occupational therapist stated she would meet with Martin prior to his discharge home to develop an intervention plan he would follow during his outpatient occupational therapy and his follow-up therapy in the school. Additionally, the occupational therapist explained to Martin that it was important for him to actively cope with his withdrawal symptoms while he was in the hospital by using a variety of relaxation techniques. She pointed out that she had read reports indicating that those who used these techniques actually stayed in recovery longer. She gave Martin relaxation tapes and a tape recorder and a list of instructions. They went to his room and she supervised one session of using the tapes.

Prior to going home, Martin and the occupational therapist developed a plan where he was expected to attend daily occupational therapy groups for the purpose of examining his daily routine to assess the way in which his day was organized around his drinking. The plan reinforced that Martin was in the action stage of change and needed to be responsible for making decisions regarding the important actions that would lead to his recovery. Martin noted during this assessment that as his drinking progressed, he stopped seeing many of his friends, he only interacted with other boys who drank, he refused to participate in family activities, and he stopped regularly attending school or any extracurricular activities. Martin also identified the current stressors in his life that might cause his desire to drink to become out of control. With the help of the occupational therapist and the group members, Martin also identified the cues in his environment that might exacerbate a craving for alcohol. The occupational therapy group sessions focused on coping skills development to reduce the stressors and on methods to decrease his reactivity to drinking cues. Martin also developed a daily routine that included spending time with his nondrinking friends, going to church with his family, taking pictures and developing his photographs, and completing his schoolwork. Martin was encouraged to share his experiences in these daily activities with the group so that they could give him positive feedback regarding his ability to use coping strategies. The idea that even during enjoyable activities, it is normal to experience cravings and daily hassles was discussed.

As Martin progressed, he returned to school and his outpatient groups were discontinued. In their place, Martin attended follow-up groups at school with the same occupational therapist. The purpose of the follow-up programming was to support positive behavioral changes made within the school environment, assist him in gradually learning to cope with the normal stress of being in school and coming into contact with those with whom he drank, and monitor any signs of relapse. Martin did enter the relapse stage of change as he had a slip where he drank a beer with an old friend after school. Through the help of the occupational therapist, he was able to implement his recovery strategies of calling his group members for support, going to an AA meeting immediately following the slip, and engaging in an enjoyable activity that helped him experience satisfaction and relaxation without the use of alcohol.

 ## CONCLUSION

Occupational therapy practitioners working in community settings have a tremendous potential to provide an occupation-focused perspective on helping individuals who struggle with substance use disorders by enhancing their occupational performance in environments that support their health and meaningful occupational roles.

Occupational therapy intervention includes the following main approaches:

- Targeting change in occupational performance of the individual using substances and of the family members affected by the substance use of others
- Identifying occupations that are satisfying and that can compete with the positive affect previously attributed to use of the substance
- Removing barriers that interfere with abstinence, such as methods for resolving the financial problems typical for persons with substance use disorders
- Helping the individual make environmental changes that are conducive to abstinence and that compensate for performance component impairments
- Developing coping skills that assist the individual in responding to temptations and cravings and to typical daily hassles and frustrations with occupational performance

 ## STUDY QUESTIONS

1. Define the following terms: substance dependence, tolerance, withdrawal, compulsive drug-taking behavior, substance abuse, and problem drinking.

2. Describe the impact of substance use disorders on occupational behavior.

3. Explain the stages of change and how they impact intervention in substance use disorders.

4. Identify three types of community-based interventions for substance use disorders and describe the benefits and limitations of each type.

5. What unique contributions can occupational therapy provide in community-based programs for substance use disorders?

REFERENCES

Alcoholics Anonymous World Services. (1976). *Alcoholics Anonymous* (3rd ed.). New York: AA.

Alcoholics Anonymous World Services. (1970). *A member's-eye view of Alcoholics Anonymous.* New York: Author.

Alcoholics Anonymous World Services. (1996). *Alcoholics Anonymous 1995 membership survey.* New York: Author.

American Occupational Therapy Association. (1994). *Uniform terminology* (3rd ed.). Bethesda, MD: Author.

American Psychiatric Association. (1994). *Diagnostic and statistical manual of mental disorders, fourth edition (DSM IV).* Washington, DC: Author.

Babor, T.F., Ritson, E.B., and Hodgson, R.J. (1986). Alcohol-related problems in the primary health care setting: A review of early intervention strategies. *British Journal of Addiction, 81,* 23–46.

Christiansen, C., Clark, F., Kielhofner, G., and Rogers, J. (1995). Occupation: A position paper. *American Journal of Occupational Therapy, 49,* 1015–1018.

Christopher, J. (1989). *Unhooked. Staying sober and drug free.* New York: Prometheus Books.

Clark, F., Wood, W., and Larson, E. (1998). Occupational science: Occupational therapy's legacy for the 21st century. In M.E. Neistadt and E.B. Crepeau (Eds.), *Willard and Spackman's occupational therapy* (9th ed., pp. 13–21). Philadelphia: Lippincott.

Cooney, N.L., Zweben, A., and Fleming, M.F. (1995). Screening for alcohol problems and at-risk drinking in health-care settings. In R.K. Hester and W.R. Miller (Eds.), *Handbook of alcoholism treatment approaches: Effective alternatives* (2nd ed., pp. 45–60). Boston: Allyn and Bacon.

Dickey, B., and Azeni, H. (1996). Persons with dual diagnoses of substance abuse and major mental illness: Their excess costs of psychiatric care. *American Journal of Public Health, 86,* 973–977.

Doweiko, H.F. (1993). *Concepts of chemical dependency* (2nd ed.). Pacific Grove, CA: Brooks/Cole.

Emrick, C., Tonigan, J.S., Montgomery, H., and Little, L. (1993). Alcoholics Anonymous: What is currently known? In B.S. McCrady and W.R. Miller (Eds.), *Research on Alcoholics Anonymous: Opportunities and alternatives* (pp. 41–76). New Brunswick, NJ: Alcohol Research Documentation, Rutgers, the State University of New Jersey.

Ewing, J. (1984). Detecting alcoholism: The CAGE questionnaire. *Journal of the American Medical Association, 252,* 1905–1907.

Finney, J.W., and Monahan, S.C. (1996). The cost-effectiveness of treatment for alcoholism: A second approximation. *Journal of Studies on Alcohol, 57,* 229–243.

Finney, J.W., and Moos, R.H. (1992). The long-term course of treated alcoholism: II. Predictors and correlates of 10-year functioning and mortality. *Journal of Studies on Alcohol, 53,* 142–153.

Grinspoon, L. and Bakalar, J.B. (1990). Alcohol abuse and dependence. *Harvard Medical School Mental Health Review, 2,* 1–20.

Heather, N. (1995). Brief intervention strategies. In R.K. Hester and W.R. Miller (Eds.), *Handbook of alcoholism treatment approaches: Effective alternatives* (2nd ed., pp. 105–122). Boston: Allyn and Bacon.

Hester, R.K. (1995). Behavioral self-control training. In R.K. Hester and W.R. Miller (Eds.), *Handbook of alcoholism treatment approaches: Effective alternatives* (2nd ed., pp. 148–159). Boston: Allyn and Bacon.

Hubbard, J.R., Everett, A.S., and Khan, M.A. (1996). Alcohol and drug abuse in patients with physical disabilities. *American Journal of Drug and Alcohol Abuse, 22,* 215–231.

Humphreys, K., and Moos, R.H. (1996). Reduced substance-abuse-related health care costs among voluntary participants in Alcoholics Anonymous. *Psychiatric Services, 47,* 709–713.

Chapter 16 / Community-Based Approaches for Substance Use Disorders

341

Humphreys, K., Moos, R.H., and Cohen, C. (1997). Social and community resources and long-term recovery from treated and untreated alcoholism. Journal of Studies on Alcohol, 58, 231–238.

Humphreys, K., Moos, R.H., and Finney, J.W. (1996). Life domains, Alcoholics Anonymous, and role incumbency in the 3-year course of problem drinking. Journal of Nervous Mental Disorders, 184, 475–481.

Jackson, J., Carlson, M., Mandel, D., Zemke, R., and Clark, F. (1998). Occupation in lifestyle redesign: The well elderly study occupational therapy program. American Journal of Occupational Therapy, 52, 326–336.

Johnston, L.D., et al. (1997). Monitoring the future study. East Lansing, MI: Institute for Social Research, University of Michigan.

Kaplan, H.I., and Sadock, B.J. (1996). Concise textbook of clinical psychiatry. Baltimore: Williams and Wilkins.

Kielhofner, G. (1995). A model of human occupation: Theory and application (2nd ed.). Baltimore: Williams and Wilkins.

Kwapil, T.R. (1996). A longitudinal study of drug and alcohol use by psychosis-prone and impulsive-nonconforming individuals. Journal of Abnormal Psychology, 105, 114–123.

Marlatt, G. A. (1985). Cognitive assessment and intervention procedures for relapse prevention. In G.A. Marlatt and J.R. Gordon (Eds.), Relapse prevention: Maintenance strategies in the treatment of addictive behaviors (pp. 201–279). New York: Guilford.

Mattingly, C., and Fleming, M. (1994). Clinical reasoning: Forms of inquiry in a therapeutic practice. Philadelphia: F. A. Davis.

McCrady, B.S., and Miller, W.R. (1993). Research on Alcoholics Anonymous: Opportunities and alternatives. New Brunswick, NJ: Alcohol Research Documentation, Rutgers, the State University of New Jersey.

Miller, W.R. (1995). Increasing motivation for change. In R.K. Hester and W.R. Miller (Eds.), Handbook of alcoholism treatment approaches: Effective alternatives (2nd ed., pp. 88–104). Boston: Allyn and Bacon.

Miller, W.R. (1998). Researching the spiritual dimensions of alcohol and other drug problems. Addiction, 93, 979–990.

Miller, W.R., and Cooney, N.L. (1994). Designing studies to investigate client-treatment matching. Journal of Studies on Alcohol, Supplement, 12, 38–45.

Miller, W.R., and Munoz, R.F. (1982). How to control your drinking (Rev. ed.). Albuquerque, NM: University of New Mexico Press.

Miller, W.R., and Sanchez, V.C. (1994). Motivating young adults for treatment and lifestyle change. In G. Howard (Ed.), Issues in alcohol use and misuse by young adults (pp. 55–82). Notre Dame, IN: University of Notre Dame Press.

Miller, W.R., Zweben, A., DiClemente, C.C., and Rychtarik, R.G. (1992). Motivational enhancement therapy (MET): A clinical research guide for therapists treating individuals with alcohol abuse and dependence (DHHS Publication N. ADM 92-1894). Washington, DC: U.S. Government Printing Office.

Moos, R.H., Finney, J.W., and Cronkite, C. (1990). Alcoholism treatment: Context, process, and outcome. New York: Oxford University Press.

Moyers, P.A. (1991). Occupational therapy and treatment of the alcoholic's family. Occupational Therapy in Mental Health, 11, 45–64.

Moyers, P.A. (1992a). Substance abuse: A multidimensional assessment and treatment approach. Thorofare, NJ: Slack.

Moyers, P.A. (1992b). Occupational therapy intervention with the alcoholic's family. American Journal of Occupational Therapy, 46, 105–111.

Moyers, P.A. (1997). Occupational meanings and spirituality: The quest for sobriety. American Journal of Occupational Therapy, 51(3), 207–214.

Moyers, P.A., and Barrett, C.E. (1992). Neurocognition and alcoholism: Implications for occupational therapy. In S.C. Merrill (Ed.), Occupational therapy and psychosocial dysfunction (pp. 87–115). Binghamton, NY: Haworth.

Moyers, P.A., Jones, B.E., Mirchandani, T., and Sherwood, E. (1993). Working in the school system with children whose parents are alcoholic. Occupational Therapy Practice, 4(2), 39–60.

Moyers, P.A., and Stoffel, V.C. (1999). Alcohol dependence in a client with a work-related injury. American Journal of Occupational Therapy, 53(6), 640–645.

National Institute on Alcohol Abuse and Alcoholism. (1994). Alcohol Health and Research World AHRW, 18(3), 243, 245.

National Center for Health Statistics. (1991). Advance Data, USDHHS, No. 205, September 30, p. 1.

Ouimette, P.C., Moos, R.H., and Finney, J.W. (1998). Influence of outpatient treatment and 12-step group involvement on one-year substance abuse treatment outcomes. *Journal of Studies on Alcohol, 59*, 513–522.

Pinger, R.R., Payne, W.A., Hahn, D.B., and Hahn, E.J. (1998). *Drugs: Issues for today.* Boston: McGraw-Hill.

Pollack, E.J. (1996, September 9). HMOs push cheaper, short-term rehab. *The Wall Street Journal,* pp. B1, B8.

Prochaska, J.O., and DiClemente, C.C. (1982). Transtheoretical therapy: Toward a more integrative model of change. *Psychotherapy: Theory, Research, and Practice, 19,* 276–288.

Prochaska, J.O., and DiClemente, C.C. (1986). Toward a comprehensive model of change. In W.R. Miller and N. Heather (Eds.), *Treating addictive behaviors: Process of change* (pp. 3–27). New York: Plenum.

Roehrich, L., and Goldman, M.S. (1993). Experience-dependent neuropsychological recovery and the treatment of alcoholism. *Journal of Consulting and Clinical Psychology, 61,* 812–821.

Rollnick, S., and Bell, A. (1991). Brief motivational interviewing for use by the nonspecialist. In W.R. Miller and S. Rollnick (Eds.), *Motivational interviewing: Preparing people to change addictive behavior* (pp. 203–213). New York: Guilford.

Rotunda, R.J., Scherer, D.G., and Imm, P.S. (1995). Family systems and alcohol misuse: Research on the effects of alcoholism on family functioning and effective family interventions. *Professional Psychology: Research and Practice, 26,* 95–104.

Rumpf, H.J., Hapke, U., Erfurth, A., and John, U. (1998). Screening questionnaires in the detection of hazardous alcohol consumption in the general hospital: Direct or disguised assessment? *Journal of Studies on Alcohol, 59,* 698–703.

Selzer, M.L. (1971). The Michigan alcoholism screening test: The quest for a new diagnostic instrument. *American Journal of Psychiatry, 127,* 1653–1658.

Sobell, L.C., Cunningham, J.A., and Sobell, M.B. (1996). Recovery from alcohol problems with and without treatment: Prevalence in two population surveys. *American Journal of Public Health, 86,* 966–972.

Soderstrom, C.B., and Cowley, R.A. (1987). A national alcohol and trauma center survey. *Archives of Surgery, 122,* 1067–1071.

Stoffel, V.C. (1992). The Americans with Disabilities Act of 1990 as applied to an adult with alcohol dependence. *American Journal of Occupational Therapy, 46,* 640–644.

Stoffel, V.C. (1994). Occupational therapist's roles in treating substance abuse. *Hospital and Community Psychiatry, 45,* 21–22.

Stoffel, V.C., and Moyers, P.A. (1997). *Occupational therapy practice guidelines for substance use disorders.* Bethesda, MD: The American Occupational Therapy Association.

Tarter, R.E., and Vanykov, M. (1994). Alcoholism: A developmental disorder. *Journal of Consulting and Clinical Psychology, 62,* 1096–1107.

Trimpey, J. (1992). *The small book: A revolutionary alternative for overcoming alcohol and drug dependence* (3rd ed.). New York: Delacorte.

U.S. Department of Health and Human Services Public Health Service. (1998). *National household survey on drug abuse.* Washington, DC: U.S. Department of Health and Human Services.

U.S. Department of Health and Human Services Public Health Service. (1999). *National household survey on drug abuse.* Washington, DC: U.S. Department of Health and Human Services.

Weisner, C.J. (1995, June). Distinctive features of the alcohol treatment system. *Frontlines: Linking Alcohol Services Research and Practice,* 1–2.

Wilcock, A. (1998). *An occupational perspective of health.* Thorofare, NJ: Slack.

Wilcock, A. (1993). A theory of the human need for occupation. *Occupational Science: Australia, 1,* 17–24.

Women for Sobriety. (1976). *AA and WFS.* Quakertown, PA: Women for Sobriety.

Zweben, A., and Rose, S.J. (1999). Innovations in treating alcohol problems. In D. Biegel and A. Blum (Eds.), *Innovations in practice and service delivery with vulnerable populations* (pp. 197–227). New York: Oxford University Press.

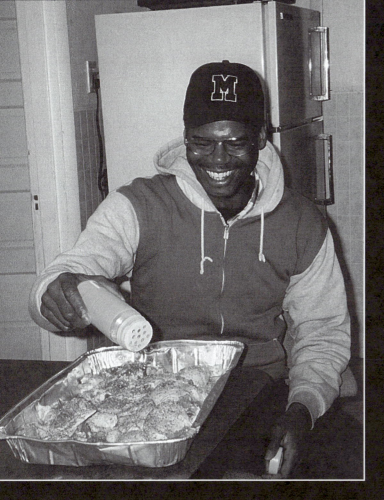

SECTION

Looking Ahead

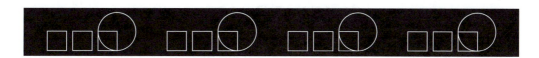

17

CHAPTER

Future Directions in Community-Based Practice

Marjorie E. Scaffa, PhD, OTR, FAOTA
Vanessa Russell, OTR
Carol A. Brownson, MSPH

■ OUTLINE

Assisted living
Aquatic therapy
Case management
Community foundation
Contract
Corporate foundation
Ecological worldview
Entrepreneur
Ergonomics
Family foundation
Forensic medicine

Four P's
Funding
Grant
Hippotherapy
Horticulture therapy
Integration
National general purpose
    foundation
Reimbursement
Self-assertion
Special purpose foundation

LEARNING OBJECTIVES

This chapter is designed to enable the reader to:
- Discuss the principles of futurist thinking.
- Describe the characteristics of an ecological worldview, applying it to community-based practice.
- Identify strategies that occupational therapy practitioners can use to develop ideas for community-based practice.
- Describe the role of occupational therapy in each of the different types of community-based programs.
- Compare and contrast the terms "funding" and "reimbursement."
- Discuss the potential sources of funding for community-based programs.
- Describe how the "four P's" of marketing apply to community practice.

> What we see depends on how we look.
>
> Capra and Steindl-Rast (1991)

 ## INTRODUCTION

In ancient Greece and Rome, an oracle was a place where, or a medium by which, deities were consulted for advice or prophecy about the future. The modern futurist movement, which began in the 1960s, was fueled by the desire to understand and shape the future and is guided by three basic principles (Cornish, 1980). The first principle, or conviction, is the unity or interrelatedness of reality. It is the perception that the whole is greater than the sum of its parts, an insistence on the interconnectedness of everything in the universe (Cornish, 1980).

The second principle that directs futurist thinking is the crucial importance of time. The world of the future is shaped by the decisions made today and the determinations made in the past (Cornish, 1980). Futurists believe that almost anything can be accomplished in a period of 20 years.

The third principle on which futurists rely is the importance and power of ideas, particularly ideas about the future. The future is created out of ideas, the tools of thought. Without them, change is not possible. Futurists believe that human achievement is constrained more by conceptual restrictions or limitations in our ideas than by our access to material resources (Cornish, 1980).

346

Some advocate that the profession should *re-create* or *re-invent* itself. However, this is not the only available choice of action. An alternative is to embrace a vision that incorporates the fundamental principles of the profession, with its focus on occupation and one that *expands* the scope of practice to include populations not typically served in settings not commonly utilized. The profession would not be where it is today if it had not survived the challenges of the past century. Thus, it is not possible or desirable to discard what has been part of the profession's heritage.

What occupational therapy needs most to move forward in the 21st century is creative ideas and thoughtful decisions put into action. Only in this way can the profession fulfill its destiny as "health agent" (Finn, 1972), enhance community health, and facilitate "community occupational development" (Bockhoven, 1968).

 ## AN ECOLOGICAL WORLDVIEW

To become health agents, occupational therapy practitioners must make a paradigm shift from a holistic perspective to an **ecological worldview.** "An ecological worldview is holistic, but it's more than that. It looks not only at something as a whole, but also how this whole is embedded into larger wholes" (Capra and Steindl-Rast, 1991, p. 69). Ecological awareness recognizes the interrelatedness and interdependence of all phenomena.

The root of the word "ecological" comes from the Greek "oikos," which means house. In a broader context, it refers to "the inhabited world, the house of humanity" (Capra and Steindl-Rast, 1991, p. 70). The house of humanity includes the biological, psychological, and spiritual aspects of life embedded in a physical, social, and cultural reality. The shift to an ecological paradigm reflects not only a change in thinking but also a change in values. Overall, the shift in values is characterized by a shift from *self-assertion* to *integration* (Capra and Steindl-Rast, 1991). **Self-assertion** is a living system's tendency toward domination in an effort to preserve and protect itself, while **integration** is the tendency to partner with other systems in order to fulfill the greater good. Table 17–1 provides a synopsis of the changes in values required by the ecological paradigm.

Self-assertion is not completely lost in the ecological paradigm because it is essential for survival. However, left unchecked, self-assertion can become destructive, evidenced by the variety of community health problems, such as violence, poverty, racism, homelessness, substance abuse, and destruction of the environment, experienced today. Self-assertion must be tempered with integration to be useful and healthy. Koestler (1978) speaks of this dichotomy as the *Janus* nature. A living system is an integrated whole that asserts itself to protect its individuality. However, as part of a larger whole, the living system is required to integrate itself into the larger system. "It is important to realize that those are opposite and contradictory tendencies. We need a dynamic balance between them, and that's essential for physical and mental health" (Capra and Steindl-Rast, 1991, p. 74).

 ## CREATING OPPORTUNITIES IN THE COMMUNITY

To develop creative ideas for community-based practice, one must simply be observant, open-minded, and reflective. Opportunities are abundant, but one must know *where* to look and *how* to see potential. Getting to know the community and becoming involved in community affairs are necessary first steps. Volunteering one's time and talents begins the networking process. Communities typically have a variety of

TABLE 17–1

CHANGE IN PARADIGM, CHANGE IN VALUES

From a Holistic Perspective with an Emphasis On	To an Ecological Paradigm with an Emphasis On
Self-assertion	Integration
Rational thought	Intuitiveness
Analysis	Synthesis
Competition	Cooperation
Expansion	Conservation
Quantity	Quality
Domination	Partnership
Individuality	Community

groups, organizations, and agencies that need volunteers and may be potential recipients of occupational therapy services. Table 17–2 identifies a number of types of community groups that may benefit from occupational therapy expertise.

To be successful in community-based practice settings, practitioners must see themselves providing a wide range of interventions. Direct service to individuals is only a small part of what occupational therapy has to offer. In community-based practice, the client is often not an individual but rather a group, organization, agency, or collective. Potential interventions may include case management, training, consulting, program coordination, policy development, and advocacy. These levels of intervention and their strategies and goals are described in Table 17–3.

After selecting a target agency and identifying appropriate levels of intervention, the practitioner must develop a proposal for providing services. The proposal is a formal communication between the service provider and the potential recipient and/or funding source. A successful proposal typically:

● Addresses a significant problem
● Defines specific objectives
● Uses a creative, innovative approach
● Details well-conceived methods
● Requests funds in proportion to the scope of the project
● Establishes the credibility of the applicant
● Meets the deadline
● Is appropriate to the interests of the funding source
● Is written clearly and concisely
● Addresses what happens after funding ends

Effective community-based interventions share some characteristics in common with effective occupational therapy treatment for individuals. Both are client centered, involve the recipient of services in the planning and implementation of the intervention, utilize existing environmental resources, and prepare clients to become self-managers and self-advocates. Occupational therapy practitioners can learn much from the professional literature in health education and public health regarding the design and implementation of community health interventions. Basic principles of effective community interventions are listed in Box 17–1.

TABLE 17–2

SEARCHING FOR OPPORTUNITIES

Community Resource	Examples
Artistic organizations	Choral, theatrical, writing
Business organizations	Chamber of Commerce, neighborhood business associations, trade groups
Charitable groups and drives	Red Cross, Cancer Society, United Way
Church groups	Prayer groups; men's, women's, youth, and seniors' groups; religious social services
Community support groups	"Friends" of the library, nursing home, hospital auxiliaries
Elderly groups	Senior citizens centers, assisted living centers
Health and fitness groups	YMCA, YWCA, health clubs
Interest clubs	Garden clubs, Audubon Society, conservation clubs, pet owners
Local government	Town, township, fire department, emergency units, area agency on aging
Local media	Radio, newspaper, local-access cable TV
Mutual support (self-help) groups	Alcoholics Anonymous, Epilepsy Self-Help, Alzheimer's Association
Political organizations	Democrats, Republicans, caucuses
School groups	Printing club, PTA, child care
Service clubs	Kiwanis, Rotary, Lions, Shriners, Junior League, American Association of University Women
Social cause groups	Peace, rights, advocacy, service groups
Sports leagues	Bowling, swimming, baseball, fishing, volleyball
Veteran groups	American Legion, Amvets
Youth groups	4H, Future Farmers, Scouts

Source: McKnight and Kretzmann, in *Mapping Community Capacity* [1990, p. 39]. Institute for Policy Research, Northwestern University. With permission.

 INNOVATIVE IDEAS PUT INTO ACTION

Occupational therapy practitioners have begun to put some innovative ideas into action. These ideas and actions *expand* the scope of practice. Each of these examples, taken from recent literature, is described briefly. Some involve expansion of professional roles, some include populations not typically served, and others describe practice in settings not typically utilized.

CASE MANAGEMENT

Occupational therapy and case management share a common goal. They both seek to promote function. However, the way in which the goal is achieved differs somewhat. Occupational therapy practitioners typically work in a clinic or hospital while

TABLE 17-3

STRATEGIES, GOALS, AND LEVELS OF OCCUPATIONAL THERAPY INTERVENTION

Intervention Type	Strategy or Process	Goals/Outcomes	Target/Level
Direct service	Providing occupational therapy treatment	Improved occupational performance	Individual
Counseling	Helping people learn how to achieve personal goals, resolve problems, make decisions, or change behaviors	Goal attainment, healthy behaviors, empowerment	Individual, interpersonal
Case management	Coordinating care plans	Improved client outcomes, comprehensive, coordinated care	Individual, interpersonal, organizational
Education	Providing information and employing the methods, strategies, and tools that facilitate learning	Positive change in knowledge, attitude, or behavior	Individual, interpersonal, organizational, societal/ community, governmental/ policy
Training	Providing information to enhance a skill or process	Competence in targeted skills, processes, techniques	Individual, interpersonal, organizational
Consulting	Using the knowledge and experience of an "expert" to help a person or organizational leaders make better decisions or deal more effectively with situations	Problem solving in area of concern	Individual, interpersonal, organizational, societal/ community, governmental/ policy
Program development	Assessing the need for, planning, and evaluating programs and services	Improved services/ care for target population	Organizational, societal/ community
Program coordination	Managing the resources (staff, materials, space, finances, etc.) to accomplish the objectives of a program	Effective and efficient use of resources	Organizational, societal/ community, governmental/ policy

Intervention Type	Strategy or Process	Goals/Outcomes	Target/Level
Policy development	Formulating rules, laws, policies, procedures	Laws, rules, policies, and procedures that are favorable to area of concern	Governmental/policy
Advocacy	Using the power of persuasion to alter public opinion and mobilize resources in favor of a policy or issue	Favorable change in policies, regulations, resource allocation	Organizational, societal/community, governmental/policy
Research	Building knowledge through systematic study	Improved practice, evidence-based practice	Organizational, governmental/policy

Source: Washington University community practice model.

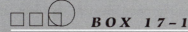

BOX 17-1

Principles of Effective Community Interventions

- Tailor to a specific population within a particular setting.
- Involve the participants in planning, implementation, and evaluation.
- Integrate efforts aimed at changing individuals, social and physical environments, communities, and policies.
- Link participants' concerns about health to broader life concerns and to a vision of a better society.
- Use existing resources within the environment.
- Build on strengths found among participants and their social networks and communities.
- Advocate for the resources and policy changes needed to achieve the desired health objectives.
- Prepare participants to become self-managers and self-advocates.
- Support the diffusion of innovation to a wider population.
- Seek to "institutionalize" successful components and to replicate them in other settings.

Source: Freudenberg, N., Eng, E., Flay, B., Parcel, G., Rogers, T., and Wallerstein, N. (1995). Strengthening individual and community capacity to prevent disease and promote health: In search of relevant theories and principles. *Health Education Quarterly, 22*(3), 290–306.

providing short-term treatment that focuses on physical abilities, cognition, perceptual-motor skills, and psychosocial function. On the other hand, **case management** uses a more generalized approach by combining occupational therapy concerns with much larger issues of the client's employment, financial situation, health status, and rehabilitation prognosis. Case managers are responsible for organizing all aspects of the person's care, from the onset of the disability, with no apparent termination date for services (Collins, 1998).

Jane Mattson, PhD, OTR/L, president of Mattson Associates in Connecticut, suggests that occupational therapy practitioners are often attracted to case management because it allows a long-term relationship with the client. Although case managers are typically nurses, other professionals, such as occupational therapists, are becoming more involved. The main disadvantage to nurse case managers is their lack of rehabilitation knowledge. Health maintenance organizations that currently use nurse case managers could hire occupational therapy practitioners who are more familiar with disabilities and traumatic injuries. Because the ultimate goal is to promote function, occupational therapists are equipped with a wide range of skills that could be advantageous in case management (Collins, 1998).

ENTREPRENEURS

Entrepreneurs are individuals who are willing to assume the risk of starting new business ventures without the guarantee of success. Effective entrepreneurs combine futuristic thinking with a reality-based orientation and good organizational and planning skills. Occupational therapy entrepreneurs are typically motivated to provide services that improve the quality of life of their clients.

Paging Services

Occupational therapy is a very rewarding field because practitioners are able to assist clients in reaching their optimal goals. As an entrepreneur, Dottie Halfaker, OTR, notes that she still experiences the satisfaction of helping others. Halfaker is the director of operations and co-owner of PageMinder, Inc., a service that sends messages to clients by pager (Johansson, 1999d). The clients taking advantage of the service range from 10 to 82 years of age. The PageMinder can serve the client as a reminder for scheduling medication dosing, daily living skills such as incontinence programs or medical appointments, and adherence to postsurgical recommendations.

This service attempts to provide the client with the opportunity for independent function, improved quality of life, and cost savings. PageMinder fees are about the same as a monthly cable service. Some insurers will cover the cost since the pager aids in maintaining self-care activities. While PageMinder services are advantageous to clients with memory deficits, they may also benefit clients who require adherence to complicated medical protocols such as those with brain injury, diabetes, human immunodeficiency virus/acquired immunodeficiency syndrome (HIV/AIDS), dementia, or stroke. The only limitation in using this pager system is that the client must be able to read and follow simple instructions (Johansson, 1999d).

Environmental Redesign Consultant

Karen Earith, OTR/L, who developed her own business in Dayton, Ohio, now enjoys helping people redesign their environments. About 75 percent of her clients are referred by the vocational rehabilitation department, which uses state funds to pay for the services. As the "baby boomers" age, the need for more supportive, "user-friendly" home environments will continue to increase. According to researchers at the University of Buffalo's Rehabilitation Engineering Research Center, those most in need of supportive services include adults with disabilities, family members providing care for aging relatives, and a growing older population who increasingly want to "age in place." While the future looks promising for Earith, the growth of her business is a result of excellent marketing strategies and community outreach (Johansson, 1999b).

Horticulture Center

Horticulture therapy is another option being explored by occupational therapy practitioners who are seeking new job opportunities. When Brenda Jesse, COTA/L, left her last job, she began creating her own nonprofit corporation and designing a gardening center for people with disabilities. Jesse uses horticulture therapy with her clients "to introduce and facilitate leisure and occupational skills to help people regain maximal function" (Diffendal, 1999, p. 30). The gardening center also offers welfare recipients the opportunity to volunteer and develop gardening, retail, and business skills. Future projects will provide job training and placement, therapeutic services, and opportunities for professional development (Diffendal, 1999).

Successful businesses and organizations share certain characteristics, including the ability to anticipate change, innovative thinking, and excellence (Barker, 1992). Some strategies for optimizing one's success as an entrepreneur, private practice, or business owner are outlined in Box 17–2.

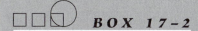

BOX 17–2

Tips for the Budding Entrepreneur

The experience of successful business owners provides some tips for OT practitioners thinking about following in their footsteps:

- Gain at least five years of clinical experience before you start.
- Take business and advanced practice courses and become an expert on payment and billing systems.
- Work for a year or two as an independent contractor or in another private practice in either another field or different geographic region.
- Seek out a business mentor and be prepared to mentor others in turn.
- Find an unmet need or unfilled niche.
- Plan to appeal to private and nonmedical payers, as well as traditional health insurance.
- Put aside a sufficient nest egg to carry you through at least the first year of the business.
- Start small and grow from there, perhaps keeping a salaried job while you get underway.
- Be prepared to put in long hours for as long as you remain in business.
- Establish an impeccable reputation and maintain visibility in the community.
- Network with other OT business owners to keep current and share ideas.
- Never rest on your laurels and never stop learning.

Source: Joe, B.E. (1998). Becoming an OT entrepreneur. *OT Week, 12*(46), p. 13. Copyright © 1998 by the American Occupational Therapy Association, Inc. Reprinted with permission.

CRIMINAL JUSTICE SYSTEM

Forensic medicine refers to the interface between health-care and the criminal justice system. Within the criminal justice system, state or federally operated prisons have mandated requirements to provide basic medical and psychiatric services. The type and amount of psychiatric services vary widely and may be provided by state mental health and/or correctional departments. As many as two-thirds of prison inmates are estimated to need psychiatric care at some point during incarceration. Psychiatric services may include prison-based inpatient units, day treatment, intermittent outpatient services, and special mental health prison programs (Dressler and Snively, 1998).

Occupational therapists may provide services in a variety of forensic facilities, including forensic hospitals, correctional institutions, and community programs for newly released prisoners. Forensic state hospitals are typically maximum security psychiatric facilities that serve individuals incompetent to stand trial, those found not guilty by reason of insanity, and those held criminally responsible but who are mentally ill. The state correctional institution in Vacaville, California, houses 3000 men, 400 of whom are psychiatric inmates. The psychiatric unit at Vacaville provides occupational therapy services. Its goal is to assist inmates to function effectively and productively within the restricted environment of the prison. To function safely in prison, inmates need to be hypervigilant to environmental cues, develop a high frustration tolerance, and be cautious about how they interact with other inmates and prison guards. The average length of stay in the psychiatric unit is four and a half months. Diagnoses seen by occupational therapists include schizophrenia, polysubstance abuse, bipolar disorder, depression, personality disorders (particularly borderline and antisocial), and mental retardation (Dressler and Snively, 1998).

Community-based correctional programs are designed for newly released prisoners, those on probation or parole, and individuals in conditional release programs. Riverside and San Bernardino counties in California have conditional release day treatment programs with an occupational therapy component. The average length of stay in these conditional release programs is two and a half years. Community-based forensic programs are designed to prevent relapse and/or reoffense and to enhance stabilization in the community. The role of the occupational therapy practitioner in these programs is to develop independent living skills and job skills and to assess the level of supervision required (Dressler and Snively, 1998).

Occupational therapists working in forensic settings need some specialized skills. Practitioners must understand the environmental demands of prison life, including its unique culture and norms. They must pay special attention to personal safety and security issues and store occupational therapy tools and supplies carefully and securely to prevent dangerous misuse. Due to the high rates of HIV, tuberculosis, and hepatitis in the prison population, infection control procedures must be followed stringently, particularly when engaging in some activities of daily living such as grooming and food preparation. In addition, occupational therapy practitioners must learn the jargon of the criminal justice system to develop effective relationships with nonmedical staff such as sheriffs, prison guards, and parole officers who do not share a therapeutic orientation (Dressler and Snively, 1998).

Sharon Dishongh, MBA, OTR, is a Texas native currently working as the senior warden at a correctional facility in Rusk, Texas. She is the director of a program designed to provide both security and rehabilitation for inmates with mental illness and/or mental retardation. Dishongh reports many behavioral similarities between patients in a state hospital and the offenders she works with in the prison. About 85 percent of the inmates have committed drug-related offenses, and many have been gang members. Inmates who improve may be sent to a regular prison or a state hospital to complete their sentences. Inmates are encouraged to participate in music, recreation, education, and work therapy in addition to attending occupational therapy sessions (Joe, 1999).

ASSISTED LIVING FACILITIES

Assisted living, a trend that is becoming more common with the ever-aging population of baby boomers, is generally defined as "group residential programs—not licensed as nursing homes—that provide scheduled and unscheduled assistance with activities of daily living" (Haggerty, 1998, p. 21). Assisted living facilities (ALFs) were created for elderly individuals in need of some assistance but who did not yet require 24-hour nursing care. Residents have the opportunity to rent their own apartment or share one with a spouse or friend while being allowed to remain in a favorable, home-like environment. Currently, more than 1 million senior citizens are taking advantage of the services offered by ALFs such as daily meals, assistance with basic activities of daily living, transportation to doctors and community outings, and planned recreational activities. The resident may also need or decide to contract for additional health-care services, including occupational therapy (OT), physical therapy (PT), speech therapy, skilled nursing, hospice, and specialized interventions.

The National Investment Conference (NIC) estimates that 9 million Americans will be in need of long-term care services in the year 2000 (Zuckerman, 1998). Unlike nursing homes that are regulated by the federal government and may be paid for by Medicare and Medicaid, consumer-driven ALFs are licensed by the states and are primarily a private-pay industry. State regulations mandate the level of care ALFs may render and under what conditions specialized services may be provided by therapists. To meet this challenge, rehabilitation professionals must create a system that enables them to maximize services to multiple ALFs within a specific geographic region. With more senior citizens seeking "to age in place," rehabilitation professionals must design their services to appeal to managed-care providers and establish successful partnerships with ALFs (Zuckerman, 1998).

APARTMENT PROGRAMS

With today's managed-care and economic demands, occupational therapy practitioners are encouraged to seek new opportunities in community-based settings that provide rehabilitative services in outpatient, day treatment, and residential settings. Occupational therapists could offer services to individuals with chronic physical and mental illnesses who reside in apartment programs.

Harvest Homes

The Prairie Harvest Human Services Foundation (PHF) of Grand Forks, North Dakota, serves citizens living within the community by offering part-time assistance with activities of daily living, transportation, shopping, and budgeting as needed. The PHF received funding from the U.S. Department of Housing and Urban Development to build a 12-plex apartment building called Harvest Homes (HH). This complex houses individuals who need a more protective housing situation and require 24-hour services. Both direct and indirect occupational therapy services are provided to meet the needs of the residents (Zimmerman, 1999).

Occupational therapy needs are determined through an evaluation process that includes the Kohlman Evaluation of Living Skills (KELS) and the Allen Cognitive Level Test (ACL). The KELS determines if the client is able to function independently in his or her environment. The ACL evaluates cognitive ability as it relates to independent functioning in ADLs. The primary goal of occupational therapy intervention was to improve independent living skills of the clients. In addition to providing direct treatment, the occupational therapy practitioner could also render case consultation, specifying the need for occupational therapy services through an evaluation summary. With the skills necessary to be leaders in the delivery of community mental health services, practitioners must seek out new opportunities and become involved with community projects such as the Prairie Harvest Human Services Foundation and Harvest Homes (Zimmerman, 1999).

Vanderbilt Apartments

Jenny Womack, MS, OTR/L, serves as the resident services coordinator at the Vanderbilt Apartments in downtown Asheville, North Carolina. The complex, home to 150 elderly individuals, consists of 158 units, primarily efficiency apartments that include kitchenettes and bathrooms. Many of the residents in this program have physical and mental disabilities and fall below the income guidelines for housing. Grant monies provided by three local philanthropic foundations and two national foundations fund the program. Efforts are focused in three areas: (1) community programming, (2) individual needs evaluation and intervention, and (3) program development. Community involvement and individual intervention are directed by the needs and interests of the residents themselves using a client-centered approach. According to Womack (1999, p. 3), overall program development has consisted of providing:

- direct involvement in community groups working to address the needs of senior citizens,
- visiting home health care providers to offer collaboration with their staff members who are serving the residents,
- networking with other community agencies in order to access their services, and
- forming an advisory group to develop and implement methods of evaluating the program.

One advantage for occupational therapy practitioners working in this type of setting is the lack of institutional reimbursement structures and policies. Womack states that she is able to prioritize her time with residents based on the problem to be addressed and follow up as necessary without the constraints of reimbursement found in other settings.

ERGONOMICS

The challenge for occupational therapy practitioners is to discover unique ways to utilize their skills, abilities, and training and enter into new practice arenas, as noted by the American Occupational Therapy Association president, Karen Jacobs (Johansson, 1999a). **Ergonomics,** the science of equipment and environmental design to enhance productivity, is a field where occupational therapists are gaining ground and becoming a vital resource. However, if a therapist is interested in the field of ergonomics, special training is required and available through continuing education courses (Le Postollec, 1999). "Occupational therapy combines the necessary skills of interviewing workers, analyzing activities, understanding symptoms and then putting together the whole picture in terms of roles, performance components, and functional impairment" (Johansson, 1999a, p. 8). Occupational therapy programs can be established to aid in the prevention of repetitive motion injuries in certain on-the-job tasks. Most businesses are willing to spend the money on programs that will reduce their workers' compensation costs. California companies that have implemented ergonomic programs have witnessed the benefits of fewer injuries and lower workers' compensation rates (Johansson, 1999a).

Many individuals work at jobs that require a great deal of strenuous physical activity. Therefore, a workplace fitness program may be instituted to help workers avoid developing cumulative trauma disorders (CTDs). CTDs are typically neuromusculoskeletal in nature, for example, lumbar disk herniation, carpal tunnel syndrome, and tendonitis. Practitioners can teach workers simple flexibility, strengthening, and stretching exercises that can be performed at the job site. In many cases, fitness activities can be incorporated into the employees' daily routine, performing the exercises at their workstations. Evidence supports that healthier, fit individuals are less likely to develop CTDs and other injuries. Consultation services can also be provided to a company through in-service training on body mechanics and posture, stress management, stretch breaks and relaxation, and job-specific strengthening programs (Blaz, 1998).

Ergonomics consultant Audrey Morris, of Carmel, California, began her own business as a result of her disappointment with the therapy services patients were receiving in hospitals. She also noticed that the workers' compensation system failed to address the prevention of work-related injuries. Morris now provides consultations with managers and workers, work-site assessments, and assistance in determining reasonable accommodations for employees with special needs. In addition, she offers workshops that emphasize posture and exercise programs and stress management for office workers and manual laborers (Johansson, 1999a).

Sallie Taylor, MEd, OTR, and Donna Hoelscher, OTR, joined forces and started an ergonomics consulting business in Missouri called Safesite. Services offered by Safesite do not require a physician's referral and are usually paid for by the businesses. In addition to providing consultation to area businesses, Taylor and Hoelscher are also devoted to helping other therapists start their own consultation services. Ergonomics consulting is a great option for practitioners in search of new job opportunities because it involves evaluation, activity analysis, goal setting, and problem-solving skills (Johansson, 1999a).

DRIVING PROGRAMS

The overall concern about safety and mobility has significantly increased in recent years due to the aging population. According to the American Association of Motor Vehicle Administrators (AAMVA), one in five drivers will be over the age of 65 by the year 2020 (Johansson, 1999c). State agencies have a responsibility to guarantee that elderly or disabled drivers who can safely remain on the road are not prohibited from doing so. Some states have already begun to change their policies toward older drivers by requiring more frequent testing. Connecticut was the first state to introduce the "voluntary graduated license," which allows the elderly or disabled person to continuing driving with certain restrictions. Restrictions may include day driving only, use of corrective lenses, or operating vehicles equipped with special controls or devices (Johansson, 1999c).

John Eberhard, a U.S. Department of Transportation research psychologist, suggests that there are many opportunities for intervention due to the increase in the number of older drivers and their dependence on the automobile (Berg, 1998). A qualified occupational therapist can perform an evaluation and provide driver training to ensure the safety of the individual. Medicare and most automobile insurance companies do not cover these services. However, funding may be available through various grants or by family members paying out of pocket on a fee-for-service basis.

Bert Sorkin was faced with the possibility of never driving again when he suffered a stroke. Sorkin was able to regain 80 to 90 percent of his old abilities through rehabilitation. Sorkin enrolled in a program designed by Linda Hunt, OTR/L, to retrain elderly drivers. After a few weeks in the program and a number of times behind the wheel of the training car, Sorkin was ready to return to driving using a steering wheel knob, or "spinner," adaptation. Hunt started the program with funding from General Motors under a settlement agreement between the car manufacturer and the U.S. Department of Transportation (Berg, 1998).

AQUATIC THERAPY

Water activities provide the client with an opportunity to achieve a wide variety of occupational therapy goals in a playful yet relaxing atmosphere. **Aquatic therapy** uses the unique properties of water as a therapeutic environment. When provided by an occupational therapist, the following are characteristic: a holistic approach, an individual treatment plan that incorporates functional and occupational goals, and the use of sensory integration techniques (Joe, 1998a). However, to provide aquatic therapy, specialized training is required. This training may be obtained through workshops provided by the American Occupational Therapy Association (AOTA). Currently more than 400 individuals are involved in AOTA's aquatic therapy network (Joe, 1998a). Aquatic therapy is useful with a wide variety of clients, including breast cancer survivors, individuals with physical disabilities, and persons with developmental delay.

Aquatic therapy can help breast cancer survivors return to normal activities by improving range of motion, strength, and confidence. A successful aquatic therapy program for breast cancer survivors should address the following goals:

1. Improved cardiovascular fitness
2. Increased range of motion in the shoulder
3. Prevention or reduction of lymphedema
4. Decreased stress and promotion of wellness
5. Provision of a positive social environment (Essert, 1998)

The occupational therapy practitioner should provide a supportive group atmosphere and promote openness within the group. The therapist working with breast cancer survivors fulfills a variety of roles such as educator, motivator, and listener.

Aquatic therapy is very useful in treating clients with a wide range of physical disabilities, including arthritis, neuromuscular disorders, and spinal cord injury. Caryn Johnson, MS, OTR/L, FAOTA, who practices aquatic therapy in the Philadelphia area, instituted a swimming program for adults with physical disabilities called WETSwim (Joe, 1998a). This program provides its clients with the opportunity to enhance socialization skills, independence, self-esteem, and physical fitness, as well as decrease pain and pursue leisure goals. In Hampton Roads, Virginia, Gwendolyn Garrett, MA, OTR, established a private practice called Aquatic Therapy of Virginia. In addition to general aquatic services for children, Medicare beneficiaries, and workers' compensation cases, she provides scuba diving instruction for adults with disabilities. Garrett states, "It (water) opens up a whole new range of treatment possibilities" (Joe, 1998a, p. 13). The heat and weightlessness of the water provides clients with a new therapeutic environment.

Aquatic therapy is also a beneficial therapeutic environment used in the treatment of children with developmental disabilities. A developmentally disabled individual may display signs of self-abuse and self-restraint. This type of behavior often results in self-inflicted injury to the body. Water provides a fun, nonthreatening environment, allowing natural participation in activities. The primary goal when treating this population is to re-establish positive movement patterns and decrease or eliminate destructive behaviors. Carryover into the home environment has been successful when the individual displayed little or no abusive behaviors in the pool (Westerfield, 1998).

HIPPOTHERAPY

Hippotherapy, meaning "with the help of a horse," is commonly known as the practice of therapeutic ridings. The primary treatment tool in hippotherapy is the movement of the horse. A child or an adult with a disability uses the horse's movements as a treatment modality, rather than trying to control the horse. While the client is riding the horse, the occupational therapy practitioner incorporates traditional therapy techniques to facilitate muscle tone, vestibular function, sensorimotor integration, communication skills, and trunk control. By successfully maintaining balance on a moving horse, a client may gain a sense of fulfillment and demonstrate functional improvements that cannot otherwise be achieved by traditional interventions (Haugen, 1999).

The first university-based graduate program in hippotherapy was started by the occupational therapy department at Western Michigan University and the Cheff Therapeutic Riding Center of Augusta, Michigan. This program provides therapists with the opportunity "to learn how to screen, select and evaluate appropriate clients; select and train horses for hippotherapy; and develop a hippotherapy program and management plan" (Haugen, 1999, p. 36). Claudia Morin, MHE, OTR/L, an instructor in the program suggests, "This academic program is an important step leading to creating national standards for educating students in the practice of hippotherapy" (Haugen, 1999, p. 36).

WELFARE-TO-WORK PROGRAMS

The welfare reform plan that became a law in August 1996 requires recipients to find a job after receiving two years of assistance. At least half of the welfare recipients must be involved in work-related activities by the year 2002 or states will incur financial penalties (Johansson, 1998). Studies indicate that when welfare recipients do get jobs, they often lose them within a few months due to lack of job-support resources or inadequate job training. In addition, a significant percentage of welfare recipients experience learning problems, domestic violence, and mental health and substance use disorders hindering their sustained employability. Susan Fine, MA, OTR, FAOTA, states that "occupational therapy has a long history of preparing people to re-enter the workplace" (Johansson, 1998, p. 14) and therefore could make significant contributions in welfare-to-work programs. Occupational therapy practitioners can assist clients in setting goals, exploring vocational opportunities, and linking them to community resources to achieve the ultimate goal—successful return to work and continued employment (Johansson, 1998).

VIOLENCE PREVENTION

Littleton, Colorado's Columbine High School shooting on April 20, 1999 sparked an intense campaign to initiate more violence prevention programs in public schools across the nation. Occupational therapists could play a vital role in psychosocial screening, violence prevention efforts, and facilitating the "occupations" of adolescence. Michael Faenza, the president of the National Mental Health Association, stated that "children's mental health needs must be addressed where children are in schools" (American Occupational Therapy Association, 1999, p. vi). Because occupational therapy services are well established in the school system, the knowledge and skills of school-based practitioners can be used to address the ever-increasing social behavior problems, violence, and suicide among children and adolescents. Young people are at risk for developing these behaviors if they are unsuccessful in fulfilling the developmental occupations of adolescence. These developmental occupations include making friends, participating in group and extracurricular activities, and developing career plans. To prevent circumstances like the one at Columbine, occupational therapy practitioners with mental health training and experience could serve as consultants to school systems (Johansson, 1999e; Johansson, 1999f).

For a violence prevention program to be successful, school administrators, teachers, community leaders, parents, and students must take an active role. Occupational therapy practitioners can educate parents about child and adolescent development so they will better understand their children and strengthen the parent/child bond. In addition, the practitioner can advocate for and design occupation-based programs in the community for children and adolescents. Opportunities for occupational therapy involvement may be available through programs such as the Boys and Girls Club, Scouts, or Midnight Basketball Leagues (Johansson, 1999e; Johansson, 1999f).

The opportunities for occupational therapy creativity and innovation are endless if practitioners take a perceptive look at the needs of society. Many of our contemporary social problems, including mental illness, substance abuse, homelessness, violence, abuse, and inadequate day care, have implications for occupational performance (Baum and Law, 1998). The profession and individual practitioners have the responsibility to identify community problems, design effective and appropriate interventions, and seek funding for community health programs.

 ## FUNDING COMMUNITY-BASED PROGRAMS

Occupational therapy practitioners are accustomed to working on a fee-for-service or **reimbursement** basis. Patients are treated and third-party payers reimburse the provider for the services rendered. The primary third-party payers that reimburse for occupational therapy services include Medicare, Medicaid, workers' compensation, health maintenance organizations, and private insurance companies such as Blue Cross/Blue Shield.

Community-based programs rarely operate on a reimbursement basis. Most community-based programs receive **funding,** often in the form of grants or contracts through local, state, or federal governments. The United Way and philanthropic foundations are also sources of funding for community-based health and education programs. These funds, sums of money, or other resources set aside for specific purposes can be dispersed in a variety of ways. **Grants** are funds awarded for a specific purpose, typically for research or a service project, based on the submission of a creative original proposal. Grants must be viewed as temporary funds, sometimes referred to as "soft money." This means that the grant funding is only available for a specified time period. Some grants are for one year, while some are for multiple years. However, no grant provides a permanent revenue source. **Contracts** are similar to grants in that they provide funding for research and service projects. However, contracts differ in that the funding agency (usually local, state, or federal) has already defined the scope of the project to be completed and is requesting competitive bids from organizations in the community.

Exploring funding options outside of the medical model "requires a clear understanding of health from a socioecologic perspective and a belief that occupational therapy practitioners can effectively and appropriately intervene at any level" (Brownson, 1998, p. 62). Networking is probably the single most important strategy for identifying funding sources. Getting a program funded may mean networking with "local boards and foundations, voluntary health organizations, sororities, businesses, service agencies, lawyers, insurers, self-insured companies, and government" (Brownson, p. 64).

GOVERNMENT FUNDING

The federal government provides large amounts of funding for research and program demonstration projects. However, competition for these funds is usually intense. Federal funds are difficult to receive unless the grant proposal represents a collaborative effort among many agencies within a community. The Catalog of Federal Domestic Assistance is a primary source of information about federal funding opportunities.

The catalog can be accessed through the Internet at *www.gsa.gov:80/fdac/* (Dusseau, 1998). Federal government agencies that may have an interest in funding occupational therapy projects include the Departments of Education, Health and Human Services, Housing and Urban Development, Labor, and Transportation.

Some federal funds are provided to the states in the form of "block grants." Here, individual states determine how the resources are distributed and which programs will be funded. Some of the block grant funds are designated for specific state agencies, while other funds remain available for competitive proposals from community programs. In addition, governors may have discretionary state funds to distribute to worthwhile community programs.

Local governments sometimes receive state funds to distribute in their respective jurisdictions. Some of these funds are designated for specific purposes, while other funds remain available for distribution through a "mini" grant mechanism. State and local funds are frequently administered through organizations known collectively as regional planning commissions.

FOUNDATION FUNDING

Foundations represent the major source of funding for community-based programs. These foundations are operated by philanthropic families, corporations, or community agencies that have reserved significant amounts of money for the purpose of supporting charitable organizations and programs to address specific community needs. Foundations usually accept program grant proposals on a specified schedule. Some accept proposals quarterly, some biannually, and others only once a year (Dusseau, 1998).

Local foundations typically support only local initiatives. Therefore, they are an excellent place to begin searching for funding. In general, the goal of foundations is to support as many worthwhile projects as possible. Thus, the amount of funds awarded to any one particular organization tends to be small (Dusseau, 1998). Ascertaining what motivates the foundation decision makers, how much they typically spend annually, and what types of projects and agencies they tend to fund is important. Tailoring requests within those parameters will optimize success.

The Foundation Center is a useful source of information on grant writing and for identifying appropriate foundations from which to seek funds. The center publishes *The Foundation Directory,* the premier source for information on local, state, regional, and national foundations. The Foundation Center can be accessed through the Internet at *www.fndcenter.org.* The Council on Foundations is another reputable source for information and can be found at *www.cof.org.* In addition, most public and university libraries have foundation funding directories available in their reference sections (Dusseau, 1998).

Foundations can be grouped into five major types: (1) community foundations, (2) family foundations, (3) corporate foundations, (4) special purpose foundations, and (5) national general purpose foundations (Bauer, 1995).

Community Foundations

Typically, **community foundations** are created by local philanthropic individuals for the purpose of managing a number of named funds and servicing a specific geographic area. Community foundations generally prefer to fund needs assessments of community problems and replications of effective programs demonstrated in other similar communities (Bauer, 1995).

Family Foundations

Many of the **family foundations,** numbering over 30,000 nationwide, were set up to memorialize and honor deceased family members. Therefore, the types of projects they fund tend to reflect the life and interests of the person for whom the fund is named. Typically, funding decisions are made by family members and/or appointed board members. Family foundations often fund only a specific geographic region and may change priorities regularly. The makeup of the board and their current interests are important aspects to consider (Bauer, 1995).

Corporate Foundations

Corporate foundations, a very valuable resource, often use their funds to enhance their business image by funding important projects in the community. Available dollars from corporate foundations tend to fluctuate from year to year, depending on the financial status of the company. Corporate foundations fund a variety of types of projects, including educational programs, health and human services, community enhancements, and culture and arts programs (Bauer, 1995).

Special Purpose Foundations

Special purpose foundations, as the name implies, consistently fund projects in a specified area of interest. These foundations may be local, regional, or national in scope. The Robert Wood Johnson Foundation is one of the best known in this category. This foundation's purpose is to provide grants for the improvement of health and health care in the United States. Although the types of programs funded and the strategies used may vary, the underlying intent of the special purpose foundation always remains constant (Bauer, 1995).

National General Purpose Foundations

National general purpose foundations, small in number, account for over two-thirds of the funds held in foundations. These foundations support a wide range of activities without geographic limitations. It is not the amount of grants dispersed, but rather the scope of the foundation's interests that places it in this category. National general purpose foundations tend to fund innovative ideas with the potential of capturing national attention (Bauer, 1995).

OTHER FUNDING SOURCES

In addition to government and foundation funding, many associations and civic groups provide funding for community projects (see Table 17–4). Most associations fund projects in their particular interest area. For example, the American Cancer Society may provide funds for an educational program on breast self-examination. Civic groups may also have specific interests but typically are more flexible in what they will fund. Demonstration of community need is usually the primary criterion.

Pharmaceutical companies are an often overlooked source of funding. These businesses typically fund research projects related to their products. On occasion, they may also fund community health projects that provide some public relations benefit such as screening for diabetes, hypertension, and/or mental health problems. In addition, colleges and universities may have services or resources available for community programs. Individuals and community agencies may write grants jointly with college and university faculty to fund community projects of mutual interest.

Community-based programs must not depend on a single source of funding. Developing a broad financial base, with multiple funding sources, is critical if the program is to survive and thrive in the long term. Fundraising activities, donations from local businesses, and in-kind contributions of facilities, goods, and services from other agencies can supplement grant funding.

TABLE 17–4

POTENTIAL FUNDING SOURCES FOR COMMUNITY PROGRAMS

Associations	Civic Groups	Religious Organizations
Alzheimer's Association	Elks Club	Catholic Social Services
American Business Women's Association	Jaycees	Jewish Family Services
American Cancer Association	Junior League	Lutheran Social Services
American Diabetes Association	Kiwanis Club	
American Head Injury Foundation	Knights of Columbus	
American Hospital Association	Lions Club	
American Heart Association	Masons	
American Lung Association	Rotary Club	
American Red Cross	Shriners	
Area Agency on Aging		
Arthritis Foundation		
Chamber of Commerce		
Easter Seals		
Home Builders' Association		
March of Dimes		
National Down's Syndrome Society		
National Mental Health Association		
National Multiple Sclerosis Society		
United Cerebral Palsy		
United Way		

MARKETING COMMUNITY-BASED PROGRAMS

To effectively promote occupational therapy in community-based programs, practitioners should utilize marketing principles described in the business literature. Marketing theory attempts to classify and describe those variables impacting consumer behavior. In everyday language, the term "consumer" is often construed to mean an individual purchaser. However, in this context, consumer refers to any individual, group, or agency that is in the position of making decisions about which products and services will be purchased or funded. One marketing model that has stood the test of time is referred to as the **"four P's"**: (1) product, (2) place, (3) price, and (4) promotion (Kotler and Armstrong, 1991).

Product refers to the service to be provided: what *form* this product takes, the expected outcome or *benefits* of the service, and the *choices* available to the consumer. Occupational therapy practitioners must be able to explain in clear, commonsense terminology what the service consists of and how it fits within the mission of the community organization.

Place refers to how and where the product or service will be delivered to the consumer. Will the program be provided at a specific site, at multiple sites, or in the consumer's home or place of business? In what geographical area will services be provided? Are any special qualifications required to be eligible for services? Occupational therapy practitioners must carefully assess the needs, wants, and desires of consumers to develop and present their services using the consumers' preferred delivery mechanisms.

Price refers to the cost of the service to the consumer. Setting a price for the product or service is affected by a number of variables, including consumer demand, market competition, legal constraints, general economic factors, costs of program development and delivery, and company expectations of financial profits and losses (Burch and Davis, 1992). Realistic pricing of occupational therapy services in community programs is probably the most difficult aspect of marketing for practitioners.

Promotion refers to the process by which potential recipients are made aware of the availability of the service. If a service is purchased by an agency and underutilized, the service is in danger of being terminated. A sound marketing plan or service proposal always includes multiple promotion strategies.

All marketing efforts should be consumer centered rather than product centered. A consumer-oriented approach is consistent with occupational therapy philosophy and ensures that the service:

● Addresses an identified consumer need
● Is effective and cost-efficient
● Is accessible and appropriately utilized (Burch and Davis, 1992)

 ## CONCLUSION

The American Occupational Therapy Association has been gathering information on new markets for occupational therapy services and has identified 10 emerging practice areas:

1. Ergonomics consulting
2. Driver rehabilitation and training
3. Design and accessibility consulting and home modification
4. Low vision services
5. Private practice community health services (particularly for assisted living facilities)
6. Technology and assistive device development and consulting
7. Welfare-to-work services for welfare recipients
8. Health and wellness consulting
9. Ticket-to-work services for Supplemental Security Income (SSI) and Social Security Disability Insurance (SSDI) beneficiaries
10. Services addressing the psychosocial needs of children and youth (Johansson, 2000)

This list provides a catalyst to stimulate further dialogue and the dissemination of community practice models on these emerging practice areas and others described in this text. Successful entry into community practice will require occupational therapy practitioners to *expand* their:

● Conceptualization of the usefulness of occupation
● Perspective on the role of occupational therapy
● View of the profession
● Identification of potential opportunities
● Capabilities as program planners, consultants, advocates, and grant writers

The only real barriers are the limits of one's creativity. Occupation is fundamental to human life. It improves physical and mental health, contributes to a sense of well-being, enhances life satisfaction, and provides meaning to everyday existence. Opportunities for professionals with expertise in occupational performance are evident in all spheres of human endeavor. One need only look with fresh eyes and an open mind.

 STUDY QUESTIONS

1. Identify a need in your community and describe how occupational therapy could address that need.
2. Develop a program idea to address the need identified in the preceding question and outline the basic occupational therapy program components.
3. Describe three potential sources of funding for your program idea.
4. Discuss the strategies you would use to market your idea.

REFERENCES

American Occupational Therapy Association. (1999). A role for OT in preventing school violence. *OT WEEK, 13*(17), i, vi. American Occupational Therapy Association.

Barker, J.A. (1992). *Future edge: Discovering the new paradigms of success.* New York: William Morrow.

Bauer, D.G. (1995). *The complete grants sourcebook for higher education* (3rd ed.). Phoenix: American Council on Education, Oryx Press.

Baum, C., and Law, M. (1998). Community health: A responsibility, an opportunity and a fit for occupational therapy. *American Journal of Occupational Therapy, 52*(1), 7–10.

Berg, J. (1998). On the road again. *OT WEEK, 12*(6), 16–17.

Blaz, J. (1998). Keeping fit for duty. *OT WEEK, 12* (7), 12–13.

Bockhoven, J.S. (1968). Challenge of the new clinical approaches. *American Journal of Occupational Therapy, 22,* 23–25.

Brownson, C.A. (1998). Funding community practice: Stage 1. *American Journal of Occupational Therapy, 52*(1), 60–64.

Burch, E.A., and Davis, Q.M. (1992). Marketing, health promotion, and injury prevention programs. In J. Rothman and R. Levine, *Prevention practice: Strategies for physical therapy and occupational therapy.* Philadelphia: Saunders.

Capra, F., and Steindl-Rast, D. (1991). *Belonging to the universe: Explorations on the frontiers of science and spirituality.* San Francisco: HarperCollins.

Center for Urban Affairs and Policy Research, Northwestern University. (1988). *Mapping community capacity.* Evanston, IL: Northwestern University.

Collins, L.F. (1998). Is case management for you? *OT PRACTICE, 3*(6), 42–44.

Cornish, E. (1980). Toward a philosophy of futurism. *Health Education, 11,* 10–12.

Diffendal, J. (1999). The center of living, growing and gardening. *ADVANCE for Occupational Therapy Practitioners, 15*(5), 30.

Dressler, J., and Snively, F. (1998). Occupational therapy in the criminal justice system. In E. Cara and A. MacRae (Eds.), *Psychosocial occupational therapy: A clinical practice* (pp. 527–552). Albany, NY: Delmar.

Dusseau, S.B. (1998). Grant writing. In R.J. Bensley and J. Brookings-Fisher, *Community health education methods.* Kalamazoo, MI: Balance Group.

Essert, M.B. (1998). The healing power of water. *ADVANCE for Occupational Therapy Practitioners, 14*(42), 36–37.

Finn, G.L. (1972). The occupational therapist in prevention programs. *American Journal of Occupational Therapy, 26,* 59–66.

Freudenberg, N., Eng, E., Flay, B., Parcel, G., Rogers, T., and Wallerstein, N. (1995). Strengthening individual and community capacity to prevent disease and promote health: In search of relevant theories and principles. *Health Education Quarterly, 22*(3), 290–306.

Haggerty, M. (1998). Side by side: Partnering with assisted living facilities. *ADVANCE for Occupational Therapists, 14*(4), 21.

Haugen, J. (1999). It's not just horsing around. *ADVANCE for Occupational Therapy Practitioners, 15*(1), 36.

Joe, B.E. (1998a). Aquatic rehab: The great equalizer. *OT WEEK, 12*(33), 12–13.

Joe, B.E. (1998b). Becoming an OT entrepreneur. *OT WEEK, 12*(46), 12–13.

Joe, B.E. (1999). This warden is an OT. *OT WEEK, 13*(1), 9.

Johansson, C. (1998). New opportunities in mental health. *OT WEEK, 12*(43), 14–15.

Johansson, C. (1999a). The business of ergonomics. *OT WEEK, 13*(20), 8–9.

Johansson, C. (1999b). Crafting user friendly environments. *OT WEEK, 13*(21), 8–9.

Johansson, C. (1999c). Driver training: Can OT claim the franchise? *OT WEEK, 13*(6), 8–9.

Johansson, C. (1999d). Independent living through technology. *OT WEEK, 13*(32), 8–9.

Johansson, C. (1999e). Let's take a stand on school violence. *OT WEEK, 13*(19), 8–9.

Johansson, C. (1999f). OT prescription for school violence. *OT WEEK, 13*(30), 8–10.

Johansson, C. (2000). Top ten emerging practice areas. *OT Practice, 5*(3), 7–8.

Koestler, A. (1978). *Janus.* London: Hutchinson.

Kotler, P., and Armstrong, G. (1991). *Principles of marketing* (5th ed). Englewood Cliffs, NJ: Prentice-Hall.

Le Postollec, M.L. (1999). Holding a seat in the field of ergonomics. *ADVANCE for Occupational Therapy Practitioners, 15*(2), 23–24.

Westerfield, V. (1998). New people in the pool: What aquatics can do for your DD clients. *ADVANCE for Occupational Therapists, 14*(1), 21–22.

Womack, J. (1999). The Vanderbilt apartments: An example of occupational therapy in a community-based setting. *AOTA Home and Community Health Special Interest Newsletter, 6*(2), 1–4.

Zimmerman, S.S. (1999). Occupational therapy service delivery to an apartment program. *AOTA Home and Community Health Special Interest Section Newsletter, 6*(1), 1–3.

Zuckerman, D. (1998). It's home sweet home—at the right price. *OT WEEK, 12*(9), 12–13.

18

Implications for Professional Education and Research

Marjorie E. Scaffa, PhD, OTR, FAOTA
Carol A. Brownson, MSPH
Anne Shordike, MOT, OTR

■ OUTLINE

LEARNING OBJECTIVES

This chapter is designed to enable the reader to:
- Identify the trends and events that affect occupational therapy education.
- Demonstrate understanding of the history of community-based fieldwork in occupational therapy.
- Discuss potential curricular and fieldwork options for teaching community-based practice concepts.
- Describe the benefits to students, educators, the profession, and the community of the faculty-facilitated fieldwork model.
- Discuss the process by which innovations are diffused in a profession.

> Only people who see the big picture . . . are the ones who step out of the frame.
>
> S. Rushdie (1999, p. 43)

 ## INTRODUCTION

The world is ever changing, and professional education must respond to the demands of the current practice environment and also to anticipated future needs. Educational planners need to incorporate a view of the future into the design of curriculum content, process, and outcomes.

This chapter highlights the past and current influences on professional occupational therapy education and presents creative strategies for integrating community practice content and experiences into educational programs. Several examples of training and fieldwork are presented. Occupational therapy, to be successful, requires excellence, innovation, and anticipation.

 ## PROFESSIONAL EDUCATION: THEN AND NOW

Some predictions can be made about the future of occupational therapy education based on current trends. The following statements reflect the authors' beliefs regarding the future of occupational therapy and are offered as "food for thought." We anticipate:

- An increased role for occupational therapy in prevention and health promotion
- A significant shift in services from medical institutions to decentralized, coordinated, community-based settings

- An increased focus on the consumer as the driving force in health care
- Changing demographics, including increased cultural diversity of the population requiring a need for increased cultural competence among practitioners
- Increased numbers of elderly with a full range of health, illness, and disability
- Health-care reform that includes increased emphasis on mental health and quality of life
- A developing role for occupational therapy in preventing and reducing social problems such as violence, crime, and alcohol and drug abuse

PAST INFLUENCES

The need for occupational therapy educational programs to integrate community practice content and experiences into the curricula is clearly emphasized by the authors' predictions. However, this mandate is not new. In 1974, Grossman (p. 591) stated:

> If occupational therapists are to take leadership roles in community programs, training must begin at the student level. Curricula should include courses in description and assessment of community needs and resources, systems theory, and program development.

However, the question still remains, What do students and practitioners need to know to practice effectively in community programs?

McColl (1998) believes that the application of the existing knowledge base for biomedical clinical practice is inappropriate and will be ineffective in community-based practice. To be successful in community settings, students and practitioners need a basic understanding and appreciation of history, cultural anthropology, sociology, organizational psychology, economics, business management, epidemiology, public health, politics and policy, and systems theory. This demands an increased emphasis on the social sciences in professional preparation programs. In addition, McColl outlines some basic content knowledge to be incorporated into occupational therapy courses (see Box 18–1).

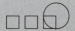 **BOX 18-1**

What Students and Practitioners Need to Know to Participate Effectively in Community Programs

- What a community is
- How organizations and communities form
- How organizations and communities are governed
- How to identify community resources
- How to identify community needs
- How to facilitate change
- How persons with disabilities live in the community
- How persons develop and pursue occupations in the community
- What supports and barriers to participation in occupation exist in the community

Source: McColl, M.A. (1998). What do we need to know to practice occupational therapy in the community? *American Journal of Occupational Therapy, 52*(1), 11–18.

Community-based fieldwork education is also not merely a contemporary phenomenon. In 1976, Cermak described a community-based fieldwork experience for senior occupational therapy students at Boston University. This community service-learning project provided prevention and early intervention services for children and their parents in local day-care facilities. According to Cermak (1976, p. 157),

> The program was designed to meet five objectives: to provide students with an effective integration of theory and practice; to allow an application of theoretical concepts to early intervention and prevention programs; to enable students to confront complexities of community service delivery; to allow students to learn new roles in community programs; and to demonstrate the role of occupational therapy within a public health model of service delivery.

Students designed perceptual-motor activities, screened children for developmental delays and learning disabilities, and provided seminars for day-care staff and parents. The program was funded by a grant from Maternal and Child Health Services (Cermak, 1976).

A similar strategy for training students in community practice was used at the University of Southern California (USC). The goal of the USC program was to prepare students to feel comfortable moving into community-based practice by providing them with program development and high-level problem-solving skills. The grant-funded project provided opportunities for students and faculty to design and implement occupational therapy services in a wide range of public agencies. Students were organized into teams that included occupational therapy assistant students and bachelor's level and graduate occupational therapy students. This provided the added advantage of learning collaboration and supervision skills (Cromwell and Kielhofner, 1976).

At the University of Florida, a faculty member and several graduates published an article in the *American Journal of Occupational Therapy* in 1977 describing an outreach activity group for elderly persons with mental illness residing in rural areas of Florida. The activity group, sponsored by a community mental health center, was held at a high school over a period of nine weeks. Church volunteers transported participants to the program. By the end of the program, the elderly persons experienced a number of physical, cognitive, and psychological benefits from their participation. Students also learned about the structure and function of a community agency. In addition, the students were able to develop administrative and consultation skills and identify potential roles for occupational therapy practitioners in community programs (Menks, Sittler, Weaver, and Yanow, 1977).

Although community-based fieldwork is an excellent tool for preparing students to enter new areas of practice, it is not without its limitations. Both level I and level II fieldwork in community settings has been a lively topic of discussion at numerous meetings of educational program directors and fieldwork coordinators. Box 18–2 illustrates some of the comments, both pro and con, expressed at these meetings.

CURRENT INFLUENCES

The convergence of three important and notable events has had a significant impact on the education of future occupational therapy practitioners. The first event occurred in September 1997 with the publication of the *National Study of Occupational Therapy Practice: Executive Summary* by the **National Board for Certification in Occupational Therapy (NBCOT).** NBCOT is the organization responsible for the initial certification of occupational therapists and occupational therapy assistants through the development and administration of the certification examination. The national study document outlined the tasks routinely performed by registered occupational therapists (OTRs) and certified occupational therapy assistants (COTAs) and the content knowledge required to accomplish those tasks. In the survey of practice, a significant percentage of time (8.3

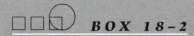

BOX 18-2

Comments Regarding Community-Based Fieldwork

Advantages:
- Promotes creative problem solving
- Increases opportunities for students to develop independence
- Breaks down stereotypes and sociocultural barriers
- Educates the public/community about occupational therapy

Disadvantages:
- Provides only limited supervision
- Is less predictable
- Provides limited occupational therapy role modeling
- Requires more work for fieldwork coordinator/faculty in designing models
- Requires more comprehensive screening of students and supervisors
- Has liability concerns

Recommendations:
- Start with level I fieldwork; develop site for level II as the program stabilizes.
- Send pairs or small groups of students, depending on the size of the community program.
- Spend adequate time developing the fieldwork plan.
- Communicate regularly with agency personnel and students on site.

percent for OTRs and 9.7 percent for COTAs) was reportedly spent providing services for populations. In addition, a small number of survey respondents indicated "an increased emphasis on community outreach and prevention as well as consultation" (National Board for Certification in Occupational Therapy, 1997, p. 30). As a result of the practice analysis data, the new test specifications for the certification examination include a focus on population-based services.

In December 1998, the **Accreditation Council for Occupational Therapy Education (ACOTE),** the organization responsible for accrediting entry-level occupational therapy educational programs, adopted new standards for both occupational therapist and occupational therapy assistant preparation programs. One entire section of the **accreditation standards** (the minimum essential requirements for accreditation of educational programs) is devoted to the context of service delivery. This section describes, in some detail, the competencies required for practicing in a variety of environments, with a major emphasis on community and social systems. Community-related competencies also can be found as minor components in other sections of the standards, including:

- Foundational content requirements
- Basic tenets of occupational therapy
- Intervention plan: formulation and implementation
- Management of occupational therapy services
- Professional ethics, values, and responsibilities
- Fieldwork education

Box 18–3 provides examples of statements that emphasize community and social systems from the *Standards for an Accredited Educational Program for the Occupational Therapist* (Accreditation Council for Occupational Therapy Education, 1998).

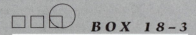

BOX 18-3

Section B: Specific Requirements for Accreditation

1.0   Foundational Content Requirements

   1.7   Demonstrate knowledge and appreciation of the role of sociocultural, socioeconomic, diversity factors, and lifestyle choices in contemporary society.

   1.8   Appreciate the influence of social conditions and the ethical context in which humans choose and engage in occupations.

2.0   Basic Tenets of Occupational Therapy

   2.6   Understand and appreciate the role of occupation in the promotion of health and the prevention of disease and disability for the individual, family, and society.

   2.7   Understand the effects of health, disability, disease processes, and traumatic injury to the individual within the context of family and society.

   2.9   Demonstrate appreciation for the individual's perception of quality of life, well-being, and occupation to promote health and prevention of injury and disease.

5.0   Intervention Plan: Formulation and Implementation

   5.6   Develop and promote the use of appropriate home and community programming to support performance in the client's natural environment.

   5.17 Plan for discharge, in collaboration with the client, by reviewing the needs of client/family/significant others, resources, and discharge environment. This includes, but is not limited to, the identification of community, human, and fiscal resources, recommendations for environmental adaptations, and home programming.

6.0   Context of Service Delivery

   6.1   Understand the models of health care, education, community, and social systems as they relate to the practice of occupational therapy.

   6.2   Understand the current policy issues in the previously mentioned systems that influence the practice of occupational therapy.

   6.3   Understand the current social, economic, political, geographic, and demographic factors that promote policy development and the provision of occupational therapy services.

   6.4   Understand the role and responsibility of the practitioner to address changes in service delivery policies and to effect changes in the system.

   6.5   Understand the trends in models of service delivery and their effect on the practice of occupational therapy, including, but not limited to, medical, educational, community, and social models.

7.0 Management of Occupational Therapy Services

7.1 Understand a variety of systems and service models, including, but not limited to, health-care, education, community, and social models, and how these models may affect service provision.

7.2 Demonstrate knowledge of the social, economic, political, and demographic factors that influence the delivery of health care in the United States.

7.8 Demonstrate an understanding of the resources a practitioner can use to respond to changes in the marketplace.

7.19 Develop fundamental marketing skills to advance the profession.

9.0 Professional Ethics, Values, and Responsibilities

9.12 Be able to assist the consumer in gaining access to occupational therapy services.

9.13 Demonstrate knowledge of advocacy for the benefit of the consumer and the profession.

10.0 Fieldwork Education

10.9 Recognize that level II fieldwork can take place in a variety of traditional settings and emerging areas of practice. The student can complete level II fieldwork in a minimum of one setting and maximum of four different settings.

10.13 In a setting where there is no occupational therapist on site, the program must document that there is a plan for the provision of occupational therapy services. On-site supervision must be provided in accordance with the plan and state credentialing requirements. The student must receive a minimum of six hours of occupational therapy supervision per week, including direct observation of client interaction. Additionally, the occupational therapy supervisor must be readily available for communication and consultation during work hours. Such fieldwork shall not exceed 12 weeks.

Source: American Occupational Therapy Association. (1998). Standards for an accredited educational program for the occupational therapist. *American Journal of Occupational Therapy, 53*(6), 578–582. Copyright © 1998 by the American Occupational Therapy Association, Inc. Reprinted with permission.

The third important event occurred in April 1999 when the Representative Assembly of the American Occupational Therapy Association (AOTA) passed **Resolution J,** which mandated entry-level education at the postbaccalaureate level. This mandate became official upon approval by the Accreditation Council for Occupational Therapy Education in August 1999. Resolution J was the culmination of two separate processes converging on the same conclusion.

ACOTE and the AOTA Commission on Education (COE) Entry Level Task Force held numerous open forums to solicit input and comments on the proposed accreditation standards, which were described as being "best met at the postbaccalaureate level," and the task force proposal of moving the profession toward postbaccalaureate entry.

While the NBCOT practice study focused on current practice, ACOTE and the COE task force were planning for the future of the profession. Part of the rationale for this change in entry-level education is the need for therapists to be more autonomous professionals, with highly evolved reasoning and program development skills. In addition, post-baccalaureate education better prepares graduates to conduct outcomes research and function effectively as members of interdisciplinary teams.

FUTURE IMPLICATIONS

To respond to these changes and fulfill its mission to produce competent practitioners for the future, professional education must develop some new curricula and fieldwork models. A primary challenge will be to balance the need to prepare students for traditional biomedical practice with the new demands of community health roles.

A number of educational approaches should be developed, implemented, and evaluated for effectiveness. The accreditation standards allow the flexibility to create a variety of curricular models that qualify for accreditation. As every community is different, so too may educational programs differ in how they meet the need to produce a new type of occupational therapy practitioner.

CREATIVE STRATEGIES IN PROFESSIONAL PREPARATION

Some educational programs are meeting the challenge by infusing community practice content throughout the curriculum, while others are creating new courses that focus entirely on community health concerns. Some programs are using community-based sites in creative ways for level I fieldwork. Other programs place students in community programs for both level I and level II fieldwork. The program descriptions that follow represent only a few examples of educational programs that have responded to the challenge. As Lao Tsu, an ancient Chinese philosopher, is credited with saying "A journey of a thousand miles begins with a single step," so too must educational programs advance in small steps toward a comprehensive curriculum which includes community practice content, skills, and models for students and faculty.

EASTERN KENTUCKY UNIVERSITY: FACULTY-FACILITATED FIELDWORK MODEL

The occupational therapy department at Eastern Kentucky University has initiated and expanded the use of nontraditional, community-based, level I fieldwork education since the beginning of the program. This was due to the shortage of occupational therapists in the state and the rural nature of the university's service area (Rydeen, Kautzmann, Cowan, and Benzing, 1995). Students complete three level I fieldwork assignments during their studies. In these fieldwork experiences, students spend 40 to 60 hours at a site during academic terms or over breaks in the school year. The placements follow the curriculum design, based on concepts of human adaptation across the life span.

The first fieldwork experience is with children, occurring in conjunction with pediatric and adolescent occupational therapy assessment and treatment courses. The second fieldwork experience is with the adult population and the third with an elderly population. Each of these experiences also occurs within the context of supportive coursework.

The settings used in this program have been diverse, including Head Start programs, adult day programs, senior citizen centers, and outpatient mental health programs. Initially, these programs required collaboration of an on-site supervisor who was not an occupational therapist and the faculty supervisor who was responsible for all course-related activities, including documentation and student observation. As fieldwork placements, particularly mental health placements, have become more difficult to find, faculty members have become increasingly involved in level I fieldwork. Several innovative, faculty-facilitated programs have been described by Rydeen et al. (1995). These community-based fieldwork placements are typically initiated by an involved faculty member and then carried out by on-site faculty members with a group of six students either one day a week for a 12-week period or for a shorter, more intensive residential experience. The faculty-facilitated fieldwork at the Hope Center, a homeless shelter for men in Lexington, Kentucky, continues to develop this model.

The Homeless Project

The increase in the homeless population and the shortage of health-care services for this growing population are well documented. Statistics on the actual number of homeless people and the reported percentages of homeless persons with mental illness vary widely. In 1994, the Interagency Council on the Homeless found that 12 million adults in the United States have been homeless at some time in their lives. Substance abuse and mental illness have been identified as contributing to homelessness. Approximately 56 percent of people who are homeless have substance abuse problems, and 12 to 25 percent of these individuals are considered to be dually diagnosed (Cnaan and Blankertz, 1993).

Occupational therapy involvement with the homeless has begun to emerge in practice and the literature during this decade. Barth (1994) describes occupational therapy intervention in a community agency for the homeless. She discusses the roles occupational therapy practitioners can assume beyond direct treatment. Marks (1997) suggests a consultation role for occupational therapists working with agencies involved with the homeless. Kavanagh and Fares (1995) use the model of human occupation as a way to design interventions for homeless individuals. Heubner and Tryssenaar (1996) describe a level I fieldwork placement that supports the transition of occupational therapy to community-based mental health service delivery. These models and phenomenological studies begin to demonstrate the effectiveness of occupational therapy with this population and explore the effect of homelessness and the homeless culture on students during their fieldwork experiences.

CONCEPTUALIZATION. Given the need for services and the benefit of occupational therapy for this population, this fieldwork was designed to provide students with an experience that involves persons who are homeless and roles that an occupational therapist could perform in the community. The students were prepared to initiate occupational therapy programming where none had existed before, with the intention of educating clients and staff regarding what services could be offered. This placement was conceived as the start of a university/community partnership that could provide a variety of types of student and faculty involvement, including research. Faculty and students regard this fieldwork as a learning community where all are resources for each other as well as for the clients and the agency.

One of the difficulties with using a level I fieldwork experience for program development is that with consecutive semester-long placements, each group of students starts at essentially the same place and makes similar progress and discoveries. Therefore, assignments and projects were created that would lay groundwork for future students and support development of the occupational therapy program. Thus, a program has been created and implemented over the past three years that allows incoming students to engage the clients more fully in the occupational therapy process.

SITE DEVELOPMENT. The Hope Center offers food and shelter to homeless men in Lexington, Kentucky. A number of programs within the center also are available to address their varying needs, including: (1) a recovery program for substance abuse, (2) a mental health program, (3) a mobile outreach program, and (4) an Hispanic program. There is an on-site clinic and a nonmedical detoxification unit.

The staff consists of social workers, case managers, and support personnel. The University of Kentucky nursing department staffs the on-site clinic. No occupational therapists were employed at the Hope Center. The staff initially knew very little about occupational therapy, with most assuming that it was similar to physical therapy. Their perception was that occupational therapy occurred in hospitals and rehabilitation clinics and involved treatment of physical injury. Most of the program directors were reluctant to supervise students from a discipline about which they had little knowledge and understanding.

This fieldwork placement began as what the American Occupational Therapy Association Commission on Education (COE) terms a nonoccupational therapy supervisor model (Privott, 1998), where the students had a "related professions" supervisor working with the faculty supervisor. With extensive in-service training and, most importantly, superior performance by the occupational therapy students, this placement became what COE would identify as a community-based and collaborative model. For the past two years, seven level I fieldwork students have been present for one day each week, involved in five programs at the Hope Center, and receiving supervision by an on-site faculty member. The success of the level I fieldwork students created the opportunity for a level II student placement to be initiated.

PROGRAMS

The Recovery Program. The recovery program at the Hope Center houses up to 30 individuals. The men live in a dorm in the center and attend classes and Alcoholics Anonymous (AA) meetings throughout most of their highly structured days. They have jobs to perform, such as working in the laundry or kitchen, doing housekeeping, or providing security services, as a way to support the center and their own recovery process. Initially, occupational therapy students were requested to provide physical exercise. However, these duties have evolved to include this and other services described later.

Because of the positive participant response, the occupational therapy students were given a formal class time with the men. For the past several semesters, this class has been well attended and quite popular. Between 20 and 35 men participate in the group. Men in the motivational track waiting to get into the recovery program and men in the dual-diagnosis program may attend. The clients identified communication skills, anger management, coping skills, humor, and the physical activity components of the occupational therapy groups as being beneficial to their recovery process.

Faculty and students are working to develop a fitness center where the men can experience both exercise and relaxation as healthy coping methods. In preparation, one team of students completed a literature review on exercise and mental health, particularly as it relates to the recovery process. A grant from the Candle Foundation is providing funding for equipment and educational materials. The Hope Center also has provided space to use for this ongoing project. It is hoped that future students will use the fitness center for wellness-related research.

The Mental Health Program. Twenty-five percent of the Hope Center's clients receive mental health treatment services provided through three programs: (1) an outreach program that serves clients in the community, (2) an eight-bed permanent housing program for those unable to live in the community, and (3) a dual-diagnosis program. The occupational therapy students have been involved with activities of daily living skills assessment and intervention, working with the clients both in the shelter and in the community. One team of students initiated a living skills program for the men in permanent housing. These men are the most impaired at the center, with all having a debilitating axis I diagnosis and severe functional problems. This group has been well attended by clients and well received by the staff.

The dual-diagnosis program serves men with both an axis I and a substance abuse diagnosis. These men take part in some of the recovery program classes. The students attend these classes with the clients and assist and support them as needed. They have started a group exclusively for the dual-diagnosis population that addresses living skills, cognitive skills, and interpersonal skills.

The Mobile Outreach Program. The Hopemobile, a converted recreational vehicle that is visible in a different church parking lot each weekday, is staffed by case managers and a nurse. It offers coffee, food, blankets, and any other services that the consumers may need or want. Participation in therapy and compliance with medication are not required. Although persons who are intoxicated are not allowed on the Hopemobile itself, sobriety is not a prerequisite to receiving services. Students on the Hopemobile assist with living skills evaluation, home-safety evaluation, and adaptation for homeless persons who are making a transition to housing. They also provide prevocational education and act as community liaisons for employment.

The Hispanic Program. The Hispanic program primarily serves the migrant population. Services include AA meetings in Spanish, English tutoring, and employment and housing assistance. Some of the men have sustained work-related injuries. Students then focus on physical rehabilitation and functional adaptation for these injuries. Although only students who could speak Spanish were initially placed in this program, staff members now seek out occupational therapy services and provide interpretation as needed.

PROGRAM EVALUATION

Student Response. The students have valued this experience highly. They note a change in their perception of persons who are homeless and those who are both homeless and mentally ill, clearly showing an "appreciation of the humanness of persons with psychiatric disorders" that Lyons and Ziviani (1995, p. 1007) consider an educational imperative. They value the intensity of the experience and the diversity of the population, as well as the direct, "hands-on" style of this fieldwork. They understand their role as ambassadors for the profession and are actively engaged in this role from the beginning. Each semester builds on the one before, so although the students change every semester, each group is able to provide targeted interventions due to the efforts of the previous students. Even though the fieldwork is short, the students understand their part in a larger program plan. They value having an on-site faculty supervisor as well as the student interaction in their own learning community. Because a number of the students have been involved in scholarly presentations, the relationship between education, community-based practice, and scholarly contribution to the profession has been modeled for all of the students in the program. These students leave this fieldwork placement more aware of the services occupational therapy can provide for this population in a community-based practice site.

Faculty Response. Participation in this program has been a rewarding experience for the faculty involved, supporting the relationship between the educational program, scholarly involvement in the profession, and practice. It has allowed the continuing development of a model that can expand the role of occupational therapy in community mental health and thus affect future practitioners. Outcome studies addressing the complete program implemented by the level II fieldwork students are in the data analysis stage.

Client Response. The clients have consistently expressed appreciation for the occupational therapy students. They appreciate the interaction and the help they receive, actively expressing this to students and faculty. They most value the relevance of the groups that the students conduct and the inclusion of all of the clients. Common comments included feeling better about themselves and learning something of value. They perceive the students as knowledgeable, committed, and caring, with many interesting and helpful ideas for intervention.

Agency Response. Over the past several semesters, the occupational therapy program at the Hope Center has increased from two to seven students and has become faculty facilitated. Faculty members are present on site and provide role modeling and assist the students with problem solving, as needed. This expansion of role occurred as the agency became aware of the potential contributions occupational therapy could provide for their clients. Each semester, all of the programs expressed a desire to have the students return. When surveyed, staff responded very favorably to the involvement of occupational therapy students with their clients. They found the students very reliable and respectful and highly effective. They also noted an increase in the clients' ability to do routine tasks and activities of daily living. They were appreciative of the interaction the students had with the clients and the access clients had to occupational therapy services.

FUTURE DIRECTIONS. This community service-based fieldwork has achieved success and will continue to grow in its vision. The community agency now values occupational therapy and the services it can provide. Brownson (1998) suggests that occupational therapists become more involved in the community by participating on community boards and committees and providing their unique professional perspectives through written proposals that describe potential occupational therapy services. Occupational therapy practitioners must be able to articulate the unique contribution of the profession in meeting the needs of the population (Brownson, 1998). This student program has demonstrated the effectiveness of occupational therapy with this population. Although the ability of the faculty to articulate the potential role of occupational therapy and the provision of in-service training got us "in the door," the consistent student involvement over time in each of the programs has been the most effective promoter of occupational therapy services.

Although there is still no occupational therapist on staff at the Hope Center, the agency has developed an occupational therapy position and is recruiting and interviewing applicants. Since this agency is primarily grant funded, the occupational therapist will need to be active in procuring funding to support their services. The occupational therapy students at this fieldwork are gaining experience working with grants and understanding that this is part of their professional responsibility. They have used this site and these populations as the basis for literature review, program development, and outcomes research. Students have explored potential roles for occupational therapists as case managers or program directors. Through these accomplishments in the educational setting, they will be better prepared to consider these options in their future practice. At the conclusion of a recent semester, one student remarked to faculty, "Maybe I'll come back after level II fieldwork and write a grant to fund myself a job here."

WASHINGTON UNIVERSITY IN ST. LOUIS: COMMUNITY PRACTICE PROGRAM

The Washington University program in occupational therapy (WUOT) formalized its community practice program in 1995 by establishing a community practice division headed by an associate director of community health. The "community practice team" is comprised of occupational therapists who teach in the program and maintain a community practice, generally through a contractual arrangement between an agency and the program.

When the community practice division was formed, a great deal of time and effort went into discussions of mission, goals, needed skills, the scope and characteristics of this initiative, and how it fit into the research and education missions of the program. The mission of the community practice initiative was to develop funded, innovative models of community-based occupational therapy practice that support the teaching and research missions of the program and foster the professional development of the therapists working in community practice.

The team recognized differences in the definitions and perceptions of the meaning of the term, "community practice." The roles being carried out by the respective members varied, ranging from direct service in the school systems, to case management in community mental health, to health promotion (exercise) classes for people with Parkinson's disease.

In general, the role of the community practice therapist at WUOT was defined as consisting of three interrelated components: (1) service, (2) education, and (3) research (see Box 18–4). *Service* refers to practice in a variety of settings and roles. The education component is carried out in the classroom, where the community practice occupational therapists teach or assist with classes, and in the community, where they supervise students completing fieldwork and/or community service assistantships. Community practice therapists support the research mission of the program through participation in master's research projects, supervising or assisting with student projects, collaborating with faculty research projects, and assisting with grant writing to help fund their work in the community.

The team came to view community practice in terms of location and philosophy. In a location perspective, anything that happens outside a health-care setting is "community." In the case of community practice at WUOT, locations have included homeless shelters, residential facilities for children with emotional and behavioral disorders, community mental health agencies, early childhood/day-care settings for children with developmental disabilities, congregate meal sites for seniors, client homes, community agencies, work settings, and more. However, the WUOT community practice team also defined "community" as a philosophy of practice that is client centered, promotes social/community integration, generally involves intervention beyond the individual level to include the systems and environments in which people participate and focuses on health and health promotion.

Goals for the community practice division were established and incorporated into the program's strategic plan. The broad goal is as follows: *To develop self-supporting, innovative models of rehabilitation and community-based occupational therapy practice that promote optimal health and independence for people with (or at risk of acquiring) disabilities.* The broad goal has four subgoals:

● Create community-based models of occupational therapy practice in collaboration with research faculty, community organizations, and consumers. Evaluate the efficacy of these interventions.
● Apply core knowledge and key skills for community practice to the planning, implementation, and evaluation and support of community practice programs. Assure education and training of community practice occupational therapists in all phases of community program development.
● Develop a peer consultation plan for each community practice therapist to assure state-of-the-art occupational therapy practice and explore the development of a mentoring plan for therapists in community practice.
● Increase awareness and understanding of community practice programs and models among occupational therapy students, the occupational therapy profession, the larger health community, and program partners.

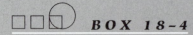

BOX 18-4

Components of the Washington University Community Practice Program

Overview:
Community practice therapists may focus on mental health, child and family health, older adult health, worker health, and/or independent living, including accessibility. They may practice in a variety of settings, including schools, day care, community centers, housing units, homeless shelters, places of worship, worksites, health-care settings, or community agencies. The community practice role may involve provision of direct service, consultation, case management, program coordination, training, and/or supervision. The job consists of three interrelated components.

Service:
● Conduct needs assessments; plan, implement, and evaluate programs and services.
● Identify and build alliances with community agencies and service providers.

Education:
● Teach labs, give guest lectures, and assist with classes as needed by the course master.
● Participate in faculty meetings and discussions.
● Serve on program committees.
● Supervise OT students doing community service and/or field work.
● Disseminate program information through oral presentations and papers.
● Participate in relevant continuing education programs.

Research:
● Help identify potential funding sources for community programs.
● Coordinate and/or assist with grant writing.
● Participate in program-sponsored research projects at community sites.
● Supervise and/or assist with supervision of master's projects.

When this initiative was undertaken, the team also spent some time discussing necessary knowledge and skills for being effective in new areas of practice. Initial brainstorming resulted in a list of essential personal characteristics and traits such as initiative, willingness to take risks, and comfort with multiple (and changing) roles. As the various practices evolved and the team gained experience, the list expanded to include areas of knowledge and skills beyond that which they had learned in their occupational therapy programs. Important areas identified included systems theory, qualitative research methods, program planning and evaluation, needs assessment, leadership, epidemiology of disability, health behavior change theory, grant writing, and advocacy/policy and legislative approaches to change. The continuing challenge is the recognition that practicing therapists need to learn new skills and, at the same time, model and teach them to students to better prepare them for future practice areas.

Initially, the community practice division focused on developing relationships and contracts for service with community agencies. Factors that were considered when negotiating with agencies included having similar client philosophies and goals, a willingness to work together to create a program, and their acceptance of student involvement. In many instances, there was also the need to work together to access funding.

The next step was to develop these practices as fieldwork sites. The team worked closely with the program's fieldwork coordinator to offer both level I and level II fieldwork opportunities at the community practice sites. In addition, the fieldwork coordinator collaborated with other occupational therapy schools and community practice sites on a mutual goal of having fieldwork students on site year round.

In addition to fieldwork, the program prepares students for community practice through ongoing evaluation and enhancement of the curriculum. The core course for learning the skills of needs assessment, program planning, and evaluation is "Health and Education: Foundations for Community Practice," taught in the summer after the students' first year. This course builds on concepts taught in the first year, providing a foundation for additional program planning work occurring during the second year. "Threads" of theory, evidenced-based practice, cultural awareness and competence, and learning styles are content areas carried throughout the educational program. In addition, the program continues to look for ways to incorporate concepts into existing classes. For example, "community health" is an option for first-year students as a topic choice for an issue paper. Grant writing has been offered as a seminar. Establishing relationships with community agencies has been offered in the form of guest lectures in the "Organization and Management" course. In addition, independent study options are offered.

Another aspect of working in the community is learning to work in service organizations with clients who are not "patients." The first-year course, "Community Service Assistantship," gives students the experience of serving as volunteers with an agency serving high-risk populations or people with disabilities. Based on a service-learning model, this course emphasizes volunteerism; awareness of organizational structure, function, and funding; working with people in community contexts; and an understanding of the health and social policies that affect the populations they serve.

Community Practice Initiatives

The community practice program faculty and staff have spent large amounts of time contacting, courting, and developing sites for the program. Descriptions of a few past and current community programs and the role of occupational therapy in each are presented here.

AMERICAN PARKINSON DISEASE ASSOCIATION (APDA). Fun 'N Fit exercise classes are offered to people with Parkinson's disease at two community sites, Windsor Community Center and Barnes Extended Care. A new video was recently produced in collaboration with the APDA to educate nursing home staff about the care of people with Parkinson's disease. Fieldwork students assist with the program.

COMMUNITY ALTERNATIVES. Community Alternatives, using an assertive community treatment model, serves persons with mental illness and/or substance abuse problems who are living in the community. Occupational therapy is involved in treatment planning, functional living skills assessment and training, and leisure activities. Fieldwork level I and level II students are also involved in the team.

DEVELOPMENTAL SERVICES OF JEFFERSON COUNTY. Developmental Services serves children between the ages of 0 to 3 years and their families. They offer both center-based and natural environment programs. The early intervention services team consists of occupational therapy, physical therapy, speech, and early-childhood special educators. Direct and consultative occupational therapy services are provided at the center and in client homes. Fieldwork students assist.

DRIVING EVALUATIONS. Clients with cognitive and/or visual deficits are referred by physicians for driving evaluations. Evaluations include laboratory tests of mental, visual, and physical status and a road test to assess driving skill. If indicated, the therapist may send a report to the state licensing bureau, indicating that the individual's current license should be evaluated. Counseling is provided to the client and his or her family as appropriate.

EDGEWOOD CHILDREN'S CENTER. Edgewood Children's Center is a residential and day-treatment/education program for children and adolescents with severe social, psychological, and behavioral problems. Occupational therapy services include individualized evaluation and treatment of children's sensorimotor, social, school-related, and daily living skills. For most children, therapy consists of group sessions, where skills, values, and concepts are learned through activities such as crafts, games, cooking projects, and role-play discussions.

HAZEL BLAND PROMISE CENTER. The Hazel Bland Promise Center serves severely developmentally disabled children ages 0 to 3 years in the home, as an outpatient and at the center; and children ages 3 to 21 years in the center. Direct and consultative occupational therapy services are provided. Steps are being taken to support parents as they meet the challenges of parenting and accessing resources for their children. Fieldwork level I and level II students work with the occupational therapist in all phases of the program.

HOME ACCESSIBILITY. Home accessibility is part of a home assessment, a comprehensive evaluation of a person's home environment and his or her ability to function in the surroundings. Home assessments are performed by a community practice occupational therapist with expertise in adaptive equipment, ergonomics, analyzing and grading tasks and activities, and designing living space. The goal is to help maximize a person's function, reduce risk and injury, and minimize the need for ancillary services or institutionalization. Services are provided upon referral from individuals or partner agencies.

LABRE CENTER. The Benedict Joseph Labre Center, a transitional housing facility, provides occupational therapy services to men with psychiatric disabilities who are homeless. The goal of occupational therapy is to support the development of living skills among clients to help achieve greater independence and integration into the community. This program is an expansion of the concept begun at Shalom House. Fieldwork level I and level II students work with the occupational therapist in all phases of the program.

MEMORY AND AGING PROJECT SATELLITE (MAPS) ACTIVITY GROUP. The memory and aging project satellite (MAPS) activity group is held weekly for clients with a diagnosis of Alzheimer's disease and for those with signs of early memory loss or confusion. The group is held to combat social isolation, improve or maintain cognitive functioning, provide exercise (physical activity), and participate in educational activities. The goal of the group is to improve or maintain the client's ability to remain in his or her own home. Students are involved with MAPS at all levels: community service assistantships and level I and level II fieldwork.

MARY RYDER HOME FOR THE AGED. The Mary Ryder Home is a residential facility serving low-income older adults. An occupational therapist who is a member of the community practice team facilitates therapeutic activity groups three times per week. Students who are completing their community service assistantships and/or fieldwork assist the therapist. The goal is to improve quality of life through meaningful occupation.

MULTIPLE SCLEROSIS (MS) WELLNESS. A wellness course developed by the WUOT program and the Gateway Chapter MS Society teaches self-management skills to people with MS. A leadership training program and manual are being developed to support the expansion of wellness programs throughout the midwest. The program was originally taught by the occupational therapy faculty who developed it. Currently, they are training MS Society staff and peer volunteers to teach the program.

OLDER ADULT SERVICE INFORMATION SYSTEM (OASIS)/HEALTH STAGES. OASIS is a national education organization dedicated to enhancing quality of life for older adults. The community practice program is working with OASIS to develop health curricula for older-adult members. The goal is to develop, offer, and evaluate programs on a comprehensive array of topics at levels that are appropriate for people at various stages of behavior change.

ST. LOUIS CONNECTCARE. St. Louis ConnectCare provides outpatient rehabilitation services to low-income and indigent residents of St. Louis, both the city and the county. The clients are referred to the program by area clinics. The community practice team provides occupational therapy services. Clients also receive physical therapy and speech therapy.

ST. LOUIS AREA AGENCY ON AGING. The "Getting to Know Life" health promotion class was developed for older adults who participate in congregate meals offered by the St. Louis Area Agency on Aging at a number of sites across the city. The seven-week class, developed by community practice therapists, was piloted at the midtown senior center. A trainer's manual is being finalized and a train-the-trainer program will be offered to volunteers identified by the agency. Occupational therapists and students will continue to provide support to the program and volunteers.

SHALOM HOUSE. Shalom House is a homeless shelter for chronically mentally ill women. A member of the community practice team acts as a consultant for the transitional housing day program and the emergency shelter. Programs, services, and treatment are based on each client's individual goals and community placement needs. Participants receive training in daily living skills, prevocational skills, and leisure skills, all toward the goal of independent community living.

SPECIALIZED TRANSITIONAL AND REHABILITATION TRAINING (START). START is a community-based agency whose mission is to enable people with severe physical disabilities to take part in the larger community. It provides supported living, employment, recreation, and education. The focus is on encouraging participants to assume responsibility for their own behavior. Community practice services include occupational therapy evaluations and follow-up intervention with participants and sites to facilitate maximum participation by clients. START also serves as a level I and level II fieldwork site for students.

VOCATIONAL REHABILITATION. Occupational therapy services provided to the state of Missouri vocational rehabilitation division include rehabilitation engineering consultation and computer training. Activities involve a functional assessment and recommendation of equipment, services, and modifications that meet the client's needs and facilitate entry or re-entry into the workforce. Services are provided upon referral.

WORK PERFORMANCE CLINICAL LABORATORY. The Work Performance Clinical Laboratory evaluates individuals with disabilities that interfere with the ability to work. Evaluations can identify accommodations needed at the work site and techniques to be used by the client to optimize work performance. Vocational exploration may be performed if a new career choice is necessary. Fieldwork level I students assist.

UNIVERSITY OF SOUTH ALABAMA: A COMMUNITY SERVICE-LEARNING APPROACH

The bachelor of science degree program at the University of South Alabama admitted its first class of students in June 1994. From the outset, faculty recognized the need to train future professionals to work effectively in community-based service sites. As part of this commitment, a specific course in community-based practice was developed and a service-learning component was infused into the curriculum.

Much research has been conducted on the effects **of community service learning.** The effects appear to be broad based and enduring, many of which are congruent with occupational therapy's history and philosophical base. Regardless of the discipline, service-based learning appears to:

- Develop open-mindedness
- Increase awareness of one's own values, beliefs, and attitudes (an essential aspect of therapeutic use of self)
- Increase problem-solving ability
- Increase empathy
- Be as effective as traditional instruction in conveying knowledge
- Increase self-efficacy and enhance a belief that a person can make a difference in other peoples' lives
- Increase social and personal responsibility (an important aspect of ethical behavior)
- Enhance communication skills
- Reinforce the development of professional behaviors (good practice for students early in their academic program)
- Instill a healthy work ethic
- Enable students to assess their strengths and weaknesses (Conrad and Hedin, 1982; Conrad and Hedin, 1991; Giles and Eyler, 1994; Markus, Howard, and King, 1993; Sankaran, Cinelli, McConatha, and Carson, 1995)

In addition, several potential benefits specific to the discipline of occupational therapy also are evident. Community service learning can increase the students' understanding of the role of occupational therapy in community-based settings, providing an opportunity to integrate theory with practice and networking opportunities with professionals in a variety of disciplines. Community service learning also allows community-based organizations, which currently may not have occupational therapy services, to experience occupational therapy firsthand, thereby increasing the potential development of new job opportunities for occupational therapy practitioners in community-based programs.

Community service learning also increases the probability that students might choose a community-based setting for future practice. It has been demonstrated that practitioners who are trained in institutions want to work in institutions (Weissert, Knott, and Steiber, 1993). What students learn in school is most likely how they will practice. Providing students, early in their academic career, with opportunities to experience the potential for community-based practice is one of the goals of this community service-learning approach to level I fieldwork.

Program Goals and Objectives

The overall goal of the community service-learning program is to develop students' skills and competencies in the provision of community-based occupational therapy services to agencies and organizations in the local community, which have typically been underserved. The program is designed to:

- Respond to actual community needs
- Provide community-based organizations with the opportunity to experience occupational therapy services firsthand
- Increase the potential for the development of new job opportunities in community-based programs
- Increase the probability that students will choose a community-based setting for future practice

Program Components

A community service-learning component was included in three required courses. In each of these courses, students were assigned to various community agencies and organizations for a half day per week throughout the semester. Each student completes approximately a total of 100 hours at three to five different sites upon completion of the curriculum. Students engage in a variety of learning activities and complete a project that addresses the needs of the community organization and its service recipients.

Learning activities completed by the students have included weekly entries in reflective journals, observation summaries, interviews of program participants, and the development and implementation of group activities. Projects that serve community needs have included in-service presentations to agency staff, needs assessment activities, development of program activities, construction of positioning devices and adaptive equipment, and environmental assessment and modification.

Collaborative Structure

The Department of Occupational Therapy has collaborated with Volunteer Mobile and the university's Office of Community Involvement in identifying sites that can provide appropriate student learning experiences and which are in need of occupational therapy services. Students are placed in a variety of community agencies, including:

- Child development centers, early-intervention programs, a preschool for the sensory impaired
- YWCA/YMCA, United Cerebral Palsy, Easter Seal Centers, Association for Retarded Citizens
- Senior citizen centers, adult day-care programs, assisted living centers
- Work rehabilitation programs, home health agencies, public schools
- AIDS support services, hospice programs, homeless shelters
- Mental health center facilities, substance abuse programs, Alzheimer's services

Program Evaluation

The program is evaluated on a number of levels. The site supervisor, using a standardized format that addresses the student's skills and professional behavior, evaluates student performance. Students evaluate the site in terms of learning opportunities available and the quality of supervision provided. In addition, faculty members keep in contact with the on-site supervisors by telephone and site visits to offer support and handle any concerns that arise. These exchanges often provide valuable insights regarding the performance of the students and the overall effectiveness of the service-learning program.

Lessons Learned

Initiating such a comprehensive service-learning component in the curriculum was more labor intensive than had been anticipated. Cultivating community-based sites is more time intensive than using traditional medical sites that employ occupational therapists. Personnel at community agencies need to be educated about what occupational therapy is and what the profession can offer to their service recipients. This approach requires a great deal of time spent in telephone contacts, site visits, and correspondence.

Planning extra time into faculty workloads is important for setting up and maintaining community contacts. We have found it preferable for the faculty teaching these courses to have direct contact with community organizations, agencies, and student supervisors rather than working through an intermediary.

The success of this community service-learning fieldwork I model is dependent on a number of factors, including the students' attitudes and motivation; good communication among the academic fieldwork coordinator, individual faculty members, and the supervisors on site; and the clarity of the objectives and assignments.

Program Successes

In the six years this program has been in operation, there have been many small but significant success stories. Two larger successes, however, are worth mentioning. Two facilities, where no occupational therapy services had been previously provided, decided to create an occupational therapy staff position as a result of experiencing the students' contributions to their program and their clients. In addition, the service-learning program in the Department of Occupational Therapy was selected as a model program by the Campus-Community Partnerships for Health and showcased in their publication titled *A Guide for Developing Community-Responsive Models in Health Professions Education* (1997).

Clearly, this approach has been a win-win-win situation. The occupational therapy department has gained positive visibility within the university and community. Students have had the opportunity to explore a variety of roles for occupational therapy practitioners in community sites. The collaborating agencies and programs, in providing this experience, receive high-quality volunteers with some fairly sophisticated skills.

 # RESEARCH IN COMMUNITY-BASED PRACTICE

Research in community-based practice has barely begun. Some researchers have attempted to test the application of current occupational therapy theoretical approaches and models in community settings with mixed results. However, the need for research in this area is clear.

The Washington University program in occupational therapy (WUOT) has a strong focus on research. Creating stronger links between research and community practice has been one of the program's goals. Another of its goals is to evaluate the outcomes of work at all levels and develop programs based on the best evidence. Toward that end, the WUOT recently organized around specific areas of study, including aging, work, pediatrics, cognition, health promotion/chronic disease self-management, and social participation. The goal is that each practitioner and each researcher be linked through their affiliation with a concentration. Practitioners will have the support of researchers who can facilitate evidenced-based practice and evaluation of outcomes. The research faculty will have "community laboratories" with experienced community practice therapists in which to implement and test models. Students will have the opportunity to select an area of concentration and obtain a spectrum of experiences in a given area through their coursework, work with research faculty on a master's research project, and experience in the field.

Baum and Law (1998) have outlined a number of research areas relevant for community practice. Occupational therapy researchers need to:

● Identify the factors that contribute to successful employment, self-sufficiency, and social integration.

● Determine the conditions that enable persons with chronic disabilities to participate fully in their families, schools, work settings, and community.
● Identify the personal, social, and environmental circumstances that promote acceptance and use of assistive devices.
● Investigate how the interaction of biopsychosocial and environmental factors contribute to the development of functional limitations, disabilities, and impairments.
● Identify the personal, developmental, and environmental attributes that contribute to successful community living.

 ## DIFFUSION OF INNOVATIONS

Through research, publication, and entry-level and continuing education, innovations
are disseminated for implementation into practice. These innovations and changes are
diffused and perpetuated in professions through a variety of communication channels.

An **innovation** is an idea, method, practice, or object that is perceived to be new or
novel. Some innovations are not really new from an objective historical perspective
but are new to the perceiver by virtue of a lapse of time since their initial discovery or
introduction (Rogers, 1995).

Innovations often require a significant period of time for diffusion before being
adopted by practitioners, academics, and researchers in a discipline. **Diffusion** refers
to "the process by which an innovation is communicated through certain channels
over time among the members of a social system" (Rogers, 1995, p. 5). Diffusion of innovation produces changes, both planned and unplanned, in the structure and function of a social system.

The process of diffusion consists of four elements: (1) the innovation itself, (2) the
communication channels utilized, (3) the time it takes for diffusion, and (4) the social
system affected. "The characteristics of an innovation, as perceived by the members
of a social system, determine its rate of adoption. Five attributes of innovations are:
(1) relative advantage, (2) compatibility, (3) complexity, (4) trialability, and (5) ob-
servability" (Rogers, 1995, p. 36).

Whatever the innovation is, it must be communicated to be adopted. The **communication channels** (the manner through which innovation is conveyed) may be
formal or informal or both. Although mass media diffusion is typically a rapid and
efficient means of conveying information about innovations, interpersonal or face-
to-face communication is often more effective in developing favorable attitudes toward a new idea. Individuals are more likely to adopt an innovation if they perceive that the communicator is a "near peer" or someone similar to themselves
(Rogers, 1995).

Time is a factor in the diffusion process. Some individuals are early adopters of innovation, while others tend to lag behind. Some innovations are adopted very
quickly. Others may take significantly longer periods of time. In a profession, diffusion of innovation requires a "critical mass" of adopters before the innovation becomes the standard. The decision to adopt an innovation occurs in five stages:

1. Knowledge acquisition, learning about the innovation
2. Persuasion, forming a favorable or unfavorable attitude or impression of the innovation
3. Decision, choice to adopt or reject the innovation
4. Implementation of the innovation, putting the idea, method, or object to use
5. Confirmation, the reinforcement the person receives for adopting the innovation
(Rogers, 1995)

The social system is the unit affected by the innovation. The **social system** may be a group of individuals, an organization, a profession, or a society. The communication structure and function, the norms, and leadership patterns of a social system can either facilitate or impair the innovation's diffusion. Some social systems are more open to innovation than others. If consensus is required to adopt an innovation, the process can be extremely time-consuming.

The occupational therapy profession is at a critical crossroads in its history. Do we adopt the innovation of community practice and all that it entails and move ahead quickly and deliberately, or do we reinforce the status quo and work within the existing parameters of practice? While some practitioners are losing their jobs in the managed-care arena, other opportunities are becoming available in community settings. These emerging practice areas are very much in harmony with the founders' visions of the profession. Will we respond quickly and enthusiastically to these challenges? Fidler (2000) clearly supports change and suggests moving "beyond the therapy model." She advocates that practitioners become "occupationalists," who have the capability to practice and conduct research in a variety of areas, including, but not limited to (Fidler, p. 101):

- services and programs of wellness, of prevention, of learning enhancement, and lifestyle counseling;
- community planning and design;
- organizational, agency and institutional design and operations; and
- treatment, restorative interventions and rehabilitation.

 ## CONCLUSION

To paraphrase Barker (1992), the three keys to the success of the occupational therapy profession in the 21st century are excellence, innovation, and anticipation. **Excellence** refers to the ability to do whatever it is one does with the utmost quality, in a cost-effective manner, while seeking continuous improvement. **Innovation** is the ability to initiate or introduce something new and different, and in unison with excellence is a powerful and potent combination. **Anticipation** is the ability to be in the right place at the right time with an excellent, innovative product or service. Anticipation allows one to predict or foresee future needs, trends, and priorities. If, in some small way, one can anticipate the future, then there is no need to fear it. The future can be embraced as an opportunity for growth and revitalization.

> Do not follow where the path leads,
> rather go where there is no path and leave a trail.
>
> Author unknown

 ## STUDY QUESTIONS

1. What do students and practitioners need to know to practice effectively in community-based settings?
2. Generate five new researchable questions (not already described in this text) related to community-based practice.
3. Discuss how your occupational therapy educational program meets the accreditation standards related to community-based practice.
4. Describe the advantages and disadvantages of community-based fieldwork, including ways to overcome the barriers.

5. List the five attributes of an innovation that determine its rate of adoption and the process an individual or group uses to decide to accept or reject the innovation.

REFERENCES

Accreditation Council for Occupational Therapy Education. (1998). *Standards for an accredited educational program for the occupational therapist.* Bethesda, MD: American Occupational Therapy Association.

Barker, J.A. (1992). *Future edge: Discovering the new paradigms of success.* New York: William Morrow.

Barth, T. (1994). Occupational therapy interventions at a shelter for homeless, addicted adults with mental illness. *American Occupational Therapy Association Mental Health Special Interest Section Newsletter, 17*(1), 7–8.

Baum, C., and Law, M. (1998). Community health: A responsibility, an opportunity and a fit for occupational therapy. *American Journal of Occupational Therapy, 52*(1), 7–10.

Brownson, C.A. (1998). Funding community practice: Stage I. *American Journal of Occupational Therapy, 52*(1), 60–64.

Cermak, S.A. (1976). Community-based learning in occupational therapy. *American Journal of Occupational Therapy, 30*(3), 157–161.

Community-Campus Partnerships for Health. (1997). *A guide for developing community-responsive models in health professions education.* San Francisco: UCSF Center for the Health Professions.

Cnaan, R.A., and Blankertz, L.E. (1993). Serving the dually diagnosed homeless: Program development and interventions. *The Journal of Mental Health Administration, 20*, 100–112.

Conrad, D., and Hedin, D. (1982). The impact of experiential education on adolescent development. *Child and Youth Services, 4*, 57–76.

Conrad, D., and Hedin, D. (1991). School-based community service: What we know from research and theory. *Phi Delta Kappan, 72*, 743–749.

Cromwell, F.S., and Kielhofner, G.W. (1976). An educational strategy for occupational therapy community service. *American Journal of Occupational Therapy, 30*(10), 629–633.

Fidler, G.S. (2000). Beyond the therapy model: Building our future. *American Journal of Occupational Therapy, 54*(1), 99–101.

Giles, D.E., and Eyler, J. (1994). The impact of a college community service laboratory on students' personal, social and cognitive outcomes. *Journal of Adolescence, 17*, 327–339.

Grossman, J. (1974). Community experience for students. *American Journal of Occupational Therapy, 28*(10), 589–591.

Heubner, J., and Tryssenaar, J. (1996). Development of an occupational therapy practice perspective in a homeless shelter: A fieldwork experience. *Canadian Journal of Occupational Therapy, 63*, 24–32.

Interagency Council on the Homeless, U.S. Department of Housing and Urban Development (1994). *Priority: Home! The federal plan to break the cycle of homelessness.* Available from Community Connections, PO Box 7189, Gaithersburg, MD.

Kavanagh, J., and Fares, J. (1995). Using the model of human occupation with homeless mentally ill clients. *British Journal of Occupational Therapy, 58*, 419–422.

Lyons, M., and Ziviani, J. (1995). Stereotypes, stigma, and mental illness: Learning from fieldwork experiences. *American Journal of Occupational Therapy, 49*, 1002–1008.

Marks, L. (1997). Homeless program benefits from OT skills. *OT Practice, 7*, 22–23.

Markus, G.B., Howard, J.P., and King, D.C. (1993). Integrating community service and classroom instruction enhances learning: Results from an experiment. *Educational Evaluation and Policy Analysis, 15*, 410–419.

McColl, M.A. (1998). What do we need to know to practice occupational therapy in the community? *American Journal of Occupational Therapy, 52*(1), 11–18.

Menks, F., Sittler, S., Weaver, D., and Yanow, B. (1977). A psychogeriatric activity group in a rural community. *American Journal of Occupational Therapy, 31*(6), 376–384.

National Board for Certification in Occupational Therapy. (1997). *National study of occupational therapy practice: Executive summary.* New York: Professional Examination Service.

Privott, C.R. (1998). *The fieldwork anthology.* Bethesda, MD: The American Association of Occupational Therapy.

Rogers, E.M. (1995). *Diffusion of innovations* (4th ed.). New York: The Free Press.

Rushdie, S. (1999). *The ground beneath her feet*. New York: Henry Holt.

Rydeen, K., Kautzmann, L., Cowan, M.K., and Benzing, P. (1995). Three faculty facilitated, community-based level I fieldwork programs. *American Journal of Occupational Therapy, 49,* 112–118.

Sankaran, G., Cinelli, B., McConatha, D., and Carson, L. (1995). Voluntarism: An investment in preparing health professionals for the future. *Journal of Health Education, 26*(1), 58–60.

Weissert, C., Knott, J., and Steiber, B. (1993). *Health professions education reform: Understanding and explaining states' policy options*. Michigan State University: The Department of Political Science and the Institute for Public Policy and Social Research.

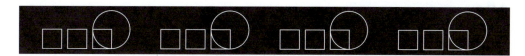

Appendix

Occupational Therapy Assessment Tools for Early Intervention

SENSORY INTEGRATION TOOLS FOR EARLY INTERVENTION

Test Name	Ages	Information	Available from
Test of Sensory Functions in Infants	Children 4 to 18 months	Twenty-four items and five subtests: reactivity to deep tactile pressure, adaptive motor functions, visual tactile integration, ocular motor control, reactivity to vestibular stimulation	Communication/Therapy Skill Builders, The Psychological Corp., 555 Academic Court, San Antonio, TX 78204-2498, 1-800-211-8378, www.hbtpc.com
Response to Sensory Input	Children with autism		*American Journal of Occupational Therapy,* 1980, *34,* 375–381
Infant Toddler Symptom Checklist	Children 7 to 30 months	Six versions, by ages, measure self-regulation, modulation of sleep/wake cycles, response to sensory stimulation, attachment, emotional functioning	Communication/Therapy Skill Builders, The Psychological Corp., 555 Academic Court, San Antonio, TX 78204-2498, 1-800-211-8378, www.hbtpc.com

(Continued)

SENSORY INTEGRATION TOOLS FOR EARLY INTERVENTION (*Continued*)

Test Name	Ages	Information	Available from
Sensorimotor Performance Analysis	Preschool children to young adults	Criterion-referenced instrument, rolling, belly crawling, bat and ball and hands and knees, kneeling balance, pellets in bottle, paper, pencil, and scissor tasks	Communication/Therapy Skill Builders, The Psychological Corp., 555 Academic Court, San Antonio, TX 78204-2498, 1-800-211-8378, www.hbtpc.com
Childhood Autism Rating Scale		Criterion-referenced behavior rating scale includes diagnostic information about ranges of autism—mild, moderate, severe	Western Psychological Services, 12031 Wilshire Blvd., Los Angeles, CA 90025, 1-800-648-8857
Sensory Integration Inventory for Individuals with Developmental Disabilities	Children to adults	Screening tool, checklist of behavioral descriptions, four sections—general reactions, tactile, vestibular, proprioceptive	Communication/Therapy Skill Builders, The Psychological Corp., 555 Academic Court, San Antonio, TX 78204-2498, 1-800-211-8378, www.hbtpc.com
Sensorimotor History		Checklist, questionnaire, tactile, auditory, olfactory, visual, gustatory, vestibular sensation, muscle tone, reflexes, coordination	Western Psychological Services, 12031 Wilshire Blvd., Los Angeles, CA 90025, 1-800-648-8857

DEVELOPMENTAL TOOLS FOR EARLY INTERVENTION

Test Name	Ages	Information	Available from
Peabody Developmental Motor Scales	Birth to 83 months	Standardized rating scales, performance based, comes with test kit and manual; norm-referenced and criterion-referenced subtests: gross-motor scales, fine-motor scales; time to administer: 45 to 60 minutes	Riverside Publishing Co., 8420 Bryn Mawr Ave., Chicago, IL 60631-9979, 1-800-767-8378 Pro Ed, 8700 Shoal Creek Blvd., Austin, TX 78757-6897, 1-512-451-3246, www.proedinc.com
Denver Developmental Screening Test II	Birth to 72 months	Standardized task performance and observation, test kit and manual; subtests: personal-social, fine-motor adaptive, language, gross motor	Denver Developmental Materials, Inc. PO Box 6919, Denver, CO 80206, 1-800-419-4729
Bayley Scales of Infant Development (2nd ed.)	Children 1 month to 42 months	Norm referenced, standardized, three-part evaluation: mental, motor, infant behavior; complete set includes manual, stimulus booklet, mental-scale forms, motor-scale forms with tracing design sheet, behavioral rating scale forms	The Psychological Corporation, 555 Academic Court, San Antonio, TX 78204-2498, 1-800-228-0752, www.hbtpc.com
Batelle Developmental Inventory	Birth to 8 years	Standardized norm-referenced test, gross motor, fine motor, cognitive, personal-social, self-help	Riverside Publishing Co., 8420 Bryn Mawr Ave., Chicago, IL 60631-9979, 1-800-767-8378

(Continued)

DEVELOPMENTAL TOOLS FOR EARLY INTERVENTION (*Continued*)

Test Name	Ages	Information	Available from
Early Intervention Developmental Profile	Birth to 3 years	Criterion referenced, developmental	University of Michigan Press, 389 Greene Street, Ann Arbor, MI 48104-1104, 1-313-764-4392
Early screening profiles	Children 2 to 6 years	Norm referenced, developmental	American Guidance Services, Inc., Publishers Bldg., Circle Pines, MN 55014, 1-800-328-2560
Hawaii Early Learning Profiles	Birth to 3 years	Criterion referenced, developmental; domains: gross motor, fine motor, self-help, cognitive, expressive language, social-emotional	VORT Corp., PO Box 60132, Palo Alto, CA 94306, 1-415-322-8282
Mullen Scales of Early Learning	Birth to 68 months	Norm referenced, developmental	American Guidance Services, Inc., Publishers Bldg., Circle Pines, MN 55014, 1-800-328-2560
Movement Assessment of Infants	Birth to 12 months	Criterion referenced, identifies motor dysfunction, muscle tone, reflexes, automatic reactions, volitional movement	Chandler, PO Box 4631, Rolling Bay, WA
Bayley II	Children 1 to 42 months	Norm referenced, population included children with prematurity, HIV antibody, prenatal drug exposure, asphyxiation, DD, otitis media, autism, Down's syndrome, mental scale, motor scale, behavior scale	The Psychological Corporation, 555 Academic Court, San Antonio, TX 78204-2498, 1-800-228-0752, www.hbtpc.com
Alberta Infant Motor Scale (AIMS)	Birth to 18 months	Observational tool, gives percentiles, prone, supine, sitting, standing	WB Saunders Co., 6277 Sear Harbor Drive, Orlando, FL 32821-9826

Test Name	Ages	Information	Available from
Miller Assessment Preschoolers (MAPS)	Children 2.9 to 5.8	Standardized task performance, developmental, sensory and motor abilities, cognitive abilities, combined abilities	Psychological Corporation, 555 Academic Court, San Antonio, TX 78204-2498, 1-800-228-0752, www.hbtpc.com
Callier Azusa Scales	Birth to 5 years	Observation-based developmental scale, criterion referenced, for severely handicapped children, motor, perceptual, daily living, cognition, communication, language, social	University of Texas at Dallas, Callier Center for Communication Disorders, 1966 Inwood Road, Dallas, TX 75235, 1-214-883-3060
Early Learning Accomplish-ment Profile (ELAP)	Birth to 36 months	Criterion-referenced assessment, establish basal and ceiling ages, gross motor, fine motor, cognitive, language, self-help, social-emotional	Kaplan School Supply, PO Box 25408, Winston Salem, NC, 1-800-334-2014
INFANIB	Children 4 to 18 months	Neuromotor assessment of infants, supine, prone, sitting, standing, suspended	Communication/Therapy Skill Builders, The Psychological Corp., 555 Academic Court, San Antonio, TX 78204-2498, 1-800-211-8378, www.hbtpc.com
Carolina Curriculum for Handicapped Infants and Infants at Risk	Birth to 24 months	Field-tested curricula includes instructions for modifications for children with impairments for extra cues, 26 subdomains, cognition, communication, social adaptation, fine motor, gross motor	Paul H. Brookes Publishing Co., PO Box 10624, Baltimore, MD 21285-0624, 1-800-638-3775, www.brookespublishing.com

(Continued)

DEVELOPMENTAL TOOLS FOR EARLY INTERVENTION (*Continued*)

Test Name	Ages	Information	Available from
Carolina Curriculum for Preschoolers with Special Needs	Children 2 to 5 years	Field-tested curricula includes instructions for modification for children with impairments for extra cues, 25 subdomains, cognition, communication, social adaptation, fine motor, gross motor	Paul H. Brookes Publishing Co., PO Box 10624, Baltimore, MD 21285-0624, 1-800-638-3775, www.brookespublishing.com
Pediatric Evaluation of Disability Inventory (PEDI)	Children 6 months to 7 years	Norm referenced, social, self-care, mobility areas rated by functional skills, caregiver assistance and modifications	Communication/Therapy Skill Builders, The Psychological Corp., 555 Academic Court, San Antonio, TX 78204-2498, 1-800-211-8378, www.hbtpc.com

MISCELLANEOUS ASSESSMENTS FOR EARLY INTERVENTION

Test Name	Ages	Information	Available from
Developmental Test of Visual Motor	Children 2.9 to 19.8 years	Printed booklets with scoring manual, screening for learning disabilities, 24 geometric designs, stop after three failures; raw score converts to percentage and standard scores	Modern Curriculum Press, 13900 Prospect Road, Cleveland, OH 44136, 1-800-321-3106
Erhardt Developmental Prehension Assessment	Birth to 15 months	Observation, task performance checklist, involuntary arm/hand patterns, voluntary movements, pre-writing skills	Communication/Therapy Skill Builders, The Psychological Corp., 555 Academic Court, San Antonio, TX 78204-2498, 1-800-211-8378, www.hbtpc.com
Erhardt Developmental Vision Test	Birth to 6 months	Observation, behavior rating scale, involuntary visual patterns, voluntary eye movements	Communication/Therapy Skill Builders, The Psychological Corp., 555 Academic Court, San Antonio, TX 78204-2498, 1-800-211-8378, www.hbtpc.com
Oral Motor Feeding Rating Scale	Children 1 year plus	Breast/bottle-feeding, spoon-feeding, cup drinking, biting, chewing, straw drinking	Communication/Therapy Skill Builders, The Psychological Corp., 555 Academic Court, San Antonio, TX 78204-2498, 1-800-211-8378, www.hbtpc.com
Test of Attention in Infants	Children 7 to 30 months	Four subdomains: visual attention, tactile attention, auditory attention, multisensory attention	Southpaw Enterprises, PO Box 1047, Dayton, OH 45401, 1-800-228-1698

(Continued)

MISCELLANEOUS ASSESSMENTS FOR EARLY INTERVENTION (*Continued*)

Test Name	Ages	Information	Available from
TIME Test of Infant Motor Evaluation	Birth to 3.6 years	Subtests: mobility, stability, motor organization, functional performance, social-emotional abilities	Communication/Therapy Skill Builders, The Psychological Corp., 555 Academic Court, San Antonio, TX 78204-2498, 1-800-211-8378, www.hbtpc.com
Transdisciplinary Play Based Assessment	Infancy to 6 years	Natural play observation assessment to assess developmental level, learning styles, temperament, motivation, interaction patterns	Communication/Therapy Skill Builders, The Psychological Corp., 555 Academic Court, San Antonio, TX 78204-2498, 1-800-211-8378, www.hbtpc.com

Index

A "b" following a page number indicates a box. An "f" following a page number indicates a figure. A "t" following a page number indicates a table.

399